Recent Advances in
PSYCHIATRY

Recent Advances in PSYCHIATRY

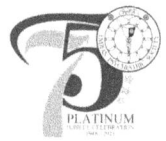

Indian Psychiatric Society Publication

Editors

Anil Kakunje
DPM MD
Professor and Head
Department of Psychiatry
Yenepoya Medical College
Mangaluru, Karnataka, India

Mrugesh Vaishnav
MD
Director
Samvedana Happiness Hospital
Ahmedabad, Gujarat, India

Sujit Sarkhel
DPM MD
Professor
Department of Psychiatry
Institute of Psychiatry
Kolkata, West Bengal, India

Dipayan Sarkar
DPM (MGIMS)
Consultant Psychiatrist
Modern Psychiatric Hospital
Agartala, Tripura, India

Foreword
Ajit Avasthi

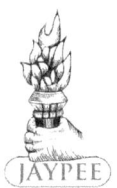

JAYPEE BROTHERS MEDICAL PUBLISHERS
The Health Sciences Publisher
New Delhi | London

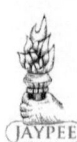

Jaypee Brothers Medical Publishers (P) Ltd

Headquarters

Jaypee Brothers Medical Publishers (P) Ltd
EMCA House, 23/23-B
Ansari Road, Daryaganj
New Delhi 110 002, India
Landline: +91-11-23272143, +91-11-23272703
+91-11-23282021, +91-11-23245672
Email: jaypee@jaypeebrothers.com

Corporate Office

Jaypee Brothers Medical Publishers (P) Ltd
4838/24, Ansari Road, Daryaganj
New Delhi 110 002, India
Phone: +91-11-43574357
Fax: +91-11-43574314
Email: jaypee@jaypeebrothers.com

Overseas Office

JP Medical Ltd
83 Victoria Street, London
SW1H 0HW (UK)
Phone: +44 20 3170 8910
Fax: +44 (0)20 3008 6180
Email: info@jpmedpub.com

Website: www.jaypeebrothers.com
Website: www.jaypeedigital.com

© 2024, Jaypee Brothers Medical Publishers and Indian Psychiatric Society

The views and opinions expressed in this book are solely those of the original contributor(s)/author(s) and do not necessarily represent those of editor(s) or publisher of the book.

All rights reserved. No part of this publication may be reproduced, stored or transmitted in any form or by any means, electronic, mechanical, photocopying, recording or otherwise, without the prior permission in writing of the publishers.

All brand names and product names used in this book are trade names, service marks, trademarks or registered trademarks of their respective owners. The publisher is not associated with any product or vendor mentioned in this book.

Medical knowledge and practice change constantly. This book is designed to provide accurate, authoritative information about the subject matter in question. However, readers are advised to check the most current information available on procedures included and check information from the manufacturer of each product to be administered, to verify the recommended dose, formula, method and duration of administration, adverse effects and contraindications. It is the responsibility of the practitioner to take all appropriate safety precautions. Neither the publisher nor the author(s)/editor(s) assume any liability for any injury and/or damage to persons or property arising from or related to use of material in this book.

This book is sold on the understanding that the publisher is not engaged in providing professional medical services. If such advice or services are required, the services of a competent medical professional should be sought.

Every effort has been made where necessary to contact holders of copyright to obtain permission to reproduce copyright material. If any have been inadvertently overlooked, the publisher will be pleased to make the necessary arrangements at the first opportunity.

Inquiries for bulk sales may be solicited at: jaypee@jaypeebrothers.com

Recent Advances in Psychiatry

First Edition: **2024**

ISBN: 978-93-5696-151-7

Contributors

Adarsh Tripathi MD
Professor
Department of Psychiatry
King George's Medical University
Lucknow, Uttar Pradesh, India

Alka A Subramanyam MD DPM DNB
Associate Professor
Department of Psychiatry
Topiwala National Medical College and
Bai Yamunabai Laxman Nair Charitable
Hospital
Mumbai, Maharashtra, India

Amulya Koneru MD
Consultant
Department of Psychiatry
Women's Wellness Clinic, Asha Hospital
Hyderabad, Telangana, India

Anamika Das MD DPM
Senior Resident
Department of Psychiatry
IQ City Medical College
Durgapur, West Bengal, India

Anil Kakunje DPM MD
Professor and Head
Department of Psychiatry
Yenepoya Medical College
Mangaluru, Karnataka, India

Anshu Prasad MD
Junior Resident
Department of Psychiatry
Himalayan Institute of Medical Sciences
Dehradun, Uttarakhand, India

Arabinda Brahma
DNB MNAMS DPC PhD
Director and Consultant Psychiatrist
Girindra Sekhar Bose Clinic
Kolkata, West Bengal, India

Aratrika Sen MD
Senior Resident
Department of Psychiatry
Institute of Psychiatry
Institute of Post Graduate Medical
Education and Research
Kolkata, West Bengal, India

Arijit Mondal MD
Assistant Professor
Department of Psychiatry
Santiniketan Medical College
Bolpur, West Bengal, India

Astha MD
Senior Resident
Department of Psychiatry
University College of Medical Sciences
Guru Teg Bahadur Hospital
New Delhi, India

Avinash De Sousa
MD DPM MS MBA MPhil PsyD
Consultant Psychiatrist and Research
Associate
Department of Psychiatry
Lokmanya Tilak Municipal Medical
College
Mumbai, Maharashtra, India

Biju Viswanath MD
Additional Professor
Department of Psychiatry
National Institute of Mental Health and
Neurosciences (NIMHANS)
Bengaluru, Karnataka, India

Dipayan Sarkar DPM (MGIMS)
Consultant Psychiatrist
Modern Psychiatric Hospital
Agartala, Tripura, India

G Prasad Rao MD
Director
Asha Hospital
Hyderabad, Telangana, India

Ganesan Venkatasubramanian
MD PhD
Professor
Department of Psychiatry
National Institute of Mental Health and Neurosciences
Bengaluru, Karnataka, India

Ganesh Kini K MD
Associate Professor
Department of Psychiatry
Yenepoya Medical College
Mangaluru, Karnataka, India

Guru S Gowda MD DNB
Assistant Professor
Department of Psychiatry
National Institute of Mental Health and Neurosciences
Bengaluru, Karnataka, India

Hareesh Angothu MD DPM
Additional Professor
Department of Psychiatry
National Institute of Mental Health and Neurosciences
Bengaluru, Karnataka, India

Henal Shah MD DPM
Professor
Department of Psychiatry
Topiwala National Medical College and Bai Yamunabai Laxman Nair Charitable Hospital
Mumbai, Maharashtra, India

Imon Paul MD DPM
Professor
Department of Psychiatry
IQ City Medical College
Durgapur, West Bengal, India

Kartik Singhai MD
Senior Resident
Department of Psychiatry
National Institute of Mental Health and Neurosciences
Bengaluru, Karnataka, India

Kishor M MD
Professor and Head
Department of Psychiatry
JSS Medical College
JSS Academy of Higher Education and Research
Mysuru, Karnataka, India

Krishna Prasad Muliyala MD
Additional Professor
Department of Psychiatry
National Institute of Mental Health and Neurosciences
Bengaluru, Karnataka, India

Malay Kumar Ghosal MD
Former Professor and Head
Department of Psychiatry
Medical College Kolkata
West Bengal, India

Malvika Nagpal MD
Consultant Psychiatrist
Amaha Mental Health Center
New Delhi, India

Mansi P Somaiya MD DNB
Consultant Psychiatrist
Department of Psychiatry
Specific Learning Disability Centre and School Mental Health Clinic
Topiwala National Medical College and Bai Yamunabai Laxman Nair Charitable Hospital
Mumbai, Maharashtra, India

Mina Chandra DNB PhD
Professor and Head
Department of Psychiatry
Atal Bihari Vajpayee Institute of Medical Sciences (ABVIMS)
Dr Ram Manohar Lohia Hospital
New Delhi, India

Mohan Raju S MPhil
Clinical Psychologist
Department of Psychiatry
Ramaiah Medical College
Bengaluru, Karnataka, India

Mrugesh Vaishnav MD
Director
Samvedana Happiness Hospital
Ahmedabad, Gujarat, India

Nimesh G Desai MD MPH MRCPsych
Former Director
Institute of Human Behaviour and
Allied Sciences (IHBAS)
New Delhi, India

Nishant Goyal MD DPM
Professor
Department of Psychiatry
KS Mani Centre for Cognitive
Neurosciences
Central Institute of Psychiatry
Ranchi, Jharkhand, India

Omkar Nayak MD
Assistant Professor
Department of Psychiatry
Lokmanya Tilak Municipal Medical
College
Mumbai, Maharashtra, India

OP Singh MD
Professor
Department of Psychiatry
West Bengal Medical Education Service
Kolkata, West Bengal, India

Pratham Ved Bhasyakarula MBBS
Intern
Department of Psychiatry
Asha Hospital
Hyderabad, Telangana, India

Prerna B Khar MD PDF (CAMH)
Consultant Psychiatrist
Department of Psychiatry
Early Intervention Centre
Topiwala National Medical College and
Bai Yamunabai Laxman Nair Charitable
Hospital, Mumbai, Maharashtra, India

Priya Ranjan Avinash MD DPM
Associate Professor
Department of Psychiatry
Himalayan Institute of
Medical Sciences
Dehradun, Uttarakhand, India

Rajarshi Chakravarty MD
Assistant Professor
Department of Psychiatry
Burdwan Medical College
and Hospital
Burdwan, West Bengal, India

Rajesh Nagpal MD
Consultant Psychiatrist
Manobal Klinik
New Delhi, India

Rajkumar Lenin Singh MD PhD
Professor
Department of Psychiatry
Regional Institute of Medical Sciences
(RIMS)
Imphal, Manipur, India

Raveesh BN MD PhD
Professor and Head
Department of Psychiatry
Mysore Medical College and Research
Institute
Mysuru, Karnataka, India

Ravichandra Karkal MD
Professor
Department of Psychiatry
Yenepoya Medical College
Mangaluru, Karnataka, India

Ravindra Neelakanthappa Munoli MD
Associate Professor
Department of Psychiatry
Kasturba Medical College
Manipal Academy of
Higher Education
Manipal, Karnataka, India

Samir Kumar Praharaj MD DPM
Professor and Head
Department of Psychiatry
Coordinator
Clinical Research Center for Neuromodulation in Psychiatry
Kasturba Medical College
Manipal Academy of Higher Education
Manipal, Karnataka, India

Sayanti Ghosh MD
Associate Professor
Department of Psychiatry
Nil Ratan Sircar Medical College
Kolkata, West Bengal, India

Senjam Gojendra Singh MD
Associate Professor and Head
Department of Psychiatry
Regional Institute of Medical Sciences
Imphal, Manipur, India

Shivangini Singh MBBS MD (Psychiatry)
Junior Resident
Department of Psychiatry
King George's Medical University
Lucknow, Uttar Pradesh, India

Sriramya Veumulakonda
MBBS MPH
Senior Research Officer
Department of Psychiatry
Asha Hospital
Hyderabad, Telangana, India

Subir Bhattacharjee MD
Assistant Professor
Department of Psychiatry
Deben Mahata Government Medical College and Hospital
Purulia, West Bengal, India

Sujit Sarkhel DPM MD
Professor
Department of Psychiatry
Institute of Psychiatry
Kolkata, West Bengal, India

Swarna Buddha Nayok MD
Senior Resident
Department of Psychiatry
National Institute of Mental Health and Neurosciences
Bengaluru, Karnataka, India

Swati B Shelke MD PDF (CAMH)
Assistant Professor
Department of Psychiatry
Early Intervention Centre
Topiwala National Medical College and Bai Yamunabai Laxman Nair Charitable Hospital
Mumbai, Maharashtra, India

Thanapal Sivakumar MD
Additional Professor
Department of Psychiatry
National Institute of Mental Health and Neurosciences
Bengaluru, Karnataka, India

Vanteemar S Sreeraj DPM DNB
Associate Professor
Department of Psychiatry
National Institute of Mental Health and Neurosciences
Bengaluru, Karnataka, India

Venu Gopal Jhanwar MD
Director
Deva Institute of Healthcare and Research
Varanasi, Uttar Pradesh, India

Message from Indian Psychiatric Society Office Bearers

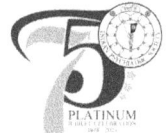 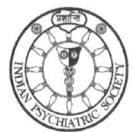

Dear Friends

Taking care of educational needs of psychiatrists in-making, has always been a priority for Indian Psychiatric Society. For the last 7 years we are more focused in identifying the needs and finding a suitable team of editors and writers to address them. It was noticed that the fourth paper of postgraduate examination, which comprises of recent advances, poses difficulty for majority of the students. Keeping this in mind, it was decided to bring out a book to cater this need. This book embodies substantial amount of recent advances in psychiatry in one binder, and this of course will be a great help to them.

We congratulate our Publication Committee, chaired by Professor Anil Kakunje, and ably advised and supported by Dr Mrugesh Vaishnav, Professor Sujit Sarkhel, and Dr Dipayan Sarkar for taking this arduous task in their hands. We highly appreciate them for conceptualizing this book so comprehensively. We are thankful to the learned contributors for finding time and taking pain to write these chapters. The Indian Psychiatric Society is grateful for your selfless service. We are sure it will help the nurturing budding psychiatrists. We express our thanks to M/s Jaypee Brothers Medical Publishers (P) Ltd, New Delhi, India, for publishing this book so well. We also thank Shri Jitendar P Vij (Group Chairman), Mr Ankit Vij (Managing Director), Mr MS Mani (Group President), Ms Chetna Malhotra (Senior Director—Professional Publishing, Marketing and Business Development), Ms Pooja Bhandari (Director—Production), and Ms Suchita Gera (Development Editor) for this beautiful production. We are sure our honorable members who are teaching faculty will motivate students to take maximum advantage from this book.

Vinay Kumar
President
Indian Psychiatric Society

Laxmikant Rathi
Vice-President
Indian Psychiatric Society

Arabinda Brahma
Hony. Secretary
Indian Psychiatric Society

Foreword

To keep abreast with the latest scientific developments, modes, trends, and practices comprise the present-day necessity for all medical practitioners, more so for psychiatrists. Spectacular advances in the field of "brain" research, evolving social demands and expectations from mental health practitioners, and easy and wider availability of scientific information made possible by telecommunication revolution have necessitated that psychiatrists remain up to date with latest developments in their area of specialization. It helps to keep pace with evolving knowledge that in turn facilitates better understanding and communication of brain mechanisms, proper choice of interventions, and delivery of finer nuances of psychiatry practice to those seeking care for their suffering.

Recent Advances in Psychiatry, a publication brought out by the Indian Psychiatric Society, is a laudable initiative to fulfill the educational needs primarily for those pursuing postgraduate training in psychiatry and has immense usefulness for academic psychiatrists and psychiatry practitioners at large.

It is a collection of diverse yet topical subjects of recent interest and research in psychiatry. Brain research pertaining to neuronal networks and communication; novel interventions such as the role of stem cells, probiotics, ketamine, and noninvasive neuromodulation techniques; emerging concerns reflected in cyber- and eco-psychiatry; and newer applications such as telepsychiatry and evolving perspectives in psychiatry teaching and training should particularly interest the psychiatry trainees. Recent advances in therapeutic challenging situations such as treatment-resistant bipolar disorder, prodrome of schizophrenia, psychiatric emergencies, and addictions have also been addressed. Issues of recent public health concerns such as mental health insurance, care of homeless populations, and recent Indian laws in relation to mental health are useful in everyday practice of psychiatry. Other topics of interest in this collection are the latest developments in psychiatry nosology as reflected in ICD-11, new products from the basket of psychopharmacology, and much hoped for prevention in psychiatry.

The eminent authors of various topics have done a painstaking job in reviewing the latest research, putting various perspectives of research in an easy communicable style and in facilitating the readers with list of "Take-Home" points. All in all, *Recent Advances in Psychiatry* is a highly recommended personal collection for psychiatry trainees and practicing psychiatrists to update their knowledge on a wide range of emerging scientific concepts and cutting-edge technologies in the subject of psychiatry. It is earnestly hoped that the Indian Psychiatric Society shall in future too periodically come out with publications pertaining to the latest developments in the science and practice of psychiatry not only for new emerging topics but also for the ones that have been addressed in this edition. I wish to complement the hierarchy of Indian Psychiatric Society led by Dr Vinay Kumar and the Publication Committee of Indian Psychiatric Society led by Dr Anil Kakunje for having conceived and delivered this seminal book.

Ajit Avasthi
Former Senior Professor and Head
Department of Psychiatry
Postgraduate Institute of Medical Education and Research
Chandigarh, India
Past President, Indian Psychiatric Society
Director, Indian Psychiatric Society
Academy for Education and Research

Preface

It was a pleasant surprise when I was selected as a publication committee *chairman* for the Indian Psychiatric Society (IPS). Until a few years back, I never thought I would be into writing books! I am thankful to the office bearers of IPS for having faith in me and the publication committee team members by entrusting us with a major responsibility.

Advisor, Dr Mrugesh Vaishnav gave valuable inputs and guidance. Dr Sujit Sarkhel with his experiences as an editor and teaching enhanced value to the team. Dr Dipayan Sarkar was enthusiastic and took up responsibilities well. It was a full teamwork!

We chose *Recent Advances in Psychiatry* as the title, as there are very few books in this area especially related to postgraduate examinations. Recent advances are a separate full theory paper and students struggle to read on this vast, changing, and dynamic topic. We selected authors of repute who have experience and interests in specific topics.

I am delighted to pen this preface for such a book, which certainly is a dream come true.

I thank the entire IPS executive committee, publication committee members, and authors for their support and cooperation. A special thanks to the team from M/s Jaypee Brothers Medical Publishers (P) Ltd, New Delhi, India. I bow to all my teachers for their efforts in training me. Last but not the least such a work is not possible without the support from family members.

Happy Reading!
Feedback is welcome

Anil Kakunje
anilpsychiatry@gmail.com

Contents

1. **Connectomics and the Brain in Relation to Psychiatry** 1
   Swarna Buddha Nayok, Vanteemar S Sreeraj,
   Ganesan Venkatasubramanian

2. **Probiotics and Psychiatry** 11
   Venu Gopal Jhanwar, Priya Ranjan Avinash, Anshu Prasad

3. **Recent Advances in the Management of**
   Prodromal Symptoms of Schizophrenia 22
   G Prasad Rao, Amulya Koneru, Sriramya Veumulakonda,
   Pratham Ved Bhasyakarula

4. **Designer Drugs** 28
   Omkar Nayak, Avinash De Sousa

5. **Telepsychiatry in India** 40
   Arijit Mondal, OP Singh

6. **Mental Health Insurance in India:**
   How far have we Progressed? 47
   Thanapal Sivakumar, Kartik Singhai, Hareesh Angothu

7. **Pharmacotherapy of Psychiatric Emergencies** 56
   Sujit Sarkhel, Aratrika Sen

8. **Newer Diagnostic Categories in ICD-11** 67
   Adarsh Tripathi, Shivangini Singh

9. **Default Mode Network and its**
   Role in Various Psychiatric Disorders 75
   Sayanti Ghosh, Malay Kumar Ghosal

10. **Role of Stem Cells and Nutraceuticals in Psychiatry** 87
    Kartik Singhai, Biju Viswanath, Krishna Prasad Muliyala

11. **Treatment-resistant Bipolar Disorder:**
    Approach to Management 101
    Alka A Subramanyam, Mansi P Somaiya,
    Prerna B Khar, Swati B Shelke

12. **Ketamine and Psychiatry** 115
    Rajesh Nagpal, Malvika Nagpal

13. **Newer Noninvasive Neuromodulatory Techniques in Psychiatry** 134
    Samir Kumar Praharaj, Nishant Goyal

14. **Mental Health Services for Homeless Populations** 143
    Nimesh G Desai

15. **Cyberpsychiatry** 156
    Rajarshi Chakravarty, Subir Bhattacharjee, Arabinda Brahma

16. **Recent Indian Laws in Psychiatry** 163
    Raveesh BN, Guru S Gowda, Ravindra Neelakanthappa Munoli

17. **Newer Drugs in Psychiatry** 170
    Imon Paul, Anamika Das

18. **Changing Perspectives in Psychiatry Training in India** 183
    Henal Shah, Kishor M

19. **Treating Addiction: Multidimensional Approach and Prevention to Relapse** 189
    Senjam Gojendra Singh, Rajkumar Lenin Singh

20. **Early Prevention in Psychiatry** 194
    Ravichandra Karkal, Ganesh Kini K, Mohan Raju S

21. **Ecopsychiatry: An Overview** 207
    Astha, Mina Chandra

Index *223*

CHAPTER 1

Connectomics and the Brain in Relation to Psychiatry

*Swarna Buddha Nayok, Vanteemar S Sreeraj,
Ganesan Venkatasubramanian*

INTRODUCTION

How does our brain work? From the basic tasks of regulating breathing and hunger to performing complex mathematical abstractions to understand black holes, the brain seems to have the astounding ability to do it all seamlessly and at the same time. Deciphering the mysterious and astonishing abilities of the human brain has been difficult. Recent advances in neuroimaging techniques have given neuroscience an enormous potential to understand our brains. We have gradually understood that while different brain areas perform different tasks, this is seldom done in isolation. The connections between various parts of the brain ultimately decide its outcome.

These days neuroimaging techniques can map the structural and functional connectivity of the brain in vivo.[1,2] Such a map of the various neural structures and their interactions with each other is called a *connectome*. At its most restrictive meaning, the connectome is "a structural description of brain connectivity", while at its broadest, it helps us to gauge how brain connections interact over time, beyond its structural boundaries.[3]

To do this, we need relatable animal models, precise but affordable neuroimaging techniques, enormous statistical computing power, and thousands and thousands of scans and repeat scans. Charting such a map is a humongous feat, as the map changes at each level of the nervous system. Till now, the connectome of a fruit fly has been mapped completely, and the size of its brain mapped is about the thickness of two hair strands (250 μm in diameter).[1,4] It contained 25,200 neurons and 20 million connections! Comparing the human brain, which has at least 65 billion neurons (about 34 lakh times more). We are right now at the starting "point" of connectomes!

How is all this related to psychiatry? By now it is quite obvious that psychiatric disorders cannot be reduced to one simple malfunctioning area or functioning of the brain.[5] From its etiopathology to its treatment, it is essentially a subject of neural interaction at different levels. Though behavioral malfunctions remain the basis of its diagnostic classifications, we have found structural abnormalities of the brain in almost all psychiatric disorders. However, the problems may lie at a different level, i.e., where different brain regions connect and interact with each other.[1,6] Understanding psychiatric illnesses based on such a paradigm opens up pathophysiological models. Moreover, these paradigms lend hypotheses to be testable, a provision that has been lacking in current diagnostic classificatory systems.

USEFUL TOOLS AND CONCEPTS REGARDING CONNECTOMES

Below we introduce important concepts and terms to understand connectome-related advances and research.[1,2,5-7] We then discuss how these will elevate our understanding of the brain in general and for psychiatric disorders in particular. For an analogy, we will compare our brain to a large city with a suburban area around.

- *Diffusion-weighted magnetic resonance imaging (DWI):* This specifically tracks the axons of the entire brain, giving the basic framework of how neurons run through the place. This is the most commonly used starting point of connectome mapping.[1] Think of it as the broad and speedy highways, and the narrow and congested slow lanes of the city.
- *Functional connectivity:* What if we want to know how the people of a city are related to each other? Who are the relatives and friends of a particular family? Relatives of the same family may be scattered throughout the town. So how do we track them? They will all look similar morphologically. One way may be to see who all gets invited to attend a family get-together! Based on a similar logic, functional connectivity is assumed when spatially separated brain areas show activity together for a certain task.[2,6] If we feel hungry, the centers for understanding hunger should function together. This is indirectly achieved through functional MRI (fMRI), which measures statistical dependencies of the different areas at rest or during a task, which means that these observations are made over a period of time (time-series).[8] In fMRI, the signals which light up with temporally statistical significance (correlated to each other) are considered to be working together, despite being spatially separated. This is not a conjecture, but is neurophysiologically stated by the Hebbian postulate of neurons that "fire together, wire together".[8,9] It sounds simple enough now, but to think about it, we mostly assume the opposite, that is, neurons that "wire together, fire together". Compare it to saying, people who eat together, form a "family" together! Isn't that a paradigm shift?
- *BOLD signal:* fMRI signal is based on the hypothesis (hemodynamic response) that blood oxygenation level increases around a neuron when it is activated, and this signal—blood oxygenation level dependent (BOLD)—is picked up by the MRI machine. The BOLD signal follows linear time-invariant properties, making it predictable. It is also a good measure spatially as compared to electroencephalograph (EEG) signals, although less robust in temporal precision.[8]

- *Voxel-based measurements:* To understand what we "see" in a picture, our brain accumulates the collective signal represented by the smallest unit of it, called the pixels. For 3D images, this becomes a *voxel.* Thus, in an fMRI scan, the voxels provide all the information for further analysis. Processing the images is therefore mathematical processing of the intensity or quantity of signals present in these voxels. Further analyses are to find a relationship (or the lack of it) between voxels (or their clusters) throughout the brain.[8] Voxel-based whole brain functional connectome studies have shown to pick up connections which are spatially far apart and temporally sparse. Compare this to taking a picture of the city at the night from above, showing only dark and bright areas, and trying to find out buildings and busy streets based on that.
- *Parcellation:* To understand the whole brain interactions, we can divide the brain into smaller functional units. This has been quite difficult, as there is no single right way to divide the brain as seen in the MRI. It is usually done by using markers, based either on local properties like cytoarchitecture, receptor density, and myelin or on global properties like resting state connectivity and structural covariance.[7] Compare this to dividing the city into parts based on the language they speak or their occupation. Neuroimaging techniques offer parcellation of the brain into even hundreds of units.
- *Region of interest (ROI):* While exploring all the voxels sounds good, it may be beneficial to select certain regions which are neuroanatomically/physiologically known to be associated with certain functions of the brain and compare these with other known areas. This makes things pragmatic (closely related to parcellation) and is called ROI-based analysis. Most commonly used ROIs are predominantly from frontal and temporal areas or limbic-amygdalo-hippocampal-striatal regions.[1,6,8]
- *Statistical inference:* At this level of neural signals, nothing is left to the naked eye. The inferences drawn are essentially statistical. It would be simple if functional connectivity needed just one scan to find all the connections. To get a time-series data, hundreds of scans are repeated in one setting. There are several ways to go about making sense of the signals. Initially, differences in the means of signals and their intensities are evaluated to find and remove artifacts. Then the data goes through several levels of preprocessing methods to make the signals "readable." Then the data is subjected to higher order statistical analyses like principal and independent component analysis (ICA). These (also called methods for matrix decomposition) essentially find out how the different signals are correlated to each other (and therefore connected to each other). Such analyses reduce the brain into meaningful "components" or clusters, based on the signals.[8]
- *Intrinsic networks:* While we often associate signals to an underlying activity, the brain is always active, even at rest. Therefore, if we analyze the

signals at their "rest", we get to know what is the basic functional structure of the brain. Resting-state, first described by Biswal et al. in 1995 (Biswal was a doctoral student at that time), shows us the fundamental network processes of our brain.[10] These networks, found through ICA, are called intrinsic connectivity networks (ICNs). Three networks seem to form the basic ICN: the Default Mode Network (DMN), the Central Executive Network (CEN), and the Salience Network (SN).[11]

The DMN shows the baseline activity of the brain, integrating self-referential mental processes. It prominently includes the posterior cingulate cortex, medial prefrontal cortex, and medial temporal lobe. Contrasting with this is the CEN, which is activated during cognitively demanding tasks, essentially rule-based problem solving, working memory, and goal-directed decision making. It includes the dorsolateral prefrontal cortex and posterior parietal cortex. However, the change of the brain state from DMN to CEN is often mediated by the SN, which detects and decides which external and internal stimuli are important. It includes the dorsal anterior cingulate cortex and frontoinsular cortex.[1,6,11]

There are many more networks detected besides the above-mentioned triple-network system, such as the Language Network (LN), Visual Network (VN), Auditory Network (AN), Precuneus Network (PN), and Sensorimotor Network (SMN).[11,12]

- *Graph theory metrics:* So, after establishing units and measuring their relationships, we will get a complex matrix of correlation among each unit. How do we coherently represent this? A way to do this is by *Graph theory*.[1,2,13] This is used essentially to understand interacting systems. Here each node represents an area and an edge attached to it represents the connection (much like how we draw a family chart, with the thickness of the lines/edges showing the strength of connection). These can then be represented in a correlation matrix, which charts the overall strengths of the connection of each node to another. Retaining the strongest connections through statistical measures gives a chart of the functional connection between brain regions.

- *Small world network:* What do we get to know from the connectivity matrices? They show a pattern that the brain follows. The brain tries to be the most energy efficient by giving importance to certain areas (*nodes*) and their connections (*edges*).[1,14] The brain tries to cluster high-functioning areas (*hubs*) and reduce the distance of their edges thus increasing the network efficiency. This is a typical characteristic of a *small-world network*.[1,2,14,15] Mathematically, it is a unique way to make each node accessible to another through a small number of steps. It is easier to understand this in today's context of social media, where any two unknown persons can be "connected" to each other through a few friends.

- *Pathoconnectomics:* While these graph theoretical measures can show us how our brain works, they can also show us what goes wrong in psychiatric disorders. This is termed *pathoconnectomics*; it not only shows us what is abnormal at that point but also informs us regarding how information is and will be processed in an abnormal setting.[2,16] Integration and segregation of information seem to be dysfunctional in most psychiatric disorders and pathoconnectomics may lead us to new ways to understand and diagnose psychiatric disorders and further treatments. These will also help us to understand various phenomena from consciousness and attention to impulsivity and aggression, from low mood and suspiciousness to anhedonia and delusions.

FINE-TUNING CONNECTOMES TO UNDERSTAND THE WHOLE BRAIN

Now that we know the basics of connectomes and the brain, we may be tempted to erroneously believe that all we need to do is map out each neural element, add them all and we get the whole brain. Just like a city is much more than the individual additions of the building, roads, and people, a brain is more than the sum of its components (close to Gestalt theory).[1,2,17] However, this comes from a statistical understanding of physical laws, which tells us that the macroscopic functioning of a system is independent of its microscopic constituents. As we understand that a living being is much more than its organic molecules, the behaviors of a neural subsystem cannot be understood by simply charting out the structural and functional connectivity of each neuron.[18]

Therefore, it may be beneficial to look at different areas of the brain based on their white matter connectivity. This may sound counterintuitive; after all, functional connectivity is to see the brain beyond its structural limitations. However, the structure is of prime importance. For example, if we want to find farmers, we cannot look at the busy offices, we have to look at the suburbs, where the topography allows fields to exist and therefore farmers to function. To understand various interactions of the brain at a macroscopic level, we have to focus on mesoscopic levels such behavior of the neuronal population.[18,19]

This line of research leads to the combination of neuronal mass models with structural connectivity and testing these models on a causal hypothesis (Granger Causality or Dynamic Causal Modeling).[1,2,18] In these large-scale models, the resting functional state of the brain is evaluated to understand synaptic activities and neural mass is then modeled statistically to obtain desired results (Conductance-based biophysical model, FitzHugh–Nagumo model, Kuramoto model, etc.). If this sounds too difficult, it is probably so, especially for psychiatrists! A fun way may be to explore using *The Virtual Brain* (http://www.thevirtualbrain.org) which is a neuroinformatics platform, making things somewhat easier.[20]

UNDERSTANDING PSYCHIATRIC DISORDERS THROUGH CONNECTOMES

We now have two important understandings: the brain works as a network based on smaller functional hubs and structural connections, and both of these are extremely important for the network to work optimally. Structural damage at the microscopic level may bring catastrophizing changes in the functional properties which is what we see in stroke and traumatic brain injuries. On the other hand, abnormalities in the central hubs and connections are implicated in schizophrenia, bipolar disorder, and other psychiatric disorders. Below we highlight a few of the current understandings of psychiatric disorders based on connectomes:[1,2,5,6,16]

- *Schizophrenia:* It is considered to be a prototype disorder to understand pathoconnectomics; the brain in schizophrenia shows a wide range of functional and structural connectivity abnormalities and network functioning.[2] Decreased or aberrant local integration and segregation are found mainly in the prefrontal, pericentral, superior parietal, temporo-occipital, thalamic, and striatal areas. The small-world properties of the brain are compromised in schizophrenia, where it is less efficient, with abnormal clustering disproportionately affecting abnormalities in the "rich-club" hubs as compared to nonhub clusters, decreased number of "shortest paths" across the nodes. Certain intrinsic networks, like the DMN, have been repeatedly shown to be disturbed in schizophrenia.[21,22] There are hints that these abnormalities change throughout the illness and also show changes after treatment.[23] A different line of investigation has targeted the psychotic symptoms like hallucinations across boundaries showing module connectivity abnormalities in intrinsic networks.[24,25]

- *Bipolar disorder:* Structural and functional connectivity abnormalities, such as reducing gray matter in prefrontal and anterior cingulate cortex, dysfunctional networks for emotion regulation, changes in amygdala and hippocampus, and aberrant activation of the frontolimbic circuitry have been found in longitudinal studies. These research lines have also proposed different courses for bipolar disorder, like childhood onset, which may have a more "malignant course."[23,26]

- *Depression:* Structural abnormalities in the medial prefrontal cortex, amygdala, anterior cingulate gyrus and hippocampus, abnormal connectivity at prefrontal-amygdalar-pallidostriatal-mediothalamic mood regulating circuit, and imbalance between network activation responsible for attentional tasks and self-reflective tasks are found in depression. Circuits involving anhedonia, apathy, and alexithymia are also of recent interest.[27]

Such structural and functional abnormalities are also being studied in dementias, childhood disorders, anxiety, and obsessive–compulsive spectrum disorders.[1,2] For instance, the triple networks-related dysfunctions seem to be prominent but different in various types of dementias, that they may be of diagnostic significance.[1,11]

FUTURE IMPROVEMENTS IN RESEARCH OF CONNECTOMES

While all of the above sounds exciting, difficulties lie at each step. DWI does not give the axon structure as it is in real but shows various indices such as fractional anisotropy, mean diffusivity, radial diffusivity, and axial diffusivity, which are thought to represent the axonal structure.[1,2] Recent advances also enable us to "track" the white matter fibers using deterministic and probabilistic methods using voxels (or seeds) through algorithms.[28]

Functional MRI, although most commonly used, has several feasibility issues. Resting-state measurement and analysis is far from being optimally standardized, repeated scans and measures are essential.[1,2,6] While we have discussed fMRI BOLD signals, EEG signals can also be used to understand brain functions, although through a different neurophysiological signal. EEG and magnetic EG feature prominently in connectome-related projects, and high-level analyses such as spectral analyses of EEG may give better temporally informed information on brain connectivity, especially when combined with white matter connectivity data.[29] However, whether EEG or BOLD signals are used, the rationale of data preprocessing, statistical analyses, and connectome-related inferences are anchored on the same principles.

Each study regarding connectomes agrees with a few previous literature and instead opens up newer information. Connectome studies are also linked to genomic studies, which provide further information on etiology and genetic architecture of psychiatric disorders.[1] Keeping in line, the Human Connectome Project is being extended to understand psychosis and shows promising potential.[30] Moreover, such complicated analysis and results may be best suited for machine learning paradigms, generating new perspectives on psychiatric disorders.

NEUROMODULATION AND CONNECTOMES

Connectomes and related abnormalities have been shown to respond to and predict pharmacological and psychotherapy treatments in psychiatric disorders. However, the specificity of such treatment modalities to alter brain connectivity continues to be questioned. To see changes in connectomes with specific areas and within a predetermined time frame, neuromodulatory techniques seem to be better suited. Transcranial magnetic stimulation and transcranial direct current stimulation techniques are used to stimulate and manipulate specific networks to evaluate the outcomes and test the hypothesis.[31,32] For example, the dysconnectivity hypothesis of schizophrenia can be tested by first determining various intrinsic network abnormalities, and then identifying the connected structures. Then neurostimulation may specifically target these regions, and fMRI analyses before and after the stimulation can show changes in network connectivity, correlating with symptom improvement. Such experiments may give compelling inputs to missing links in our understanding of brain activity, such as in the Research Domain Criteria Project framework.[32,33] Connectomics may finally lead us to see psychiatric disorders from our brain's physiological perspective rather than the present diagnostic constructs and form a core component of the emerging field of interventional psychiatry.

ACKNOWLEDGMENTS

For funding: Swarna Buddha Nayok acknowledges the support of the Indian Council of Medical Research (ICMR). Vanteemar S Sreeraj acknowledges the support of the India-Korea joint program cooperation of science and technology by the National Research Foundation (NRF) Korea (2020K1A3A1A68093469), the Ministry of Science and ICT (MSIT) Korea, and the Department of Biotechnology (India) (DBT/IC-12031(22)-ICD-DBT). Ganesan Venkatasubramanian acknowledges the support of Department of Biotechnology (DBT)—Wellcome Trust India Alliance (IA/CRC/19/1/610005) and Department of Biotechnology, Government of India (BT/HRD-NBA-NWB/38/2019-20(6)).

CONCLUSION

Viewing the brain and its functions through connectomes gives us a novel opportunity to update our knowledge of how our brain works. It unravels newer perspectives and a nuanced understanding of the integrated functions of the brain in healthy and diseased states. It opens several new lines of research and underlines exciting times ahead as psychiatric knowledge stands to benefit the most from such an enhanced understanding of our brains.

TAKE-HOME POINTS

- Connectomes describe brain connectivity and help us understand how brain connections interact over time beyond their structural boundaries.
- To do this, various imaging methods and concepts like blood oxygenation level-dependent signals, functional connectivity, diffusion-weighted magnetic resonance imaging, voxel-based measurements, parcellation, and mathematical concepts like small world network and graph theory are used.
- Mapping connectomes can show us what goes wrong in psychiatric disorders, and this is called pathoconnectomics.
- These approaches have unveiled the role of intrinsic connectivity networks within the brain, such as the default mode network, the central executive network, and the salience network, in healthy and diseased states.

REFERENCES

1. Deco G, Kringelbach ML. Great Expectations: Using Whole-Brain Computational Connectomics for Understanding Neuropsychiatric Disorders. Neuron. 2014;84(5):892-905.
2. Fornito A, Bullmore ET. Connectomics: a new paradigm for understanding brain disease. Eur Neuropsychopharmacol. 2015;25(5):733-48.
3. Sporns O, Tononi G, Kötter R. The Human Connectome: A Structural Description of the Human Brain. PLOS Comput Biol. 2005;1(4):e42.
4. Scheffer LK, Xu CS, Januszewski M, Lu Z, Takemura S-Y, Hayworth KJ, et al. A connectome and analysis of the adult Drosophila central brain. Elife. 2020;9:e57443.
5. Van Essen DC, Barch DM. The human connectome in health and psychopathology. World Psychiatry. 2015;14(2):154-7.
6. Cao M, Wang Z, He Y. Connectomics in psychiatric research: advances and applications. Neuropsychiatr Dis Treat. 2015;11:2801-10.
7. Eickhoff SB, Yeo BTT, Genon S. Imaging-based parcellations of the human brain. Nat Rev Neurosci. 2018;19(11):672-86.
8. Poldrack RA, Mumford JA, Nichols TE (Eds). Handbook of Functional MRI Data Analysis. Cambridge University Press; 2011. p. 239.
9. Stent GS. A physiological mechanism for Hebb's postulate of learning. Proc Natl Acad Sci U S A. 1973;70(4):997-1001.
10. Biswal B, Yetkin FZ, Haughton VM, Hyde JS. Functional connectivity in the motor cortex of resting human brain using echo-planar MRI. Magn Reson Med. 1995;34(4):537-41.
11. Menon V. Large-scale brain networks and psychopathology: a unifying triple network model. Trends Cogn Sci. 2011;15(10):483-506.
12. Lee WH, Moser DA, Ing A, Doucet GE, Frangou S. Behavioral and Health Correlates of Resting-State Metastability in the Human Connectome Project. Brain Topogr. 2019;32(1):80-6.
13. Farahani FV, Karwowski W, Lighthall NR. Application of Graph Theory for Identifying Connectivity Patterns in Human Brain Networks: A Systematic Review. Front Neurosci. 2019;13:585.
14. Liao X, Vasilakos AV, He Y. Small-world human brain networks: Perspectives and challenges. Neurosci Biobehav Rev. 2017;77:286-300.
15. Bassett DS, Bullmore ET. Small-World Brain Networks Revisited. The Neuroscientist. 2017;23(5):499-516.
16. Venkatasubramanian G, Keshavan MS. Biomarkers in Psychiatry—A Critique. Ann Neurosci. 2016;23(1):3-5.
17. Askenasy JJ, Lehmann J. Consciousness, brain, neuroplasticity. Front Psychol. 2013;4:412.
18. Cabral J, Kringelbach ML, Deco G. Exploring the network dynamics underlying brain activity during rest. Prog Neurobiol. 2014;114:102-31.
19. Scheffer LK, Meinertzhagen IA. A connectome is not enough – what is still needed to understand the brain of Drosophila? J Exp Biol. 2021;224(21):jeb242740.
20. Ritter P, Schirner M, McIntosh AR, Jirsa VK. The virtual brain integrates computational modeling and multimodal neuroimaging. Brain Connect. 2013;3(2):121-45.

21. Griffa A, Baumann PS, Ferrari C, Do KQ, Conus P, Thiran J, et al. Characterizing the connectome in schizophrenia with diffusion spectrum imaging. Hum Brain Mapp. 2014;36(1):354-66.
22. Narr KL, Leaver AM. Connectome and schizophrenia. Curr Opin Psychiatry. 2015;28(3):229-35.
23. Lei D, Li W, Tallman MJ, Patino LR, McNamara RK, Strawn JR, et al. Changes in the brain structural connectome after a prospective randomized clinical trial of lithium and quetiapine treatment in youth with bipolar disorder. Neuropsychopharmacology. 2021;46(7):1315-23.
24. Calhoun V, Sui J, Kiehl K, Turner J, Allen E, Pearlson G. Exploring the Psychosis Functional Connectome: Aberrant Intrinsic Networks in Schizophrenia and Bipolar Disorder. Front Psychiatry. 2012;2:75.
25. Schutte MJL, Voppel A, Collin G, Abramovic L, Boks MPM, Cahn W, et al. Modular-Level Functional Connectome Alterations in Individuals With Hallucinations Across the Psychosis Continuum. Schizophr Bull. 2022;48(3):684-94.
26. Lim CS, Baldessarini RJ, Vieta E, Yucel M, Bora E, Sim K. Longitudinal neuroimaging and neuropsychological changes in bipolar disorder patients: review of the evidence. Neurosci Biobehav Rev. 2013;37(3):418-35.
27. Wang L, Hermens DF, Hickie IB, Lagopoulos J. A systematic review of resting-state functional-MRI studies in major depression. J Affect Disord. 2012;142(1-3):6-12.
28. Voineskos AN, Lobaugh NJ, Bouix S, Rajji TK, Miranda D, Kennedy JL, et al. Diffusion tensor tractography findings in schizophrenia across the adult lifespan. Brain. 2010;133(5):1494-504.
29. Glomb K, Rué Queralt J, Pascucci D, Defferrard M, Tourbier S, Carboni M, et al. Connectome spectral analysis to track EEG task dynamics on a subsecond scale. NeuroImage. 2020;221:117737.
30. Demro C, Mueller BA, Kent JS, Burton PC, Olman CA, Schallmo MP, et al. The psychosis human connectome project: An overview. NeuroImage. 2021;241:118439.
31. Čukić M. The Reason why rTMS and tDCS are Efficient in Treatments of Depression. Front Psychol. 2020;10:2923.
32. Hallett M, Di Iorio R, Rossini PM, Park JE, Chen R, Celnik P, et al. Contribution of transcranial magnetic stimulation to assessment of brain connectivity and networks. Clin Neurophysiol Off J Int Fed Clin Neurophysiol. 2017;128(11):2125-39.
33. Sparing R, Mottaghy FM. Noninvasive brain stimulation with transcranial magnetic or direct current stimulation (TMS/tDCS)-From insights into human memory to therapy of its dysfunction. Methods San Diego Calif. 2008;44(4):329-37.

CHAPTER 2

Probiotics and Psychiatry

Venu Gopal Jhanwar, Priya Ranjan Avinash, Anshu Prasad

INTRODUCTION

The impact of probiotics on health has been studied since a long period of time. In 1908, Elie Metchnikoff observed that Bulgarian peasants who used to consume yogurt had higher average life span. The probiotics became commercial reality in 1930s.[1] The benefits of the probiotics have been recognized and explored for over a century. However, it was only since after 2013 that the studies affirming their role on mental health have started gaining momentum. Probiotics are generally defined as live microorganisms, preferentially of human origin, that upon ingestion in specific and sufficient numbers confer nonspecific health benefits to the host.[2] Our understanding of the impact of gut microbiome on gut–brain axis (GBA) has opened new avenues in the treatment.

MICROBIOME OVERVIEW

The human microbiome is a complex dynamic ecosystem. Although, commonly thought that initial colonization of gut by microbiota occurs during vaginal delivery, there is some evidence of a prenatal microbiome.[3] Maternal microbial influence is subject to change due to environmental factors such as prenatal stress, infections, and medicines. These factors induce maternal immune activation (MIA) **(Fig. 1)**. MIA has a potential to cause lifelong neuropathology by altering the microbial composition, immune responses, neurological changes, and other transcriptional pathways **(Fig. 2)**.[4] The microbial content in a fetal gut is of low diversity and shows variability with regards to age, sex, geography, genetic influences, etc. The neonatal microbiome is unstable and provides a "window of opportunity" for the development of lymphoid structures, differentiation, and maturation of T and B cells and, most importantly, establishment of immune tolerance to gut commensals.[5] Like a DNA fingerprint, even the microbiome shows interindividual variability, which stands true even for monozygotic twins. The microbiome evolves with respect to diversity, stability, and species predominance. Proteobacteria and actinobacteria species are more prevalent

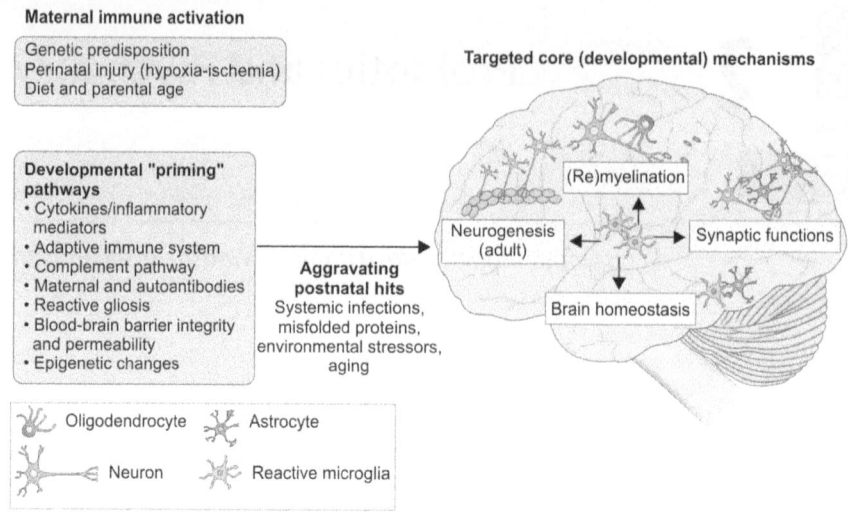

Fig. 1: Developmental priming pathways.[7]

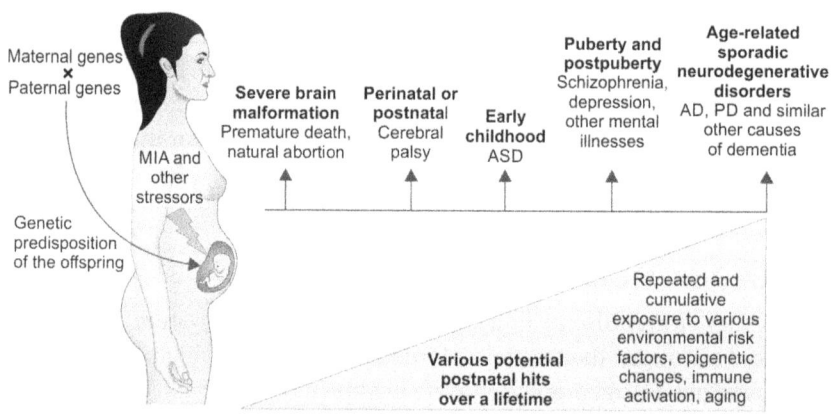

Fig. 2: Proposed causal chain of events.[7] (AD: Alzheimer's disease; ASD: autism spectrum disorder; MIA: maternal immune activation; PD: Parkinson's disease)

in a newborn infant while in adulthood, the Bacteriodetes and Firmicutes phyla, and the enterotype subtypes—*Prevotella*, *Ruminococcus*, and *Bacteroides* are more prominent. This microbiota profile continues to exist in old age and only subject to alteration when confronted with antibiotics or other insults such as disease pathology, dramatic changes in diet or medications, and other comorbidities.[6]

GUT–BRAIN AXIS

With respect to neuropsychiatric disorders, the GBA serves as a link between the central and the enteric nervous system (ENS), which altogether links

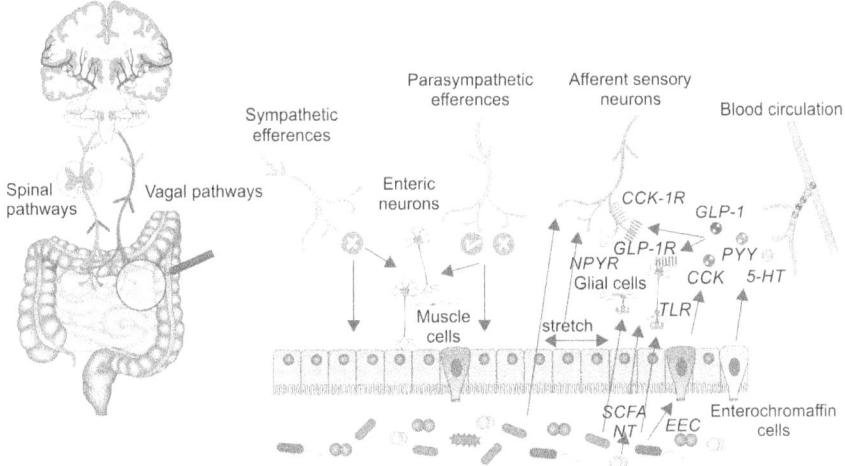

Fig. 3: The gut–brain crosstalk.[13] The gut microbiota communicates with enteric neurons and afferent sensory neurons through TLRs or indirectly with SCFAs and neurotransmitters. Conversely, the ANS controls GI functions. (ANS: autonomic nervous system; CCK: cholecystokinin; CCK-1R: cholecystokinin 1 receptor; EEC: enteroendocrine cell; GI: gastrointestinal; GLP-1: glucagon-like peptide 1; GLP-1R: glucagon-like peptide 1 receptor; NPYR: neuropeptide Y receptor; NT: neurotransmitter; PYY: peptide YY; SCFAs: short-chain fatty acids; TLR: toll-like receptor; 5-HT: serotonin)

the emotional and cognitive centers of the brain as well as the peripheral intestinal functions. The signaling from gut-microbiota to brain (GBA) and from brain to gut-microbiota (brain–gut axis) is mediated by neural, endocrine, immune, and humoral mechanisms[8] **(Fig. 3)**. The GBA through bottom-up vagal and spinal afferent signaling relay the information about gut physiology to brain. The various determinants of gut physiology such as the nutrient composition, enteric reflex, permeability of gut epithelium, and endocrine modulation are surveyed by the brain.[9] The "brain–gut" axis through vagal efferences stimulates efferent sympathetic glutamatergic brainstem neurons to control gut motility and permeability and further bacterial composition.[10,11] Like most other organs, the gastrointestinal functions are also controlled by the autonomic nervous system (ANS). Efferent parasympathetic and sympathetic communication allows top-down regulation of gut physiology via action on several effectors that include epithelial cells, enteric neurons, smooth muscle cells, interstitial cells of Cajal, and immune cells. Subsequently, the release of gut factors (neurotransmitters, hormones, and immune factors) and modulation of GI motility affect the microbiome profile of the intestine.[12]

The enteric flora releases a multitude of metabolites such as short-chain fatty acids (SCFAs), indole, secondary bile acids, and lipopolysaccharide (LPS). These metabolites bind to SCFAs or bile acid sensitive G-protein coupled receptors, LPS sensitive toll-like receptors (TLRs), and voltage-gated potassium (K_V) channels responsive to indole. Bile acids that have been deconjugated bind to G protein-coupled bile acid receptors (GPBARs) on the basolateral side of enteroendocrine L cells (such as GPBAR1). SCFAs cause the release of glucagon-like peptide 1 (GLP-1) by directly acting on the free fatty acid receptor (FFR). Additionally, SCFAs stimulate the synthesis of PYY by increasing the transcription of the human peptide YY (PYY) promoter through inhibition of histone deacetylase (HDAC). Bacterial aromatic amino acid catabolism creates indole metabolites which target K_V channels on enteroendocrine cells (EECs). These channels encourage Ca^{2+} influx and membrane depolarization. The microbiota-derived LPS can access the EECs' basolaterally situated TLR-4 where the epithelial mucosa is damaged. This starts the local production of hormones that support intestinal epithelium healing, notably GLP-2[14] (**Fig. 4**).

As aforementioned, the gut microbiota releases various metabolic products. Of these, SCFAs indirectly influence the function of enterochromaffin cells to produce serotonin. Also, gut microbiota ensures availability of monoamines directly via the degradation of amino acid and tryptophan (TPH). Other neurotransmitter molecules generated include dopamine,

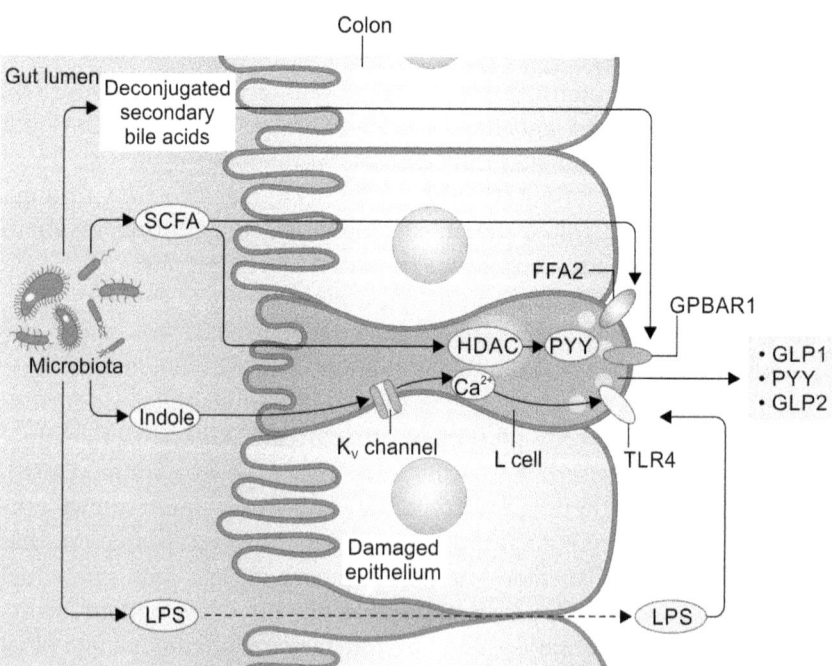

Fig. 4: Microbiota interactions with enteroendocrine cells in the colon. (FFA: free fatty acid; GLP: glucagon-like peptide; GPBAR1: G protein-coupled bile acid receptor 1; HDAC: histone deacetylase; LPS: lipopolysaccharide; PYY: peptide YY; SCFA: short-chain fatty acid; TLR: toll-like receptor)

noradrenaline, gamma-aminobutyric acid (GABA), acetylcholine, and histamine. **Table 1** summarizes the neurotransmitter-producing bacterial strains. Additionally, the ENS and other gut functions are modulated by gaseous products, such as nitric oxide (NO), methane, hydrogen, and carbon monoxide released by these microbes.[14,15] Apart from serving as a substrate

TABLE 1: Gut microbial strains that release or produce neurotransmitters.[18]

Neurotransmitters	Bacterial strains
Serotonin	• *Lactococcus lactis* subspecies *cremoris* • *L. lactis* subspecies *lactis* • *Lactobacillus plantarum* • *Streptococcus thermophilus* • *Escherichia coli* K-12 • *Morganella morganii* • *Klebsiella pneumoniae* • *Hafnia alvei*
Dopamine	• *Bacillus cereus* • *Bacillus mycoides* • *Bacillus subtilis* • *Proteus vulgaris* • *Serratia marcescens* • *Staphylococcus aureus* • *E. coli* • *M. morganii* • *K. pneumoniae* • *H. alvei*
Noradrenaline	• *B. mycoides* • *B. subtilis* • *P. vulgaris* • *E. coli* K-12
GABA	• *Levilactobacillus brevis* • *Bifidobacterium adolescentis* • *Bifidobacterium dentium* • *Bifidobacterium infantis* • *Lacticaseibacillus rhamnosus*
Acetylcholine	*L. plantarum*
Histamine	• *L. lactis* subspecies *cremoris* • *L. lactis* subspecies *lactis* • *L. plantarum* • *S. thermophilus* • *M. morganii* • *K. pneumoniae* • *H. alvei*

(GABA: gamma-aminobutyric acid)

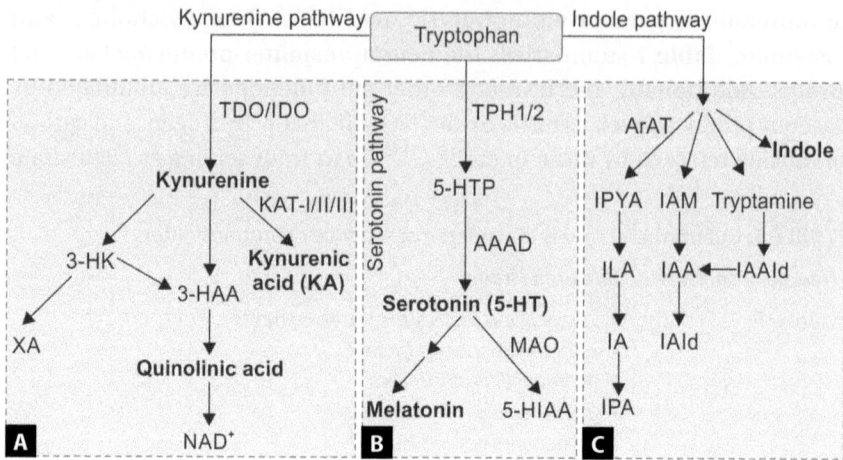

Figs. 5A to C: Tryptophan metabolic pathways. (AAAD: aromatic amino acid decarboxylase; ArAT: aromatic amino acid aminotransferase; 3-HAA: 3-hydroxyanthranilic acid; HIAA: hydroxyindoleacetic acid; 3-HK: 3-hydroxykynurenine; 5-HT: 5-hydroxytryptamine; 5-HTP: 5-hydroxytryptophan; IA: indole-3-acrylic acid; IAA: indole-3-acetic acid; IAld: indole-3-aldehyde; IAAld: indole-3-acetaldehyde; IAM: indole-3-acetamide; IDO: indoleamine 2,3-dioxygenase; ILA: indole-3-lactic acid; IPA: indole-3-propionic acid; IPYA: indole-3-pyruvic acid; KAT: kynurenine aminotransferase; MAO: monoamine oxidase; NAD^+: nicotinamide adenine dinucleotide; TDO: tryptophan 2,3-dioxygenase; TPH: tryptophan hydroxylase; XA: xanthurenic acid)

for serotonin, TPH is also involved in the kynurenine degradation pathway **(Figs. 5A to C)**. Kynurenine is further catabolized into an N-Methyl-D-Aspartate (NMDA) antagonist, kynurenic acid (KA), and a neurotoxin, quinolinic acid (QA). The metabolites mentioned above, cross the blood–brain barrier (BBB).[16] Several bacterial taxa that include Actinobacteria, Firmicutes, Bacteroidetes, Proteobacteria, and Fusobacteria and the genera of *Clostridium, Burkholderia, Streptomyces, Pseudomonas,* and *Bacillus* directly utilize TPH by expressing the enzyme tryptophanase, which converts TPH to indole, and these bacteria have been associated with the development of neuropsychiatric disorders, including autism spectrum disorders (ASDs).[16,17]

GUT DYSBIOSIS AND PSYCHIATRIC DISORDERS

"Gut dysbiosis" refers to pathology where the composition and functions of the gut microbial system are substituted from their normal beneficial state to the one that is deleterious to the host's health. There is accumulating evidence suggesting alteration of microbial composition alteration in pathogenesis of psychiatric disorders **(Table 2)**. The scope of this chapter covers the negative impact of microbiota dysbiosis on psychiatric disorders

TABLE 2: Deranged microbial profile in psychiatric disorders.

Disease (reference)		Increased	Decreased
Major depressive disorder (MDD)[21]		• Bacteroidetes • Proteobacteria • Actinobacteria phyla • Enterobacteriaceae • Alistipes	Firmicutes, Faecalibacterium
Bipolar disorder (BD)	General	• Flavonifractor genus[22] • Actinobacteria phylum • Coriobacteriia[23]	Faecalibacterium[24]
	Mania[25]	• Escherichia coli • Bifidobacterium adolescentis	
	Depression[25]	Stercoris	
Schizophrenia (SCZ)[26]		• Lactobacillaceae • Halothiobacillaceae • Brucellaceae • Micrococcineae	Veillonellaceae
Autism spectrum disorder (ASD)[27-29]		• Bacteroidetes • Proteobacteria • Firmicutes • Desulfovibrio • Sutterella • Clostridium	• Bifidobacterium • Klebsiella • Enterobacter • Prevotella • Coprococcus • Veillonellaceae
Attention deficit and hyperactive disorder (ADHD)[30]		Bifidobacterium	
Anorexia nervosa (AN)[31]		• Firmicutes • Methanobrevibacter smithii	• Roseburia • Bacteroidetes

via several intertwined pathways, collectively termed as "brain–gut–axis".[19] These pathways are as follows:

- *Leaky guts:* Disruption of intestinal epithelium
- Activation of proinflammatory cytokine pathway **(Figs. 6A and B)**
- Heightened hypothalamic–pituitary–adrenal (HPA) axis
- Decrease in absorption of beneficial nutrients, increase of deleterious compound synthesis, reduction of the antioxidant status and increase in lipid peroxidation, and increase of carbohydrate malabsorption
- Aberrant activation/deactivation of ANS
- Brain-derived neurotrophic factor (BDNF)-induced NMDA dysfunction **(Figs. 6A and B)**[20]
- Increase in intestinal pathogens (e.g., *Helicobacter pylori*)

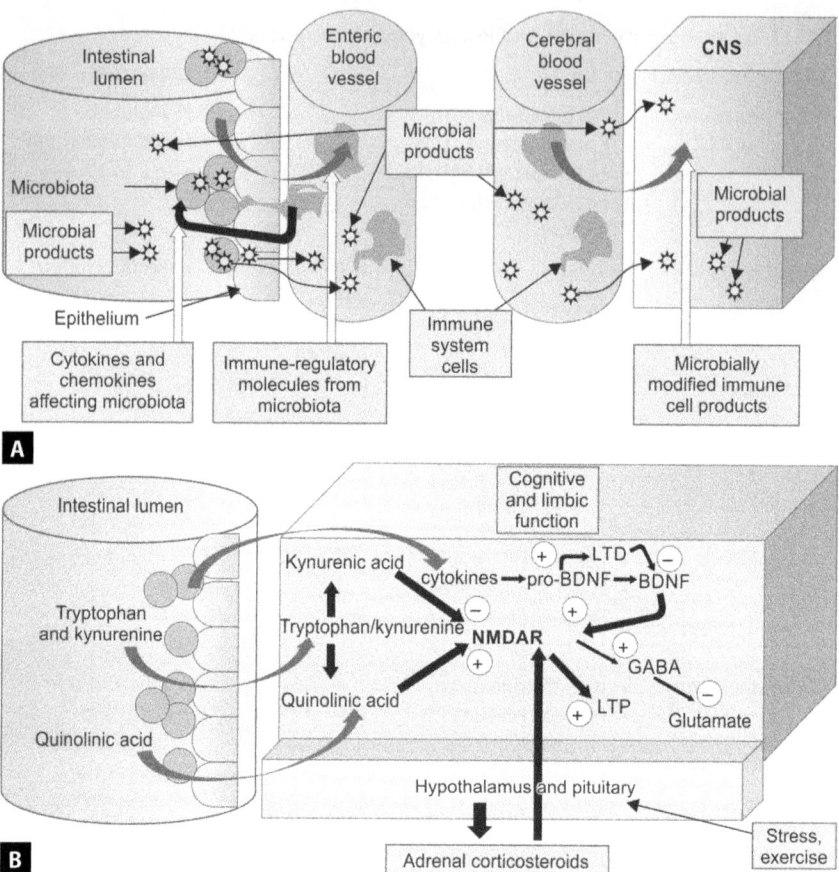

Figs. 6A and B: (A) Gut microbial products penetrate the epithelium and induce cytokine production. Conversely, cytokines released in response to stress modulate the viability and activity of the microbiota. The microbial factors reach the CNS where they are able to regulate neuronal activity and neurotransmission; (B) The tryptophan and its metabolites affect the overall concentrations of several cytokines. These cytokines in turn, modulate the synthesis of pro-BDNF and BDNF. Pro-BDNF promotes LTD while inhibiting the production of BDNF, which is a substrate in NMDAR synthesis. Conversely, NMDAR promotes LTP alongside depolarizing GABAergic neurons. Corticosteroids released via HPA axis stimulation mediates BDNF–NMDAR activity. Exercise via same pathway, increases BDNF production and cognitive function[20] (BDNF: brain-derived neurotrophic factor; CNS: central nervous system; GABA: gamma-aminobutyric acid; HPA: hypothalamic–pituitary–adrenal; LTD: long-term depression; LTP: long-term potentiation; NMDAR: N-methyl-D-aspartate receptor)

GUT MICROBIAL-BASED INTERVENTIONS

The past decade has seen a burgeoning interest in exploring the role of probiotics, both as an adjunctive and a stand-alone intervention, for psychiatric disorders. There is an accumulating data that suggests the gut microbial interventions such as probiotics, prebiotic, and fecal microbial transplant is reconfiguring the microbial composition in the gut and thereafter, the GBA. There is emerging data that administration of probiotics does not alter the relative abundance of gut microbiota, as previously believed.[32] However, these were only short-term studies. The positive outcomes of some probiotics on symptoms of depression and anxiety are consistent between the rodent and human studies. These positive effects are mediated in part by the regulation of the HPA axis and vagal nerve activity. Because of the heterogeneity of type and duration of regime, it is difficult to assess whether the positive effects were strain-specific or an interactive effect of the mixture of bacterial families.[19] The probiotics restructure the immune response possibly by the maintenance of the intestinal barrier integrity, the regulation of the inflammatory status, or the modulation of epigenetic mechanisms.[33] The effects of probiotics on different neurotransmitters and biomarkers show a temporal variation. For example, glutamate rose after 2 weeks of *Lactobacillus rhamnosus* JB-1 supplementation, but GABA rose after 4 weeks. These neuromodulatory effects outlast the duration of microbial intervention and ensure the longevity of treatment outcomes. The preliminary evidence demonstrates zero sum neuroregulatory effects (i.e., changes in excitation–inhibition balance in one brain region may be offset by those in another) of probiotics. For example, increase in both GABA and glutamate expression, control neural inhibition and excitation, respectively.[34]

CONCLUSION

There has been a renewed interest in the GBA and the role of probiotics and prebiotics in treatment of psychiatric conditions lately. The connection is a complex one and appears to be nonlinear. However, the role of gut microbiomes as a biomarker for various psychiatric disorders has been consistently explored. The gut microbial based interventions for treatment of mental health conditions are still in nascent stage and require further evidence to become mainstream.

TAKE-HOME POINTS
- The effects of maternal immune activation (MIA) are transduced to the fetus which are then embedded in the epigenetic architecture of the brain and the peripheral immune system, hence modulating the propensity of the offspring to develop neurodevelopmental disorders.
- Gut brain axis is a dynamic bidirectional signalling pathway, disruption of which has been implicated in several neurobehavioral disorders.
- Given the abundance of literature, several gut microbiome based interventions are being tailored to target brain health by reconfiguring microbial composition.

■ REFERENCES

1. Vasiljevic T, Shah NP. Probiotics—From Metchnikoff to bioactives. Int Dairy J. 2008;18(7):714-28.
2. Caselli M, Cassol F, Calò G, Holton J, Zuliani G, Gasbarrini A. Actual concept of "probiotics": Is it more functional to science or business? World J Gastroenterol. 2013;19(10):1527-40.
3. Wassenaar TM, Panigrahi P. Is a foetus developing in a sterile environment? Lett Appl Microbiol. 2014;59(6):572-9.
4. Lombardo MV, Moon HM, Su J, Palmer TD, Courchesne E, Pramparo T. Maternal immune activation dysregulation of the fetal brain transcriptome and relevance to the pathophysiology of autism spectrum disorder. Mol Psychiatry. 2018;23(4):1001-13.
5. Zhao Q, Elson CO. Adaptive immune education by gut microbiota antigens. Immunology. 2018;154(1):28-37.
6. Dinan TG, Cryan JF. Microbes, Immunity, and Behavior: Psychoneuroimmunology Meets the Microbiome. Neuropsychopharmacology. 2016;42(1):178-92.
7. Knuesel I, Chicha L, Britschgi M, Schobel SA, Bodmer M, Hellings JA, et al. Maternal immune activation and abnormal brain development across CNS disorders. Nat Rev Neurol. 2014;10(11):643-60.
8. Carabotti M, Scirocco A, Maselli MA, Severi C. The gut-brain axis: interactions between enteric microbiota, central and enteric nervous systems. Ann Gastroenterol. 2015;28(2):203.
9. Mayer EA. Gut feelings: the emerging biology of gut–brain communication. Nat Rev Neurosci. 2011;12(8):453-66.
10. Rhee SH, Pothoulakis C, Mayer EA. Principles and clinical implications of the brain–gut–enteric microbiota axis. Nat Rev Gastroenterol Hepatol. 2009;6(5):306-14.
11. Muller PA, Schneeberger M, Matheis F, Wang P, Kerner Z, Ilanges A, et al. Microbiota modulate sympathetic neurons via a gut–brain circuit. Nature. 2020;583(7816):441-6.
12. Browning KN, Travagli RA. Central Nervous System Control of Gastrointestinal Motility and Secretion and Modulation of Gastrointestinal Functions. Compr Physiol. 2014;4(4):1339-68.
13. Fried S, Wemelle E, Cani PD, Knauf C. Interactions between the microbiota and enteric nervous system during gut-brain disorders. Neuropharmacology. 2021;197:108721.
14. Cani PD, Jordan BF. Gut microbiota-mediated inflammation in obesity: a link with gastrointestinal cancer. Nat Rev Gastroenterol Hepatol. 2018;15(11):671-82.
15. Pimentel M, Mathur R, Chang C. Gas and the microbiome. Curr Gastroenterol Rep. 2013;15(12):356.
16. Roth W, Zadeh K, Vekariya R, Ge Y, Mohamadzadeh M. Tryptophan Metabolism and Gut-Brain Homeostasis. Int J Mol Sci. 2021;22(6):2973.
17. Roager HM, Licht TR. Microbial tryptophan catabolites in health and disease. Nat Commun. 2018;9(1):1-10.
18. Clarke G, Stilling RM, Kennedy PJ, Stanton C, Cryan JF, Dinan TG. Minireview: Gut microbiota: the neglected endocrine organ. Mol Endocrinol. 2014;28(8):1221-38.

19. Fond G, Boukouaci W, Chevalier G, Regnault A, Eberl G, Hamdani N, et al. The "psychomicrobiotic": Targeting microbiota in major psychiatric disorders: A systematic review. Pathologie Biologie. 2015;63(1):35-42.
20. Maqsood R, Stone TW. The Gut-Brain Axis, BDNF, NMDA and CNS Disorders. Neurochem Res. 2016;41(11):2819-35.
21. Jiang H, Ling Z, Zhang Y, Mao H, Ma Z, Yin Y, et al. Altered fecal microbiota composition in patients with major depressive disorder. Brain Behav Immun. 2015;48:186-94.
22. Coello K, Hansen TH, Sørensen N, Munkholm K, Kessing LV, Pedersen O, et al. Gut microbiota composition in patients with newly diagnosed bipolar disorder and their unaffected first-degree relatives. Brain Behav Immun. 2019;75:112-8.
23. Flowers SA, Ward KM, Clark CT. The Gut Microbiome in Bipolar Disorder and Pharmacotherapy Management. Neuropsychobiology. 2020;79(1):43-9.
24. Evans SJ, Bassis CM, Hein R, Assari S, Flowers SA, Kelly MB, et al. The gut microbiome composition associates with bipolar disorder and illness severity. J Psychiatr Res. 2017;87:23-9.
25. Huang TT, Lai JB, Du YL, Xu Y, Ruan LM, Hu SH. Current understanding of gut microbiota in mood disorders: An update of human studies. Front Genet. 2019;10:98.
26. Schwarz E, Maukonen J, Hyytiäinen T, Kieseppä T, Orešič M, Sabunciyan S, et al. Analysis of microbiota in first episode psychosis identifies preliminary associations with symptom severity and treatment response. Schizophr Res. 2018;192:398-403.
27. Coretti L, Paparo L, Riccio MP, Amato F, Cuomo M, Natale A, et al. Gut microbiota features in young children with autism spectrum disorders. Front Microbiol. 2018;9:3146.
28. Adams JB, Johansen LJ, Powell LD, Quig D, Rubin RA. Gastrointestinal flora and gastrointestinal status in children with autism—comparisons to typical children and correlation with autism severity. BMC Gastroenterol. 2011;11(1):1-13.
29. Yang Y, Tian J, Yang B. Targeting gut microbiome: A novel and potential therapy for autism. Life Sci. 2018;194:111-9.
30. Ming X, Chen N, Ray C, Brewer G, Kornitzer J, Steer RA. A Gut Feeling: A Hypothesis of the Role of the Microbiome in Attention-Deficit/Hyperactivity Disorders. Child Neurol Open. 2018;5:2329048X18786799.
31. Seitz J, Trinh S, Herpertz-Dahlmann B. The Microbiome and Eating Disorders. Psychiatr Clin North Am. 2019;42(1):93-103.
32. McNulty NP, Yatsunenko T, Hsiao A, Faith JJ, Muegge BD, Goodman AL, et al. The impact of a consortium of fermented milk strains on the gut microbiome of gnotobiotic mice and monozygotic twins. Sci Transl Med. 2011;3(106):106ra106.
33. Codagnone MG, Spichak S, O'Mahony SM, O'Leary OF, Clarke G, Stanton C, et al. Programming Bugs: Microbiota and the Developmental Origins of Brain Health and Disease. Biol Psychiatry. 2019;85(2):150-63.
34. Janik R, Thomason LAM, Stanisz AM, Forsythe P, Bienenstock J, Stanisz GJ. Magnetic resonance spectroscopy reveals oral *Lactobacillus* promotion of increases in brain GABA, N-acetyl aspartate and glutamate. Neuroimage. 2016;125:988-95.

CHAPTER 3

Recent Advances in the Management of Prodromal Symptoms of Schizophrenia

G Prasad Rao, Amulya Koneru, Sriramya Veumulakonda, Pratham Ved Bhasyakarula

▪ INTRODUCTION

Schizophrenia is a major psychiatric disorder and can be traced back to ancient times with various descriptions of the symptoms. In the 20th century, the focus was more on the identification of the symptoms that constitute this illness and the treatment of the same. In the past few decades, however, there has been a rising interest in early intervention and even prevention of the disorder. This is mainly due to the extensive research that has shed awareness into the course of the illness which showed that longer periods of untreated psychosis led to poorer outcomes in the patients.

The term "prodrome" is often used to refer to the cluster of symptoms and signs that precede the actual episode. The period of prodrome can last for days, weeks, months, and often years before the onset of diagnosable illness. The symptoms can be nonspecific ones such as mood or anxiety symptoms, sleep, and cognitive disturbances or they can be specific symptoms such as odd ideation, unusual perceptual disturbances, social withdrawal, poor functioning, odd behavior, and speech.[1]

Since the symptoms are varied, the prodrome has been categorized as follows:[2]

- *Attenuated psychosis syndrome (APS):* This is characterized by subclinical or subthreshold symptoms of psychosis such as thought, cognitive, and perceptual disturbances, odd speech and behavior, flattened affect, avolition, social withdrawal, and anxiety or mood disturbances with deterioration in functioning. Current DSM-5 (Diagnostic and Statistical Manual of Mental Disorders, Fifth edition) criteria focus mainly on positive symptoms. This should have been present once per week in the past month and should have been there in the past year.
- *Brief intermittent psychosis prodromal syndrome (BIPS):* In this syndrome, the symptoms of psychosis are fleeting and resolve spontaneously within a week.
- *Genetic risk and deterioration syndrome (GRDS):* There is family history of schizophrenia in first degree relative or patient might show symptoms

of schizotypal personality disorder along with decline in the functioning, especially in the past year.

There has been increasing interest in the specific and nonspecific neurobiological, neurocognitive, and social cognitive disturbances that have been noticed in the individuals since young, subtle though they might be. These might help us herald the psychosis in at-risk individuals and give us a window to intervene leading to better outcomes.

RISK FACTORS OF THE PRODROME SYNDROME

Genetic Factors

Recent genome-wide association studies (GWAS) have shown that several genes are involved in the causation of schizophrenia leading to the understanding that schizophrenia is a polygenic disorder. Several single nucleotide polymorphisms (SNPs) within specific genes (for e.g., *ZNF804A, DISC1, DRD2, GRIA1*, etc.) have been identified to be associated with the pathology of schizophrenia. Occurrence of Copy Number Variants (CNVs) has been noted to be increased in the patients as compared to the controls. These mutations have an effect on the neurotransmitter receptor genes related to dopamine, glutamate, and gamma-aminobutyric acid (GABA) amongst others. Genes related to N-methyl-D-aspartate receptor (NMDAR), oxidative stress regulation, and those related to immunity in the brain have been implicated. These can be used as biomarkers to identify the individuals in the prodrome phase.[3,4]

Environmental Factors

It has been shown that gene-environment interactions have a significant effect on the pathophysiology and development of the illness including the prodrome state. Infections during pregnancy in the mother, fetal hypoxia, premorbid IQ, ethnic minorities, urbanicity, abuse in childhood, poor attachment to parental figures, and social withdrawal in childhood have been shown to contribute to the prodrome syndrome and also increasing transition to proper psychosis.[5,6]

Developmental Factors

Neurocognitive deficits have been reported in the children and adolescents who will later on develop psychosis. So, these can be considered to be both risk factors and also part of the prodrome. Difficulties in visual and verbal memory, verbal fluency, word processing speed, working memory, general intelligence, attention and concentration, and executive functioning deficits in later ages are most often reported. These might contribute to differences in understanding and perceiving the environment leading to unusual thought, speech, and perceptual experiences.

Social cognition plays an important role in the development of an individual. Deficits in it might lead to poor social interaction and social withdrawal with difficulties in perceiving emotions of others leading to odd thoughts and behavior and suspiciousness. Dysfunction in the areas of social cognition such as assessing emotion perception, theory of mind (ToM), social perception, social knowledge, and adaptive attributional styles have been seen in the early ages in individuals prone to develop prodrome and schizophrenia.[7]

Neurobiological Factors

Neurophysiological abnormalities such as abnormalities in saccadic eye movement control event-related brain potentials have been noted. Abnormalities in neuroplasticity phenomena that result in changes in neural structure and function are seen. Deficits in synaptic pruning have been noted as one of the probable causative factors in schizophrenia. From a young age, individuals show alterations in structures of the brain such as reduced cortical, hippocampal, and thalamic volumes. There are also reductions seen in volumes of temporal and frontal lobes. Alterations in neural cortical circuits have been shown to be risk factors for development of schizophrenia, especially the circuits involved in cognition and reward processing.[8,9]

Being aware of the risk factors and identifying them will help us to recognize the at-risk individuals for early interventions.

■ MANAGEMENT OF PRODROME

Management of the prodrome stage includes assessment for which various scales are available.

Tools for Assessing Prodromal Syndrome

The following scales are often used to identify the symptoms of prodrome:[2]
- Bonn Scale for the Assessment of Basic Symptoms
- Scale for Prodromal Symptoms (SOPS)
- Structured Interview for Prodromal Symptoms (SIPS)
- Comprehensive Assessment of At Risk Mental States (CAARMS)
- Multidimensional Assessment of Psychotic Prodrome

These scales can identify the at risk individuals and their symptoms can also be monitored for progression to schizophrenia.

Management

The first question that arises is "why there is a need to identify and treat prodrome syndrome." This is because as noted earlier, the earlier the onset of the illness and the longer the duration, the poorer the outcome of the illness. The rates of conversion from prodrome to psychosis vary from 20 to 50% in different studies in a span of 1–2 years. Hence, earlier intervention might help in delaying the conversion to proper psychosis and better outcomes of schizophrenia, thus leading to lesser burden on the healthcare services.[10]

The adage "prevention is better than cure" has often been used in the medical field. The idea that it might help in mental illnesses has been explored quite a lot. Research has delved into primary prevention where poverty, violence, and lack of healthcare have been addressed. Knowing risk factors for the prodrome can help in targeting them and we can aim at reducing them.[11] Those with already established risk factors can be identified and have targeted interventions which will be discussed in the following paragraphs.

Therapeutic Interventions

Psychological Interventions

Current research shows cognitive behavioral therapy (CBT) as one of the promising interventions. It has been used to help patients in prodrome to identify and change maladaptive thoughts, emotions, and behaviors. It also helps in improving coping strategies. Family therapy can help in reducing the stress caused by dysfunctional dynamics.

Psychoeducation and raising awareness of the prodrome can help in earlier identification.[12]

These strategies do not prevent the illness but do help in delaying the progression.

Pharmacological Interventions

Low dose antipsychotics have been tried in various studies with varying success. Risperidone, aripiprazole, and olanzapine have been used in them. They have shown efficacy in improving the prodrome symptoms in many individuals. However, these do not prevent onset of psychosis. Long-term use of the same in these at-risk individuals is not recommended due to severe side-effect profile and the risks outweigh the benefits. Hence, they can be only used for short-term periods. Combining these medications with CBT has shown to improve efficacy of the treatment.[1,13,14]

Antidepressants have been tried in a few studies but there is no evidence supporting regular use.

Emerging Interventions

Since recent studies have shown how dysfunction in oxidative stress regulation and inflammation might contribute to the development of the illness, more focus on treatment strategies targeting these pathways has increased. D-serine and sodium benzoate have been studied for their therapeutic potential and have shown efficacy in treating both positive and negative symptoms of psychosis. Treatment with other anti-inflammatory compounds such as, 7,8-dihydroxyflavone (a TrkB agonist), sulforaphane, and TPPU (1-trifluoromethoxyphenyl-3-(1-propionylpiperidin-4-yl) urea might have an effect in delaying the psychosis onset.[4,15]

Dietary supplements have also been the focus of attention in prevention of the illness. Omega-3 polyunsaturated fatty acids such as eicosapentaenoic acid and docosahexaenoic acid have shown to decrease the positive and negative symptoms of psychosis and also delayed the transition to psychosis stage.

CONCLUSION

In the recent decades, there has been a lot of research that has focused on early identification and treatment of schizophrenia. This translates to identification of the prodrome stage and preventing the transition to schizophrenia proper. Identification of at-risk individuals and monitoring their progress will help in early intervention thus decreasing the load on healthcare services and the workers. Few treatment strategies have emerged to treat prodrome syndrome. However, they do not prevent the onset of psychosis and only delay it. Further research into biomarkers and primary and primordial prevention techniques may help in addressing the current concerns.[16]

TAKE-HOME POINTS

- It has been found that early diagnosis and management of schizophrenia decreases the morbidity levels of these patients and leads to attenuated deterioration of functioning levels in all aspects of life. Hence, management of prodrome symptoms will help in reducing the burden of the illness.
- Recognition of risk factors from prodrome such as genetic biomarkers, environmental factors, neurocognitive deficits, and neurological soft signs in young age and monitoring them could help in early intervention. Use of therapies such as CBT, family therapy, social skills training, etc has shown evidence in delaying the onset of illness.
- Short term use of low dose antipsychotics, use of antioxidants and vitamin supplementation might be of some use. This will lead to decreased cost and burden on health care services and lead to improved quality of life.

REFERENCES

1. Larson MK, Walker EF, Compton MT. Early signs, diagnosis and therapeutics of the prodromal phase of schizophrenia and related psychotic disorders. Expert Rev Neurother. 2010;10(8):1347-59.
2. George M, Maheshwari S, Chandran S, Manohar JS, Sathyanarayana Rao TS. Understanding the schizophrenia prodrome. Indian J Psychiatry. 2017;59(4):505-9.
3. Althwanay A, AlZamil NA, Almukhadhib OY, Alkhunaizi S, Althwanay R. Risks and Protective Factors of the Prodromal Stage of Psychosis: A Literature Review. Cureus. 2020;12(6):e8639.

4. Lin CH, Lane HY. Early Identification and Intervention of Schizophrenia: Insight from Hypotheses of Glutamate Dysfunction and Oxidative Stress. Front Psychiatry. 2019;10:93.
5. Oliver D, Reilly TJ, Baccaredda Boy O, Petros N, Davies C, Borgwardt S, et al. What Causes the Onset of Psychosis in Individuals at Clinical High Risk? A Meta-analysis of Risk and Protective Factors. Schizophr Bull. 2020;46(1):110-20.
6. Radua J, Ramella-Cravaro V, Ioannidis J, Reichenberg A, Phiphopthatsanee N, Amir T, et al. What causes psychosis? An umbrella review of risk and protective factors. World psychiatry. World Psychiatr Assoc. 2018;17(1):49-66.
7. Rek-Owodziń K, Tyburski E, Waszczuk K, Samochowiec J, Mak M. Neurocognition and Social Cognition-Possibilities for Diagnosis and Treatment in Ultra-High Risk for Psychosis State. Front Psychiatry. 2021;12:765126.
8. Davies EJ. Developmental aspects of schizophrenia and related disorders: Possible implications for treatment strategies. Adv Psychiatr Treat. 2007;13:384-91.
9. Robison AJ, Thakkar KN, Diwadkar VA. Cognition and Reward Circuits in Schizophrenia: Synergistic, Not Separate. Biol Psychiatry. 2020;87(3):204-14.
10. Bearden CE, Forsyth JK. The many roads to psychosis: recent advances in understanding risk and mechanisms. F1000Res. 2018;7:F1000 Faculty Rev-1883.
11. Joa I, Gisselgård J, Brønnick K, McGlashan T, Johannessen JO. Primary prevention of psychosis through interventions in the symptomatic prodromal phase, a pragmatic Norwegian Ultra High Risk study. BMC Psychiatry. 2015;15:89.
12. Kaur T, Cadenhead KS. Treatment implications of the schizophrenia prodrome. Curr Top Behav Neurosci. 2010;4:97-121.
13. Liu CC, Demjaha A. Antipsychotic interventions in prodromal psychosis: safety issues. CNS Drugs. 2013;27(3):197-205.
14. Liu CC, Sheu YH, Wu SY, Lai MC, Hwu HG. Rapid response to antipsychotic treatment on psychotic prodrome: implications from a case series. Psychiatry Clin Neurosci. 2010;64(2):202-6.
15. Hashimoto K. Recent Advances in the Early Intervention in Schizophrenia: Future Direction from Preclinical Findings. Curr Psychiatry Rep. 2019;21(8):75.
16. Mokhtari M, Rajarethinam R. Early intervention and the treatment of prodrome in schizophrenia: a review of recent developments. J Psychiatr Pract. 2013;19(5):375-85.

CHAPTER 4

Designer Drugs

Omkar Nayak, Avinash De Sousa

INTRODUCTION

Designer drugs, also known as "Legal Highs" are substances having psychotropic effects that are marketed and distributed for recreational use. Designer drug use has increased significantly in the past decade, especially among the young adults leading to significant problems for some users. The incidence of designer drug problems in emergency departments, hospitals, and other medical settings is largely unknown as per literature. Only a small percentage of those who use designer drugs, usually come into contact with the healthcare system, even in developed countries like USA. Having knowledge of designer drugs can help the clinicians to recognize common adverse reactions and life-threatening consequences. This chapter provides an overview of the main mechanisms of action and adverse effects of currently available designer drugs.[1]

STIMULANTS

Stimulants such as amphetamine, 3,4-methylenedioxymethamphetamine (MDMA), and cocaine, are among the most popular drugs of abuse of misuse. Methylphenidate and dextroamphetamine are some other examples of stimulants. Stimulants cause modulation of monoaminergic neurotransmission by interacting with norepinephrine, serotonin, and dopamine transporters. They also interact with monoaminergic receptors and other targets. Different selectivity and potency at different transporters result in different pharmacological effects, different clinical potencies, and different abuse liabilities. The number of available designer stimulants is constantly increasing and their use can cause various physiological complications and disturbances in mood.

Amphetamines

In addition to traditional amphetamines that have been used both medically and recreationally, several amphetamine drugs without approved medical uses have become available. MDMA is the most popular amphetamines designer drug. It was a first synthesized by Merck in 1912 as precursor in new chemical pathway. In 1980s, it became popular as recreational drug under the street name "Ecstasy" which led to ban of MDMA in most countries soon afterward. Currently, it is a promising agent for treatment of post-traumatic stress disorder.[2]

Mechanism of Action

Most amphetamines are substrate-type monoamine releasers, having a potent effect on the norepinephrine transporters. In addition to it, many amphetamines predominantly act at dopamine transporter and serotonin transporter (DAT vs. SERT) resulting in greater reinforcing effects and higher abuse liability. Those amphetamines like MDMA which has a more action on SERT as compared to DAT have a comparatively lesser abuse liability. Amphetamine also acts as substrates at vesicular monoamine transporters and inhibits the monoamine oxidase (MAO). These drugs have also been reported to interact with various monoaminergic receptors including serotonergic and adrenergic receptors and trace-amine-associated-receptor-1 which negatively modulates monoaminergic neurotransmission.

Adverse Effects

For traditional amphetamines, mainly sympathomimetic adverse effects can be expected. These include dry mouth, anxiety, insomnia, headache, mydriasis, bruxism, hypertension, tachycardia, hyperthermia, chest pain, palpitations, anorexia, nausea, vomiting, and abdominal pain. Hyperthermia may lead to potentially severe adverse effects like disseminated intravascular coagulation, renal failure, and rhabdomyolysis. Hepatotoxicity is a potentially fatal adverse effect that has been associated with the use of amphetamines and MDMA is a designer drug that has been most frequently linked to liver injury. Cardiotoxicity is another potential complication of amphetamine use, largely attributable to sympathomimetic activation, additionally also to hyperthermia. Monoamine depletion and reactive species contribute to neurotoxicity of amphetamines. However, despite extensive research, the extent to which different amphetamines are neurotoxic remains largely unknown.

Cathinone and Pyrovalerone Derivatives

Cathinone designer drugs are derivatives of β-keto amphetamine cathinone, an alkaloid that is found in the leaves of the *Catha edulis* plant. The large scale recreational use of cathinone's is a relatively new phenomenon, although several compounds have been known for long time. Several synthetic cathinones have been investigated for their medicinal potential mostly as antidepressants or anorectic agents but only a few were ever marketed because of concerns about abuse. Pyrovalerone derivatives represent a subgroup of synthetic cathinones based on structure of pyrovalerone, which was developed in the 1960s as a treatment option for lethargy, fatigue and obesity. As a result of their initial misleading marketing as "bath salts", synthetic cathinone's are still often referred to by that term.[3]

Mechanism of Action

The psychoactive effects of these drugs are primarily medicated by interactions with monoamine transporters. They are partially of fully effective substrate-type releasers at one or several monoamine transporters, but some compounds such as pyrovalerone derivatives are transporter inhibitors. Mephedrone has additionally been shown to mediate monoamine release via organic cation transporter 3 (OCT 3) indicating that cathinones target both high affinity and low affinity high capacity transporters. Similarly, to amphetamines, cathinone drugs also interact with several adrenergic and serotonergic receptors. Compared to amphetamines, however, cathinone designer drugs have been shown to interact less potently with trace-amine-associated-receptor-1 (TAAR-1) and vesicular monoamine transporter 2 (VMAT-2). These less potent interactions at TAAR-1 may result in higher risk of cathinone dependence compared with amphetamines.

Adverse Effects

The adverse effects include mainly sympathomimetic toxicity which manifests as agitation, tachycardia, hypertension, lower levels of consciousness, hallucinations, hyponatremia, chest pain, palpitations, and nausea. Rarely, severe adverse effects such as seizures, significant peripheral organ damage, and rhabdomyolysis have been reported. Numerous cathinone-related fatalities have been reported in literature.

Benzofuran and Indole Derivatives

Benzofuran and indole derivatives are analogs of MDMA and its metabolite 3,4-methylenedioxyamphetamine (MDA).[4]

Mechanism of Action

They cause norepinephrine uptake inhibition. They also have moderate to high selectivity in inhibiting 5-hydroxytryptamine (5-HT) vs. dopamine uptake, often with substrate activity at the transporters. Furthermore, affinity at adrenergic, serotonergic, and histaminergic receptors, and partial agonist at 5-HT2B receptors have been reported for these designer drugs.

Adverse Effects

They may cause side effects like agitation, insomnia headache, drowsiness, dry mouth, dry eyes, bruxism, hyperthermia, tachycardia, palpitations, nausea diarrhea, hot flashes, and clonus of hands and feet. They can also cause psychological symptoms including visual and auditory hallucinations, depression, anxiety, panic attacks, paranoia, and psychosis.

Aminoindanes

Aminoindanes are conformationally restricted analogs of amphetamines that were originally investigated as bronchodilators, analgesic, and anti-Parkinsonian agents and subsequently as dugs with psychotherapeutic value. The desired psychoactive effects of aminoindane designer drugs include euphoria, mild distortion of vision, time and space, a greater intensity of perceptions and colors, empathy, and arousal.[5]

Mechanism of Action

They are monoamine transporter substrates with relevant affinity for adrenergic, dopaminergic, and serotonergic receptors.

Adverse Effects

Self-reported adverse effects of aminoindane designer drugs include agitation, anxiety, panic attacks, headache, insomnia, hallucinations, and tachycardia. Three fatal cases were reported due to MDAI intake [5,6-methylenedixy-2-aminoindone], As per the literature, serotonin syndrome could have been a factor that contributed to death. The likelihood of serotonergic toxicity of aminoindanes in humans has not been investigated, but signs of serotonin syndrome were reported for a high dose of MDAI in rats.

Piperazines

Piperazine designer drugs are widely sold as legal party pills or powder and appeared as pure substances or adulterants in pills that are sold as "ecstasy" because of their somewhat MDMA-like pharmacological profile. Various therapeutic drugs have a piperazine moiety and some piperazine designer drugs have a history of medical use; for example 1-benzylpiperazine (BZP) has been investigated as an anthelminthic agent and antidepressant and meta-chlorophenylpiperazine [mCPP] is an active metabolite of different antidepressants.[5]

Mechanism of Action

Piperazine designer drugs exert mixed effects at monoamine transporters. All these substances bind to several serotonergic, adrenergic, dopaminergic and histaminergic receptors with sub micro molar or low micro molar affinity.

Adverse Effects

Adverse effects of piperazine designer drugs are mostly sympathomimetic including agitation, insomnia, headaches, dizziness, dilated pupils, hyperthermia, tachycardia, nausea, urine retention, and inducible clonus.

In addition to sympathomimetic toxicity, dissociative symptoms, visual and auditory hallucinations, and psychological symptoms (e.g., short temper, confusion, anxiety, depression, and paranoia) have been associated with the use of piperazine designer drugs. Furthermore, toxic seizures have been frequently observed in patients who were admitted to emergency department after the use of BZP-containing party pills. Seizures may also occur at lower doses as per literature. Other severe adverse effects of BZP include hyponatremia, severe combined metabolic and respiratory acidosis, hepatic injury, renal failure, disseminated intravascular coagulation, and rhabdomyolysis. A case of severe hyperthermia with resultant multiorgan failure and a case of hyponatremia that led to fatal brain edema were reported for the concomitant use of piperazine designer drugs and MDMA.

Phenidate Derivatives

Derivatives of the piperidine prescription drug methylphenidate have appeared as designer drugs with substitutions at the "phenyl ring" and different lengths of the carbon side chain phenidate derivatives may be used to induce euphoria or as cognitive enhancers. When insufflated, the pharmacological and subjective-effect profile of methylphenidate is similar to cocaine and phenidate derivatives may therefore be used as substitutes to cocaine.[6]

Mechanism of Action

Similar to methylphenidate, phenidate derivatives act as potent NET and DAT inhibitors that are avoid of any substrate activity. Some less potent interactions with SERT and adrenergic and serotonergic receptors have been reported but are not likely to play a relevant role in the psychoactive actions of most phenidate derivatives.

Adverse Effects

Adverse effects of phenidate derivatives are similar to amphetamines and include agitation, anxiety, hypertension, tachycardia, and palpitations. Because their onset of action is relatively slow when taken orally, the nasal insufflation or injection of phenidate derivatives is common, especially in heavy users. Nasal pain and septum perforations after insufflation and infections after intravenous injections may occur.

Aminorex Analogs

Various analogs of anorectic agent aminorex have become available as designer drugs. Aminorex was first marketed as an over-the-counter appetite suppressant in parts of Europe in the 1960s but was withdrawn a few years later due to an epidemic of chronic pulmonary hypertension that was associated with many fatalities. Aminorex analogs, like 4-methylaminorex (4-MAR), cause euphoria, mental and physical stimulation, sociability, empathy, arousal, and changes in visual perception.[7]

Mechanism of Action
Aminorex analogs are potent inhibitors of norepinephrine, dopamine, and serotonin reuptake.

Adverse Effects
Adverse effects of aminorex agents include agitation, dysphonia, insomnia, amnesia, panic attacks, psychosis, hallucinations, facial spasms, dilated pupils, foaming at the mouth, dry mouth, jaw clenching, elevations of body temperature, sweating, tachycardia, nausea, and restless legs. Pulmonary hypertension has been associated with recreational use of 4-MAR.

Phenmetrazine Derivatives

Phenmetrazine is a reinforcing stimulant which was previously used as an appetite suppressant before it was eventually withdrawn from the market. They represent relatively understudied class of drugs among which 3-fluorophenmetra (2-3-FPM) use appears to be the most widespread.[8]

Mechanism of Action
Phenmetrazine is a reinforcing stimulant. It is a substrate at the norepinephrine transporter (NET) and DAT with minor substrate activity at the SERT. Ring methylated phenmetrazine derivatives were reported to have greater potency at the SERT, in addition to activity at NET and DAT.

Adverse Effects
They elicit stimulatory toxicity similar to amphetamines. Clinical features include both miotic and dilated pupils, hypertension, and hypotension. Intravenous use of 3-FPM may result in severe vasoconstriction.

Thiophene Designer Drugs

Various analogs of amphetamines and cathinones with a theophany group that replaces the phenyl ring have appeared as designer drugs. To date, most pharmacological studies and toxicological reports involve methiopropamine (MPA) the thiophene analog of methamphetamine.[9]

Mechanism of Action

Methiopropamine is a quasi-equipotent inhibitor of norepinephrine and dopamine uptake and was reported to interact with various serotonergic, adrenergic, dopaminergic, N-methyl-D-aspartate, and sigma 1 receptors.

Adverse Effects

Methiopropamine use has been associated with significant acute toxicity and psychotic, cardiovascular, and gastrointestinal symptoms, including agitation, anxiety, confusion, insomnia, visual hallucinations, tachycardia, palpitations, nausea, vomiting, and chest tightness. There may be elevations in levels of creatine kinase.

SEDATIVES

Synthetic Opioids

While being essential for pain treatment, the nonmedical use of opioids has been a public health threat for centuries and includes the recreational use of illegal substances, the abuse of prescription medications, and drug adulteration with nonpharmacological opioids. Opioids induce euphoria, anxiolysis, feelings of relaxation, and drowsiness. Repeated use leads to development of dependence.[10]

Mechanism of Action

Synthetic opioids interact with G-protein-coupled opioid receptors in the brain as partial to full agonists at all, Delta and Kappa opioid receptors subtypes, with selectivity for the Υ opioid receptors. The agonist at Υ opioid receptors drives the main pharmacological effects of opioids, including euphoria, analgesia, respiratory depression, and development of dependence.

Adverse Effects

Adverse effects include dizziness, a lower level of consciousness, miosis, central nervous system depression, respiratory depression, pulmonary edema hypoxia, bradycardia, pruritus, nausea, vomiting, constipation, agitation, hypertension, and tachycardia. Serotonergic toxicity is one adverse effect that needs to be considered for opioid designer drugs when compared with other serotonergic agents. The competitive opioid receptor antagonist naloxone rapidly reverses central and peripheral effects of opioids and is thus an effective antidote for opioid toxicity. The initial care of patients who are intoxicated with designer drugs should include maintenance of airway, breathing, and circulation. Naloxone should be administered as soon as possible.

Designer Benzodiazepines

Benzodiazepine abuse is frequent. The main reasons for such abuse is to facilitate sleep, cope with stress, ease effects of stimulants, self-treat withdrawal symptoms, and get a high. When taken in combination with opioids, they enhance the euphoric effects of opioid use. Since 2007, several benzodiazepine designer drugs have become available, some of which are precursors or metabolites of prescription benzodiazepine. Their effects resemble those of prescription benzodiazepine.[11]

Mechanism of Action

They mediate their effects through interactions with (GABA) receptors, like prescription benzodiazepines. Benzodiazepines enhance the effect of GABA as positive allosteric modulators by binding to a receptor site that is different from binding site of GABA.

Adverse Effects

The concurrent use of benzodiazepines and other depressants such as alcohol and opioids may produce prolonged and potentially fatal respiratory depression. Reported adverse effects of designer benzodiazepines include agitation, hyperthermia, tachycardia, fatigue, impairment of thinking, confusion, dizziness, drowsiness, lethargy, amnesia, blurred vision, blurred speech, and palpitations. It can cause auditory and visual hallucinations, delirium, seizures, and coma at high doses. Chronic use may lead to development of tolerance and dependence. Withdrawal symptoms such as anxiety, panic attacks, restlessness, insomnia, seizures, and life-threatening conclusions may follow the abrupt cessation of chronic designer benzodiazepine use.

Gamma-aminobutyric Acid Analogs

Gamma hydroxybutyrate (GHB) is a short-chain fatty acid analog of the inhibitory neurotransmitter GABA. It has become popular among drug users because of its ability to induce feelings of euphoria and relaxation, reduce social anxiety, and increase sexual drive. Other structural analogs of GABA that have become available as designer drugs include gamma-butyrolactone (GBL), 1,4-butanediol (1,4-BD), gamma-hydroxyvaleric acid, 4-amino-3-phenyl-butyne acid (phenibut).

Mechanism of Action

The subjective benefits of GHB and its analogs outweigh adverse effects only over a narrow range of doses. Adverse events include a lower level of consciousness, hypothermia, respiratory depression, aspiration, bradycardia, and gastrointestinal upset. Some other nonsedative adverse events include agitation, seizures, and myoclonus. These adverse events typically have a relative short duration and are usually managed with supportive care. Abrupt cessation after regular use may trigger a potentially life-threatening withdrawal syndrome that can manifest as agitation, anxiety, confusion, disorientation, paranoia, aggression, insomnia, auditory and visual hallucinations, tremors, sweating, hypertension, and tachycardia. Benzodiazepines appear to be the treatment of choice for withdrawal from GHB and its analogs.

Synthetic Cannabinoids

The endocannabinoid system is involved in various physiological functions including cognition, behavior, memory, motor control, pain sensation, appetite, cardiovascular parameters, gastrointestinal motility, and immunoregulation.[12] The term "cannabinoid" refers to the class of compounds produced by *Cannabis sativa* and *Cannabis indica* and endogenous and exogenous ligands that interact with G protein-coupled cannabinoid type 1 (CB1) and CB2 receptors. CB1 receptors are mainly expressed in the brain and modulate neurotransmitter signaling, whereas CB2 receptors are abundant in immune tissues. The synthetic cannabinoids were developed to study human endocannabinoid receptor systems in the second half of 20th century. Today they represent the largest and most structurally diverse class of designer drugs and some of these compounds are similar to phyto- and endocannabinoids. Synthetic cannabinoids are often referred to as "spice" based on the first branded synthetic cannabinoid product. They are commonly applied to dried leaves that mimic cannabis. Desired effects of synthetic cannabinoids include relaxation, euphoria, and disinhibition, thus not significantly differing from desired effects of D^9-tetrahydrocannabinol (D^9THC), the main psychoactive component of cannabis.

Mechanism of Action

Various synthetic cannabinoids have been reported to bind to CB1 and CB2 receptors with higher efficiency at both receptors compared with D^9THC. Based signaling at cannabinoid receptors or the disruption of mitochondrial homeostasis may play a role in the difference between the clinical effects of D^9THC and synthetic cannabinoids, but research in this area is still in its infancy. The predominance of CB1 receptors in the central nervous system compared to CB2 receptors indicates that they (CB1 receptors) mainly mediate the psychoactive effects of synthetic cannabinoids. Possible effects of synthetic cannabinoids on noncannabinoid receptors and different signaling pathways have not yet been discovered, but cannot be ruled out.

Adverse Effects

The common adverse effects of synthetic cannabinoids include agitation, drowsiness, dizziness, confusion, hallucinations, hypertension, tachycardia, chest pain, nausea, and vomiting. They typically have short duration and require only symptomatic or supportive treatment. Severe clinical complications that have been reported to be associated with synthetic cannabinoid use include convulsions, delirium, ischemic stroke, intracranial hemorrhage, pulmonary embolism, pneumonia and pulmonary infiltrates, respiratory depression, ventricular and supraventricular arrhythmias, myocardial ischemia and infarction, takotsubo cardiomyopathy, liver injury, acute kidney injury, rhabdomyolysis, and hyperemesis syndrome. Furthermore, various psychiatric adverse effects have been reported including paranoia, psychosis, ideations of self-harm, and suicide.

PSYCHEDELICS

Serotonergic psychedelics induce alterations of perception and cognitive states in users. Traditional psychedelics such as phenylethylamine, tryptamines, and psilocybin and the ergot alkaloid LSD (lysergic acid diethylamide) have a history of being used as illicit black market drug. The psychedelic effects of these drugs are medicated mainly by 5-HT2A agonist. Affinity for 5-HT2A and 5-HT2C receptors is correlated with amount of drug that induces psychedelic effects in the humans.[13]

Phenylethylamines

Derivatives of mescaline comprise a large amount of psychedelic designer drugs. The widest spread phenylethylamines are 2,5-dimethoxyphenylethylamines.

Mechanism of Action

They interact with serotonergic receptors with highest affinity for 5-HT2A receptors. Some derivatives have higher affinity for 5-HT2A and 5-HT2C receptors and lower affinity for 5-HT1A receptors compared to their 2C analogs.

Adverse Effects

Most of the frequently reported adverse effects include agitation, hallucinations, confusion, drowsiness, mydriasis, aggression, hyperthermia, hypertension, and tachycardia. Severe adverse effects include seizure, coma, acute psychosis, cerebral edema, long lasting severe neurological impairment, serotonin syndrome, prolonged respiratory failure, renal failure, multiorgan failure, metabolic acidosis, and rhabdomyolysis.

Tryptamines

The core structure of tryptamine designer drugs contains an indole ring that is connected to an amino group by an ethyl side chain. They have recently regained interest for their therapeutic use.

Mechanism of Action

5-HT2A receptor agonist plays a key role in mediating the psychedelic effects of naturally occurring and synthetic tryptamine psychedelic. Most traditional and novel tryptamine psychedelics bind to 5-HT1A and 5-HT2A receptors with similar affinity. Some tryptamines are slightly more selective at one or the other receptor subtype. They have been also shown to bind at various other targets in vitro like the adrenergic, dopaminergic, histaminergic receptors. They have interactions at NET, DAT as well as SERT. Substrate activity at VMAT has also been described for tryptamine psychedelics. Tryptamines are prone to metabolism by MAO and MAO inhibitors counteract extensive degradation of tryptamine after oral use.

Adverse Effects

They alter the perception and can induce psychological disturbances in users, including acute psychosis. Adverse events include restlessness, disorientation, clouding of consciousness, confusion, hallucinations, amnesia, catalepsy, mydriasis, tachypnea, tachycardia, and hypertension. Some tryptamines can produce prolonged delusions. In severe cases the use of tryptomer designer drugs has resulted in acute renal failure and rhabdomyolysis.

Lysergamides

Several derivatives of LSD have been described in the scientific literature and such derivatives are increasingly emerging as designer drugs. The LSD-derived designer drugs such as 1-acetyl LSD, 1-propionyl-LSD, and 1-butyryl-LSD have been shown to be metabolized to LSD, in vitro and are thus considered precursors of LSD with very similar effects.

Mechanism of Action

5-HT2A receptor activation mediates the behavioral effects of LSD analogs. Additionally, 5-HT1A receptor activation likely contributes to the qualitative effects of lysergamide designer drugs, similar to LSD and tryptamine psychedelic.

Adverse Effects

Acute physiological effects of LSD include imbalance, difficulty concentrating, feelings of exhaustion, dizziness, headache, dry mouth, lack of appetite, and nausea.

CONCLUSION

Various types of designer drugs are available in the market. It is important to know and spread information about their effects and side effects so that their misuse and abuse can be prevented or treated accordingly.

TAKE-HOME POINTS
- Designer drugs are a new emerging class of substances that are being used and abused more and more by patients in India and all over the world.
- The number of these drugs keeps increasing as new drugs are being produced as derivatives and synthetic preparations of older existing ones.
- Clinicians must be aware of designer drugs and their types to help in the management of patients that abuse these substances.

REFERENCES

1. Weaver MF, Hopper JA, Gunderson EW. Designer drugs 2015: assessment and management. Addict Sci Clin Pract. 2015;10(1):1-9.
2. Luethi D, Liechti ME. Designer drugs: mechanism of action and adverse effects. Arch Toxicol. 2020;94(4):1085-133.
3. Carroll FI, Lewin AH, Mascarella SW, Seltzman HH, Reddy PA. Designer drugs: a medicinal chemistry perspective. Ann N Y Acad Sci. 2012;1248(1):18-38.
4. Majchrzak M, Celiński R, Kuś P, Kowalska T, Sajewicz M. The newest cathinone derivatives as designer drugs: an analytical and toxicological review. Forensic Toxicol. 2018;36(1):33-50.
5. Pourmand A, Mazer-Amirshahi M, Chistov S, Li A, Park M. Designer drugs: Review and implications for emergency management. Hum Exp Toxicology. 2018;37(1):94-101.
6. Luethi D, Kaeser PJ, Brandt SD, Krähenbühl S, Hoener MC, Liechti ME. Pharmacological profile of methylphenidate-based designer drugs. Neuropharmacology. 2018;134:133-40.
7. Abbate V, Guillou C, Schwenk M. Psychoactive Designer Drugs: Classes, Mechanisms, Regulation. Regul Toxicol. 2021:1-7.
8. Liu L, Wheeler SE, Venkataramanan R, Rymer JA, Pizon AF, Lynch MJ, et al. Newly emerging drugs of abuse and their detection methods: an ACLPS critical review. Am J Clin Pathol. 2018;149(2):105-16.
9. Wang GS, Hoyte C. Novel drugs of abuse. Paediatr Rev. 2019;40(2):71-8.
10. Klega AE, Keehbauch JT. Stimulant and designer drug use: primary care management. Am Fam Phys. 2018;98(2):85-92.
11. Williams JF, Lundahl LH. Focus on adolescent use of club drugs and "other" substances. Pediatr Clin. 2019;66(6):1121-34.
12. Zawilska JB, Wojcieszak J. An expanding world of new psychoactive substances—designer benzodiazepines. Neurotoxicology. 2019;73:8-16.
13. Greenblatt HK, Greenblatt DJ. Designer benzodiazepines: a review of published data and public health significance. Clin Pharmacol Drug Dev. 2019;8(3):266-9.

CHAPTER 5
Telepsychiatry in India

Arijit Mondal, OP Singh

■ INTRODUCTION

The United States Food and Drug Administration (US FDA) defines telemedicine as "consultative services to individual patients and the transmission of information related to care, over distance, using telecommunication technologies. It incorporates direct clinical, preventive, diagnostic, and therapeutic services and treatment; consultative and follow-up services; remote monitoring of patients; rehabilitative services; and patient education."[1] In a simple way, it refers to delivery of health care services to a distant place using multimedia technology.

Telepsychiatry is like telemedicine that allows a psychiatrist and a patient can talk to each other directly. It also includes psychiatrists who give advice and help to primary care providers about mental health care. Mental health care can be given through live, two-way communication. It could also involve taking medical data (images, videos, etc.) and sending it to a remote location so that it can be looked at later.

Telepsychiatry's benefits and necessity:
- Availability and easy access to mental health care services in remote and rural areas.
- Bring medical attention to the patient's location.
- Integration of mental health care with primary health care for better outcome.
- Reduce the need for emergency room visits.
- Reduce delay in health care delivery.
- Persistent regular care and follow-up.
- Reduce the need for time off work, childcare services, and so on to travel to distant appointments.
- Reduce the need for long transportation to avail health care services.
- Remove the stigma barrier[2]

An increase in patients experiencing their first experience of psychiatric problems such depression, anxiety, and even acute psychosis has been linked to the coronavirus disease 2019 (COVID-19) pandemic.

Acute exacerbations and relapses in people with preexisting psychiatric illnesses have also been documented.[3] The creation of a proper systemic and reliable telepsychiatry structure must urgently be escalated in light of the aforementioned emergencies. Thankfully, the lockdown that followed in many nations has opened up possibilities for teleconsultation, and within weeks, numerous authorities have suggested telepsychiatry rules.

Allely first described two types of telemedicine delivery systems:[4]

1. *Synchronous telemedicine:* By using telephone voice call, online chat communication or video call, synchronous telemedicine "provides live, two-way interactive transmission between patient and provider at remote sites."[4] It is distinguished by: (1) sending data continuously without interruptions; (2) being beneficial to remote sections of the nation in need of expert advice; (3) assisting in the swift treatment of epidemic situations.
   Disadvantage: Expensive setup; challenging to put up in underdeveloped rural areas.
2. *Asynchronous telemedicine:* "Involves collecting medical data and then transmitting this clinical information in the form of data, audio, video clips, or recordings via e-mail or web applications for subsequent review by a specialist."[4] It is distinguished by two things: (1) no need for synchronized communication between the two sides; (2) cheaper cost and fewer hardware requirements.

DIFFERENT MODELS OF TELEPSYCHIATRY IN INDIA

Schizophrenia Research Foundation Telepsychiatry in Pudukkottai Model

Schizophrenia Research Foundation (SCARF), a nongovernmental organization (NGO) operates from Chennai and provides psychiatric services. The first telepsychiatry model was published by Thara et al. in 2008 which led down a new path in the field of telepsychiatry.[5] Different components of STEP (SCARF Telepsychiatry in Pudukottai) model are:

- *Establishment of base:* Choosing a location with good communication and easy access to necessary infrastructure
- Collaboration and communication with local NGO for the training of staff
- Awareness campaign in the nearby locality about the availability of service
- Providing teleconsultations
- Supply of medicines free of cost
- Case documentation and follow-up

Mobile Telepsychiatry Model by Schizophrenia Research Foundation

Schizophrenia Research Foundation was also a pioneer in the initiation of mobile telepsychiatric unit in India. Following the success of nonmobile telepsychiatry unit, the first mobile telepsychiatry service was first started in 2010, in Pudukkottai district, Tamil Nadu, India. A mobile telepsychiatry unit is usually a bus accommodating a pharmacy and a consultation room. A psychiatrist provides consultations after interviewing with the patient and informant in the mobile unit. The advice from psychiatrist is issued as prescription and the medicines are provided at no cost. The mobile telepsychiatry unit was also used for psychosocial intervention and awareness programs.[6]

Post Graduate Institute of Medical Education and Research Chandigarh: "Psychiatrist-on-web" Model

This model entailed providing patients in remote areas with comprehensive mental health care. Due to dearth of treating psychiatrists, especially in rural and remote areas, this model was developed using software application which provides automated diagnosis and guidance to nonspecialists and attendant regarding line of management, thereby eliminating the requirement of a psychiatrist to be present for every case. Psychiatrists are required for challenging cases, psychiatric emergencies, and for specialized treatment methods, such as autism. This is known as the "tele enabling model" and it allows nonspecialists to reach diagnosis and to treat psychiatric disorders under guidance. The software application has child and adult versions as well as default diagnostic tools with good specificity and sensitivity for the majority of psychiatric illnesses.[7]

Ganiyari Model

Another telepsychiatry program is currently operating as part of the Jan Swasthya Sahyog community health program. It was created to serve the tribal population of Bilaspur and the surrounding areas of Chhattisgarh, India's central state. Since 2012, this Ganiyari program has provided collaborative service through a specialist–doctor/paramedical–personnel model using the Skype platform.[8]

National Institute of Mental Health and Neurosciences: Extension for Community Health Outcomes

The Centre for Addiction Medicine, National Institute of Mental Health and Neurosciences (NIMHANS), Bengaluru, India, has launched a new program that offers a forum for active learning, discussion, and participation for mental health care workers from different parts of the country. The concept is to disseminate knowledge and clinical experience to frontline physicians for the treatment of "chronic, common, and complex diseases" by case discussions and opinion from experts in the field. Weekly video conferences are held via multipoint video conference, which is led by subject matter experts.[9]

Balasinorwala et al. Model

This telepsychiatry model was utilized in the state of Maharashtra. The primary care physicians refer the case and the investigations to the psychiatrists via email. Psychiatrists diagnose the case and offer advice based on the content of e-mails.[10]

TELEMEDICINE PRACTICE GUIDELINES 2020

In March of 2020, the Ministry of Health and Family Welfare, Government of India issued "Telemedicine Practice Guidelines" to assist registered medical practitioners (RMPs) in incorporating telemedicine into their normal medical practice. This guideline was drafted by the Board of Governors in collaboration with the National Institution for Transforming India (NITI Aayog), which succeeded the Medical Council of India. This guideline is included in appendix V of the 2002 regulations pertaining to "professional conduct and ethics" under the Indian Medical Council Act of 1956.[11]

According to the guidelines, the RMPs should check the identity of the patient using their name, age, email ID, address, and phone number. The RMPs should also provide information for the patient to check the identity of the RMPs, including name, professional qualification, medical council registration, and contact information. The RMP should document the age of the patient. Teleconsultation should only be done in the presence of an adult and identity of the adult must be documented before starting consultation. Teleconsultation requires explicit consent, which must be documented. Consent is implied when the patient starts communication with the RMP for consultation. When a health care worker, an RMP, or a caregiver starts a teleconsultation, explicit consent must be taken and documented.

Before making any professional decisions, RMPs should give sufficient effort to gather adequate information. If more medical information is required, an in-person consultation should be considered. All records, including patient details, clinical notes, and investigation reports should be retained properly. Only after an accurate diagnosis, medications should be prescribed. The guidelines divide drugs into four categories: prohibited drug list, list-A, list-B, and list-O **(Table 1)**. If it is the first consultation, list-A drugs can only be advised after video consultation. If a prescription is sent directly to a pharmacy, it must be sent electronically to the patient and the patient must give explicit consent.

TABLE 1: Drug lists according to the type and mode of teleconsultation.

List group	Mode of consultation (video/audio/text)	Nature of consultation (first-consultation/follow-up]	List of medicines
O	Any	Any	List O[1]
A	Video	First consultation Follow-up, for continuation of medications	List A[2]
B	Any	Follow-up	List B[3]
Prohibited	Not to be prescribed	Not to be prescribed	Schedule X of Drugs and Cosmetics Act and Rules or any narcotic and psychotropic substance listed in the Narcotic Drugs and Psychotropic Substances Act, 1985[4]

[1]This list included commonly used "over-the-counter" medications such as paracetamol, oral rehydration solution (ORS) packets, and antacids.
    This list also includes medicines that may be deemed necessary during emergencies and would be notified from time to time.
[2]This list includes usually prescribed medications for which diagnosis is possible only by video consultation such as antifungal medications for tinea cruris and ciprofloxacin eye drops for conjunctivitis and refill medications for chronic diseases such as diabetes, hypertension, and asthma.
[3]This list includes "add-on" medications which are used to optimize an existing condition; for instance, if the patient is already on atenolol for hypertension and the blood pressure is not controlled, an angiotensin-converting enzyme (ACE) inhibitor such as enalapril.
[4]For instance, anticancer drugs; narcotics such as morphine and codeine.
Source: Telemedicine Practice Guidelines 2020.[11]

The guidelines do not say anything about using digital technology to do surgery or invasive procedures remotely. The guidelines also do not say anything about research, evaluation, and continuing education for health professionals who use telemedicine technology. The guidelines do not mention anything about consultations outside of India's jurisdiction or about specifications for telemedicine hardware, software, and infrastructure. The guidelines also define professional misconduct, which includes not protecting patient privacy and confidentiality, prescribing medicines without a proper diagnosis, prescribing medicines from a restricted list, advertising or offering incentives to get patients and insisting on telemedicine consultations when the patient wants an in-person consultation.

Before listing any RMP on its online portal, technology platforms that provide telemedicine consultations should conduct due diligence.

Every RMP listed on the platform should have their name, qualification, registration number, and contact information displayed on the platform. Artificial intelligence or machine learning-based technology platforms are not permitted to prescribe medications or to counsel patients. Only RMPs are permitted to consult with and prescribe medications.

TELEPSYCHIATRY OPERATIONAL GUIDELINES 2020

Indian Psychiatric Society (IPS) in collaboration with Telemedicine Society of India (TSI) and NIMHANS, Bangalore published Telepsychiatry Operational Guidelines in May 2020.[12]

By integrating provisions from the Mental Health Care Act of 2017, the operational guidelines adapt Telemedicine Practice Guidelines for telepsychiatry practice. The guidelines cover interactions with people who are breaking the law. Any type of telepsychiatry advertising is strictly prohibited. The rules also tell RMPs what precautions they should take when using social media. For setting up a telepsychiatry service, there are technical ideas, like using an electronic health record. In the guidelines, there are instructions on how to change or end a telepsychiatry consultation, such as when a person withdraws consent, when it is hard to figure out if they have the ability to consent, when they need emergency care, when they are in trouble with the law, or when they ask for a certificate or health records. The guidelines also let telepsychiatry consultations with caregivers happen without the patient's permission if they have moderate-to-severe dementia and have lost the ability to give permission. The guidelines for telemedicine practice say that psychotropics are on lists A and B. The rules say that injectable psychotropics should not be used during telepsychiatry consultations.

TELE MENTAL HEALTH ASSISTANCE AND NETWORKING ACROSS STATES

In its Union Budget 2022, the Government of India (GoI) announced the National Tele Mental Health Programme of India, Tele Mental Health Assistance and Networking Across States (Tele MANAS), and entrusted its overall implementation to the Ministry of Health and Family Welfare (MoHFW). Tele MANAS will be divided into two levels. Tier 1 will include trained counselors and mental health specialists from the State Tele MANAS cells. Tier 2 specialists will be drawn from the District Mental Health Programme (DMHP) or medical college resources for in-person consultation. The program's goal is to deliver universal access to high-quality mental health services through tele mental health program available 24 hours a day, seven days a week as a digital component of the National Mental Health Programme (NMHP) in all the states and union territories.[13]

CONCLUSION

Schizophrenia Research Foundation (SCARF), Chennai has shown the path of telepsychiatry in India. COVID-19 pandemic reintroduced telepsychiatry as an alternative healthcare delivery system which is cheap, accessible to remote place and bypasses the stigma of in person psychiatric consultation. The Government of India issued Telemedicine Practice Guidelines 2020 to promote widespread adoption of telemedicine. Indian Psychiatric Society (IPS) in collaboration with Telemedicine Society of India (TSI) and NIMHANS, Bangalore published Telepsychiatry Operational Guidelines 2020 which is an adaptation of Telemedicine Practice Guidelines 2020 to cover the need of telepsychiatry practice. In 2022, Government of India has started the Tele MANAS program to provide universal access to quality mental healthcare.

REFERENCES

1. White LA, Krousel-Wood MA, Mather F. Technology meets healthcare: distance learning and telehealth. Ochsner J. 2001;3(1):22-9.
2. AbbasyM SUH. Importance and Advantages of Telepsychiatry in Mental Health During COVID 19 Pandemic. Psychol Psychother Res Study. 2020;4(2).
3. Javed A, Mohandas E, Sousa A. The interface of psychiatry and COVID-19: Challenges for management of psychiatric patients. Pak J Med Sci. 2020;36(5):1133-6.
4. Allely EB. Synchronous and asynchronous telemedicine. J Med Syst. 1995;19(3):207-12.
5. Thara R, John S, Rao K. Telepsychiatry in Chennai, India: the SCARF experience. Behav Sci Law. 2008;26(3):315-22.
6. Thara R, Sujit J. Mobile telepsychiatry in India. World Psychiatry. 2013;12(1):84.
7. Malhotra S, Chakrabarti S, Shah R, Gupta A, Mehta A, Nithya B, et al. Development of a novel diagnostic system for a telepsychiatric application: a pilot validation study. BMC Res Notes. 2014;7:508.
8. Jan Swasthya Sahyog (JSS). [online] Available from http://www.jssbilaspur.org/ [Last accessed April, 2023].
9. Center for Addiction Medicine, NIMHANS. (2023). Building a Virtual Knowledge Network (VKN) [online] Available from https://vknnimhans.in/ [Last accessed April, 2023].
10. Balasinorwala VP, Shah NB, Chatterjee SD, Kale VP, Matcheswalla YA. Asynchronous telepsychiatry in maharashtra, India: study of feasibility and referral pattern. Indian J Psychol Med. 2014;36(3):299-301.
11. Board of Governors in supersession of the Medical Council of India. (2020). Telemedicine Practice Guidelines [online] Available from https://www.mohfw.gov.in/pdf/Telemedicine.pdf [Last accessed April, 2023].
12. National Institute of Mental Health & Neurosciences, Bengaluru. (2020). Telepsychiatry Operational Guidelines [online] Available from https://nimhans.ac.in/publication/list-of-nimhans-publications-for-sale/ [Last accessed April, 2023].
13. Ministry of Health and Family Welfare. (2023). Tele MANAS [online] Available from https://telemanas.mohfw.gov.in/#/home

Mental Health Insurance in India: How far have we Progressed?

Thanapal Sivakumar, Kartik Singhai, Hareesh Angothu

INTRODUCTION

India's expenditure on health is 2.1% of the gross domestic product (GDP): among the lowest in the world. The inadequate investment in health care is reflected by over 80% of health financing happening in the private sector. The out-of-pocket expenditure (OOPE) accounts for 58.7% of national health expenditure in India.[1]

According to National Mental Health Survey 2015–2016, families are driven into economic crisis due to expenditure incurred to access psychiatric care (about ₹ 1,000–1,500 per month for treatment and travel).[2] Health insurance is a promising strategy to enable families to utilize healthcare services without incurring catastrophic OOPE.

CONCEPT OF HEALTH INSURANCE

Insurance is a contract represented by a policy in which an insurance company offers the policyholder financial protection or reimbursement against losses. It works on the concept of "risk pooling".[3]

According to the registration of Indian insurance companies regulations 2000, health insurance or health cover is defined "as the effecting of contracts which provide sickness benefits or medical, surgical or hospital expense benefits, whether inpatient or outpatient, on an indemnity, reimbursement, services, prepaid hospital, or other plan bases, including assured benefits and long-term care".[4]

TYPES OF HEALTH INSURANCE POLICIES

Health insurance plans can be divided into individual and group health insurance policies depending on the number of people covered. They may also be divided into two broad categories: private and public, depending on whether a private company or the Government offers them. Under private, individuals, or a group of individuals purchase policy from a company. Under public, eligible beneficiaries can avail of the health insurance without any formal policy purchase from any company as in Ayushman Bharat Pradhan

Mantri Jan Arogya Yojana (PM-JAY) or by purchasing from an approved company at subsidized prices as in Niramaya health insurance scheme.

For the majority of the postindependence era, mental illness was not covered by health insurance companies which even disqualified persons with mental illness from getting benefits of treatment of physical ailments. A beginning was made when the Ministry of Social Justice and Empowerment, Government of India launched subsidized health insurance schemes for Persons with Disabilities (PwD) covered under National Trust Act (NTA), 1999 and Persons with Disabilities Act, 1995.

NIRAMAYA HEALTH INSURANCE SCHEME

The National Trust launched the Niramaya Health Insurance Scheme on March 26, 2008.[5] The scheme covers conditions under the NTA 1999, namely mental retardation, autism, cerebral palsy, and multiple disabilities. The scheme is available to all persons with disabilities (PwD) covered under NTA 1999 and there is no age limit. The premium to be paid by the beneficiary is nominal and ranges from ₹ 50 to 500 per annum, depending on whether the PwD is below the poverty line (BPL) or not. The sum insured is of ₹ 1 lakh. There is a provision for State Governments to pay the premium on behalf of PwD from BPL families.[3] The scheme offers OPD coverage of ₹ 19,000 per annum.

SWAVLAMBAN HEALTH INSURANCE SCHEME

This was the first health insurance scheme that covered mental illness. On October 2, 2015, The New India Assurance Company Limited, in association with the Department of Empowerment of Persons with Disabilities, Ministry of Social Justice and Empowerment, launched this scheme.[6] The aim was to provide affordable health insurance to seven disabilities covered under the Persons with Disabilities Act, 1995, including two psychiatric conditions: mental retardation and mental illness. Any PwD with a self-declared annual family income of ₹ 3 lakhs or below was eligible for this scheme. The premium payable by the PwD for a health insurance coverage of ₹ 2 lakhs per annum was ₹ 357. The scheme offered outpatient coverage of ₹ 3000 per annum for persons with mental illness.[3] National Institute of Mental Health and Neurosciences (NIMHANS), Bengaluru, took an initiative in 2016–2017, wherein about 643 persons with disabilities and their family members were enrolled in the scheme. However, in mid-2017, the scheme was stopped.[6]

IMPACT OF MENTAL HEALTH CARE ACT 2017 ON INSURANCE FOR MENTAL ILLNESS

The Mental Health Care Act (MHCA) 2017 is an important milestone for insurance coverage of persons with mental illness. Chapter 1 of MHCA 2017 states that mental illness "means a substantial disorder of thinking, mood, perception, orientation or memory that grossly impairs judgment, behaviour, capacity to recognise reality or ability to meet the ordinary demands of life, mental conditions associated with the abuse of alcohol and drugs, but does not include mental retardation which is a condition of arrested or incomplete development of mind of a person, specially characterised by subnormality of intelligence".[7] All mental illnesses under the F code of ICD-10 are covered under this definition, except intellectual disability.

According to Section 21 (4) of MHCA 2017, "every insurer shall make provision for medical insurance for treatment of mental illness on the same basis as is available for the treatment of physical illness".

AYUSHMAN BHARAT PRADHAN MANTRI JAN AROGYA YOJANA

In 2018, the Government of India launched the Ayushman Bharat, as recommended by the National Health Policy 2017 to achieve the vision of Universal Health Coverage (UHC).[8] Ayushman Bharat PM-JAY, the largest health assurance scheme in the world, aims to provide a health cover of ₹ 5 lakhs per family per year for secondary and tertiary care hospitalization. It covers over 10.74 crores of poor and vulnerable families (approximately 50 crore beneficiaries) that form the bottom 40% of the Indian population.

Various states are implementing the Ayushman Bharat schemes under various names. The Karnataka version, named "Arogya Karnataka" includes packages to treat mental illnesses and substance use disorders in Government hospitals.[9] In Odisha, Biju Swasthya Kalyan Yojana covers expenditure incurred to treat mental illness in Government hospitals.[2,10]

A few states do not mention coverage for mental illness, namely Swasthya Sathi (Government of West Bengal), Aarogyasri (Government of Telangana), and Quality Health for all (Government of Delhi).

STATE GOVERNMENT GROUP HEALTH INSURANCE FOR THE EMPLOYEES

A few health insurance policy documents available in the public domain for some state government employees cover mental illness. Kerala state government group health insurance policy covers mental illness treatment and provides a maximum amount of ₹ 1,750/- per day.[11] Under Employees Health Scheme, the Telanagana government offers coverage of ₹ 32,890–37,090 for the medical management of schizophrenia.[12] There is no data on the utilization of these insurance schemes.

INSURANCE REGULATORY AND DEVELOPMENT AUTHORITY OF INDIA CIRCULARS ON MENTAL ILLNESS

On August 16, 2018, after one and a half years of the passing of MHCA 2017, the Insurance Regulatory and Development Authority of India (IRDAI) issued a circular to health insurance companies to include mental illness under the ambit of insurance coverage.[13] As there was no impact on the availability of health insurance for persons with mental illness, a public interest litigation was filed in the supreme court.[14] On June 2, 2020, IRDAI issued a circular that insurance companies comply with the MHCA 2017 provisions. It also directed insurance companies to publish on their website the philosophy and approach about covering persons affected with mental illness, placing a deadline on compliance by October 1, 2020.[15] On October 18, 2022 the IRDAI released another circular making it compulsory for all insurance products to cover for mental illnesses in compliance with the MHCA 2017 and to ensure this by October 31, 2022.[16] It also stated that all the insurance products that are in force on or after the date of MHCA, 2017 coming into force shall be deemed to provide cover for mental illnesses.

The IRDAI further released a circular on 27.02.2023 that clearly states that health insurers will have to come up with a specific cover for persons with mental illness, persons with disabilities and those afflicted with HIV/AIDS. The circular mandates each insurer to have a board approved underwriting policy that ensures no one from the above stated disabilities/illnesses are denied access to insurance and that this shall come into effect immediately after release of the circular.

With this circular, health insurance policies will now have to provide cover for pre-existing mental illnesses, however, there is likely to be a waiting period. This is a step towards equalizing insurance policy benefits for mental illnesses at par with those for physical illnesses.[17]

COURT CASES INVOLVING IRDAI AND HEALTH INSURANCE COMPANIES ON COVERAGE OF MENTAL ILLNESS

A recently concluded legal case [Shikha Nischal vs. National Insurance Company Ltd. (NICL) and ANR] provides much enlightenment. In this case, the petitioner had purchased a health insurance policy with total cover of ₹ 3,95,000.[18] Later, in June 2020, the petitioner received inpatient care for a diagnosis of schizoaffective disorder for which an expenditure of ₹ 5,54,636 was incurred. However, the reimbursement application for the same was rejected by NICL on the grounds that the policy excluded cover of psychiatric disorders.

Based on the provisions of the MHCA, 2017, the petitioner then filed a complaint before the insurance ombudsman. The insurance ombudsman also rejected the claim on the basis that it would have to be settled as per the policy's terms and conditions. Subsequently, she filed a petition in Delhi High Court that such rejection violated MHCA 2017. In the further proceedings then, following the hearing on March 18, 2021, the IRDAI directed the NICL to pay the petitioner's claim. Accordingly, the maximum coverage of the health insurance policy of ₹ 3,95,000 (the entire sum insured) was paid to the petitioner. The Delhi High Court clarifies in its judgement that "mental illnesses can be treated no differently from physical illnesses. Insurance policies also cannot discriminate between these two types of illnesses. The reasons for the nondiscriminatory provisions between mental and physical illnesses are not far to seek".

Another key case (Subhash Khandelwal vs. Max Bupa Health Insurance Company) deserves mention. In this case, the Delhi High Court questioned the IRDAI as to how insurance policies that exclude mental conditions from full coverage were approved.[15] The petitioner claimed that he has been regularly paying the premium for a sum assured of ₹ 35 lakhs. However, when he claimed for the treatment and went through the fine details, a cap of ₹ 50,000 per year was present on almost all prevalent mental health conditions.

IMPACT OF COURT CASES ON HEALTH INSURANCE FOR MENTAL ILLNESS

Since the advent of the MHCA 2017, IRDAI circulars, and recent court judgments, several health insurance companies have started to include mental illnesses in their policy coverage. However, the health insurance policies have not uniformly adopted the definition of mental illness as per MHCA 2017. A salient exclusion is the treatment of substance use disorders and attempted suicide. A person with preexisting mental illness will have a waiting period ranging from 24 to 48 months. Only a few health insurance policies cover OPD treatment with the rest covering only inpatient treatment. Another issue is separate cap limits for mental illnesses compared to physical illnesses. Many policies do not provide a cashless benefit facility.

IRDAI MASTER CIRCULAR 2020: CLAUSES IN VIOLATION OF MHCA 2017

The IRDAI master circular on standardization of health insurance products (2020) states that health insurance policy should not incorporate the following exclusions in terms and conditions of the policy: treatment of mental illness, stress and psychological disorders, and neurodegenerative disorders; behavioral and neurodevelopmental disorders including disorders of adult personality and disorders of speech and language including stammering, dyslexia, etc. Paradoxically, some of these conditions have been excluded by some health insurance policies.

Another contradiction is worth mentioning. While the MHCA 2017 definition of mental illness includes "mental conditions associated with the abuse of alcohol and drugs", none of the health insurance policies follow the MHCA definition of mental illness and exclude substance use-related disorders. Furthermore, the IRDAI master circular on standardization of health insurance products (2020) permits exclusion of *"treatment for alcoholism, drug or substance abuse or any addictive condition and consequences thereof"* from health insurance coverage, which is in clear violation of the MHCA 2017, is illegal, and discriminatory.

Decriminalization of suicide and presumption of severe stress in a person who attempted suicide was one of the standout features of the MHCA 2017. The Government has a duty to provide "care, treatment and rehabilitation" to the person who attempted suicide. But the available health insurance policies do not cover self-inflicted injuries and suicide attempts. While the intention of the Government is progressive, the decision of the insurance companies to carry on with the age-old exclusion of attempted suicide is regressive.[18-20]

TELEPSYCHIATRY AND HEALTH INSURANCE

During the COVID-19 crisis and the ensuing lockdown, the Telemedicine Practice Guidelines (TPG) were released on March 25, 2020 by the board of governors in supersession of the Medical Council of India. TPG provides the legal and regulatory framework for Indian telemedicine practice.[21,22] The Telepsychiatry Operational Guidelines were formulated along similar lines.[23] Subsequently, in an encouraging move, IRDAI directed insurance companies to offer insurance coverage for teleconsultations on par with in-person consultations.[24] According to IRDAI, claims for teleconsultations should be according to the "terms and conditions" in the insurance policy contract issued to the client at the time of payment of premium.

WAY FORWARD

Indian health insurance policies have a long way to go regarding mental illness and treatment coverage compared to developed countries.[25,26] Current health policies do not treat mental illness on par with physical illness, have separate caps for expenditure incurred for treating mental illness, the number of OPD visits, and an extended waiting period to cover preexisting mental illness. Noncoverage of outpatient care by most insurance policies is a concern since it accounts for a substantial proportion of mental health services.[27] Intellectual disability and autism spectrum disorders are missing from most policies.[28] Coverage for daycare treatment such as electroconvulsive and other neuromodulatory treatments is also missing from most policies.[27] Professional bodies should interact with the IRDAI and major insurers to plug the loopholes and take the legal route, as Courts are highly supportive of such initiatives in the backdrop of MHCA, 2017.[28]

CONCLUSION

Mental illnesses are beginning to garner much-needed equity with other illnesses, and the same is now appearing in the health insurance domain. Stringent enforcement of the MHCA 2017 rules and IRDAI instructions by the health insurance policies, coupled with dissemination of the provisions to the target population, is needed. This will provides much-needed impetus in achieving universal health coverage and fulfilling the sustainable development goals.

TAKE-HOME POINTS

- According to MHCA 2017, mental illnesses are to be considered at par with other physical illnesses as far as insurance coverage is concerned.
- Many individual and group policies (Government and Private) now provide coverage for mental illnesses.
- Disparity remains in the type of coverage provided with a separate cap for mental illnesses in some policies and exclusion of OPD-based care.
- Available health insurance policies continue to exclude attempted suicide and substance use disorders in violation of MHCA 2017.

REFERENCES

1. Ambade M, Sarwal R, Mor N, Kim R, Subramanian SV. Components of out-of-pocket expenditure and their relative contribution to economic burden of diseases in India. JAMA Netw Open. 2022;5(5):e2210040.
2. Gururaj G, Varghese M, Benegal V, Rao GN, Pathak K, Singh LK, et al. NMHS collaborators group. National Mental Health Survey of India, 2015-16: Mental Health Systems. Bengaluru, National Institute of Mental Health and Neuro Sciences, NIMHANS Publication No. 130, 2016. [online] Available from https://main.mohfw.gov.in/sites/default/files/National%20Mental%20Health%20Survey%2C%202015-16%20-%20Mental%20Health%20Systems_0.pdf [Last accessed February, 2023].
3. Sivakumar T, James JW, Basavarajappa C. Health insurance schemes for children and adolescents with psychiatric disability. J Indian Assoc Child Adolesc Ment Health. 2017;13(1):1-9.
4. Mohandoss AA, Thavarajah R. An Audit of Indian Health Insurance Claims for Mental Illness from Pooled Insurance Information Bureau's Macroindicator Data. Indian J Psychol Med. 2017;39(3):254-61.
5. Ministry of Social Justice and Empowerment (MSJE). (2022). NIRAMAYA. [online]. Available from https://www.thenationaltrust.gov.in/content/scheme/niramaya.php [Last accessed February, 2023].
6. James JW, Basavarajappa C, Sivakumar T, Banerjee R, Thirthalli J. Swavlamban Health Insurance scheme for persons with disabilities: An experiential account. Indian J Psychiatry. 2019;61(4):369.
7. MOHFW. (2017). Mental Health Care Act 2017 No. V.15011/09/2017-PH-1. [online] Available from https://main.mohfw.gov.in/sites/default/files/Mental%20Healthcare%20CMHA%20and%20MHRB%20Rules%202018_0.pdf [Last accessed February, 2023].

8. National Health Authority. GOI. [online] Available from https://nha.gov.in/PM-JAY [Last accessed February, 2023].
9. Welcome Arogya Karnataka Scheme. [online] Available from https://arogya.karnataka.gov.in/ [Last accessed February, 2023].
10. Biju Swasthya Kalyan Yojana (BSKY). Government of Odisha. [online] Available from http://www.bsky.odisha.gov.in/ [Last accessed February, 2023].
11. Medical Insurance Scheme for State Employers and Pensioners. Government of Kerala. G.O.(P)No. 87/2019/Fin. [online] Available from https://medisep.kerala.gov.in/EmpanelmentHospitalView.jsp. [Last accessed February, 2023].
12. Employees Health Scheme, Telangana. [online] Available from https://pmmodiyojana.in/wp-content/uploads/2020/02/EHS-Hospital-List-PDF.pdf [Last accessed February, 2023].
13. IRDAI circular IRDA/HLT/MISC/CIR/128/08/2018 dated 16 August, 2018 on The Mental Healthcare Act, 2017. [online] Available from https://www.irdai.gov.in/adminncms/cms/whatsNew_Layout.aspx?page=PageNo3555&flag=1 [Last accessed February, 2023].
14. Gaurav Kumar Bansal vs Union Of India & Ors. on 12 October, 2020 [online] Available from https://indiankanoon.org/doc/121963272/ [Last accessed February, 2023].
15. IRDAI circular IRDA/HLT/MISC/CIR/129/06/2020 dated 2 June, 2020 on Disclosure of underwriting philosophy of offering Insurance coverage to Persons with Disability (PWD) and people affected with HIV/AIDS and mental illness diseases. [online] Available from https://www.irdai.gov.in/admincms/cms/whatsNew_Layout.aspx?page=PageNo4140&flag=1 [Last accessed February 2023].
16. IRDAI circular IRDA/HLT/MISC/CIR/129/06/2020 dated 18 October, 2022 on providing cover for mental illness under Health insurance policies. [online] Available from https://new.irdai.gov.in/web/guest/document-detail?documentId=1445610 [Last accessed February 2023].
17. IRDAI (2023). Product for Persons with Disabilities (PWD), Persons aflicted with HIV/AIDS, and those with Mental illness. [online] Available from https://irdai.gov.in/web/guest/document-detail?documentId=2865446 (last accessed 27th March 2023)
18. Shikha Nischal V. National Insurance Company Limited and ANR. [online] Available from https://www.legitquest.com/case/shikha-nischal-v-national-insurance-company-limited-anr/1E717A [Last accessed February, 2023].
19. Explain the basis for approving insurance policies excluding mental illnesses from full coverage: HC to IRDA. The Hindu; 18 April, 2021. [online] Available from https://www.thehindu.com/news/cities/Delhi/explain-basis-for-approving-insurance-policies-excluding-mental-illnesses-from-full-coverage-hc-to-irda/article3439773.ece [Last accessed February, 2023].
20. Sarkhel S. Mental health insurance and attempted suicide: Need for a reappraisal. Indian J Psychiatry. 2021;63(6):624-5.
21. Nirisha PL, Thippaiah SM, Fargason RE, Malathesh BC, Manjunatha N, Math SB, et al. Telepsychiatry and Medical Insurance: Comparative Perspectives Between India and the United States. Indian J Psychol Med. 2020;42(5 suppl):92S-97S.
22. Telemedicine Practice Guidelines. Board of governors in supersession of the Medical Council of India. [online] Available from http://egazette.nic.in/WriteReadData/2020/219374.pdf [Last accessed February, 2023].

23. Math SB, Manjunatha N, KumarCN. Telepsychiatry operational guidelines—2020. Bengaluru: NIMHANS; 2020.
24. IRDAI. (2020). Guidelines on telemedicine. Hyderabad: Insurance Regulatory and Development Authority of India. [online] Available from https://www.irdai.gov.in/ADMINCMS/cms/frmGuidelines_Layout.aspx?page=PageNo4155 [Last accessed February, 2023].
25. Ghosh M. Mental health insurance scenario in India: Where does India stand? Indian J Psychiatry. 2021;63(6):603-5.
26. Ghosh M. Mental health insurance in India: lack of parity. Lancet Psychiatry. 2021;8(10):860.
27. Singhai K, Sivakumar T, Angothu H, Jayarajan D. Review of Individual Health Insurance Policies for Mental Health Conditions. Indian J Priv Psychiatry. 2021;15(1):3-9.
28. Singh OP. Insurance for mental illness in India—Great achievement but there is need to plug the loopholes. Indian J Psychiatry. 2021;63(6):521-2.

CHAPTER 7

Pharmacotherapy of Psychiatric Emergencies

Sujit Sarkhel, Aratrika Sen

INTRODUCTION

Psychiatric emergencies by definition are sudden alterations and disturbances of thought, mood, behavior, or social relationships. Psychiatric emergencies can cause harm to patients themselves as well as other individuals in the society which is in contrast to general medical emergencies. Thus, these emergencies require immediate attention and intervention, both to improve patients' subjective symptoms as well as to prevent their harmful behavior.[1]

A large epidemiological study by Saddichha et al. showed that 11.4% of all general emergencies are actually psychiatric emergencies. Owing to the prevailing mental health treatment gap in India, majority of psychiatric emergencies are often being first attended by primary healthcare givers. Thus, a basic knowledge about management of psychiatric emergencies should be known to all. After the initial management, patient can be referred to a psychiatrist in a tertiary care hospital.[2]

TYPES

No definite classification of psychiatric emergencies exists in published literature. However, the major psychiatric emergencies that can be most commonly encountered are suicidal behavior and agitated, disruptive behavior. For the purpose of this chapter, we have classified psychiatric emergencies into the following:
- Suicidal behavior
- Agitated behavior
- Substance induced emergencies
  - Intoxication
  - Withdrawal
- Delirium
- Catatonia
- Iatrogenic
  - Acute dystonia
  - Neuroleptic malignant syndrome

Suicidal Behavior

Suicide is an act of intentionally causing one's death. Suicidal behaviors which often present as psychiatric emergencies include an attempted suicide (where there is an intent to die) or nonsuicidal self-injury (where there is no intent to kill oneself) or acute suicidal ideation. Although nonpharmacological measures are the main stay in the management of suicidal behavior, pharmacological measures are often helpful, especially in preventing recurrences.

- *Lithium:* It has established efficacy in reducing suicidality in patients with bipolar disorder and major depressive disorder. However, the immediate risk of overdosage with lithium in an actively suicidal patient has to be kept in mind. Thus, in the immediate period following a suicidal attempt, it should be prescribed for short duration and preferably under supervision of family members and caregivers.[3]
- *Antidepressants:* Antidepressant treatment is generally recommended in the treatment of suicidal behavior in cases with unipolar depression. The efficacy of fluoxetine and venlafaxine has been proved in reducing depression and suicidality in adult and geriatric population. There are concerns of antidepressant-induced suicidality for which the treating team must psychoeducate the patient and the family members wherever applicable. Particular attention to this aspect must be paid during treatment for the first one month, especially among adolescents.
- *Ketamine:* Studies have shown that ketamine is effective in rapidly reducing suicidal ideation, even with a single dose of 0.5 mg/kg. Ketamine is usually administered as an intravenous (IV) infusion. The major issue concerning ketamine is that the benefits have been found to be short-term and the trials have been carried out on small patient groups. Hence, the use of ketamine infusion in suicidal behavior still remains off-label. Ketamine needs to be used with caution due to associated side effects related to hemodynamic stability, emergent reactions like vivid dreams, hallucinations, respiratory depression, and drug-induced liver injury among others.
- *Clozapine:* It has been found to reduce suicides and suicide attempts in patients with schizophrenia. It is recommended in this group of patients with suicidal behavior.
- *Measures to control acute anxiety and agitation:* These measures are often indicated in controlling severe agitation and anxiety in actively suicidal patients and can be useful in the immediate management. Injectable antipsychotics and benzodiazepines may be used for this purpose in the emergency treatment setting. Benzodiazepines are sometimes used for treating severe anxiety associated with suicidality. These drugs may be effective in treating severe insomnia associated with suicidality.[4]

Agitated and Disruptive Behavior

When a patient presents to emergency room in an agitated state, a basic assessment should always be made to rule out any underlying medical conditions. Once the medical conditions are ruled out, focus should be made on the psychiatric disorders which can lead to such behavior. The psychiatric disorders that can cause such behavior are given below.[1]
- Acute exacerbation of psychosis or mania
- Acute anxiety or acute stress reaction
- Intoxication or withdrawal of psychoactive substances
- Delirium due to other systemic cause

The pharmacological management of the first two possibilities will be discussed here.

Acute Exacerbation of Psychosis or Mania

The goal of the pharmacological management is to calm down the patient without excessive sedation. The use of orally dissolving tablets or liquids is the least noninvasive intervention one can provide. Parenteral administration of drugs should be reserved for severe form of agitation.

First choice of drugs is generally an antipsychotic, preferably second generation alone or along with a benzodiazepine.
- *Oral second-generation antipsychotics:*
    - Orally disintegrating olanzapine (5-10 mg) with or without 2 mg lorazepam can be used as first-line therapy.
    - Liquid or mouth dissolving risperidone (2 mg) can also be used.[5]
- *Oral first-generation antipsychotics:*
    - In case of first-generation antipsychotics, haloperidol (5-10 mg) can be used.
- *Parenteral first-generation antipsychotics:*
    - Injection haloperidol (5-10 mg) can be given intramuscular along with oral or parenteral benzodiazepine.
- *Parenteral second-generation antipsychotics:*
    - Parenteral olanzapine (10 mg) can also be used intramuscular. However, caution should be taken in combining parenteral olanzapine with parenteral lorazepam due to potential risk of cardiorespiratory depression.[6]
- *Benzodiazepine:*
    - Most preferred benzodiazepine is lorazepam.[6]

The medications can be repeated every hour and given up to three or four doses in 24 hours, though most patients respond after the first dose.[7]

Side effects are common with intramuscular antipsychotics and thus should be monitored. Intramuscular promethazine (25 mg) is the drug of choice in acute dystonia while akathisia is managed by beta blockers like propranolol and benzodiazepines.[7]

Acute Stress Reaction

In case of acute stress reactions, benzodiazepines are the drugs of choice. Sublingual clonazepam (0.5-1 mg) can be given. If the severity is more, intramuscular lorazepam (2 mg) can be used.[1]

Substance Intoxication and Withdrawal

These are one of the most encountered psychiatric emergencies in emergency room. Patient can present in both intoxicated and withdrawal state **(Table 1)**.

Delirium

Delirium is defined as the acute reversible organic mental disorder characterized by confusion and some impairment of consciousness. Delirium

TABLE 1: Opioids intoxication and withdrawal in critically ill patients.

Substance	Intoxication	Withdrawal

Alcohol	• Clinical features:
	  – Euphoria, excitement, confusion, stupor, and coma in high doses
	  – No definite pharmacological agent has been approved
	  – Symptomatic management like hydration, oxygen therapy, and stomach pumping should be done
		• Seizures:
		  – Can precipitate within 12–18 hours of stopping of alcohol
		  – Parenteral benzodiazepines should be used for management
		  – Diazepam 5–10 mg intravenous (IV)
		  – Lorazepam 2–4 mg intramuscular (IM) or IV
		  – No definite role of anticonvulsant
		• Delirium tremens:
		  – Occurs within 3–4 days (72–96 hours) of alcohol withdrawal
		  – Clouding of consciousness/confusion
		  – Vivid hallucinations, particularly visual and tactile
		  – Marked tremor
		  – Medical emergency and always should be treated in critical care setup
		  – IV benzodiazepines
		  – Intramuscular thiamine
		  – Low dose antipsychotics such as haloperidol 0.5–2 mg are useful in controlling visual hallucinations.
		  – Fluid maintenance
		  – Electrolyte balance[8]

Contd...

Contd...

Substance	Intoxication	Withdrawal
Opioids	• Opioid overdose is characterized clinically by the triad of unconsciousness, a low respiratory rate (RR <12 breaths/min) and pin-point pupils • Management should be in a critical care setup • Give 400 μg naloxone injection into outer thigh or upper arm muscle[8]	Will present as muscle cramps, tremors, perspiration, rhinorrhea, lacrimation, and diarrhea: • Methadone 10–20 mg orally can reduce symptoms • Clonidine 0.1–0.2 mg orally for anxiety, restlessness, and hypertension • Antihistamines orally or intramuscularly for anxiety, restlessness, nausea, and vomiting • Baclofen 5–10 mg orally for muscle cramping • Loperamide 4 mg orally for diarrhea and stomach cramps • Nonsteroidal anti-inflammatory drugs (NSAIDs) for myalgias
Sedatives	• Similar presentation as alcohol intoxication • Managed in critical care set-up • Symptomatic management like maintaining hydration, electrolytes, and gastric lavage • Flumazenil can be used in benzodiazepine overdose • Initial dose is 0.2 mg which is to be given over 15 seconds OR to administer flumazenil in 0.1 mg doses (or 0.01 mg/kg) each over one minute, to a maximum of 1 mg, or until an effect is achieved or toxicity develops[9]	• Similar to alcohol withdrawal, can precipitate seizure • IV long-acting benzodiazepine like diazepam can be used • Later switching to an equivalent dose of oral diazepam

is almost invariably multifactorial, and it is often difficult to pinpoint a single causative factor.

Pharmacological management of delirium includes benzodiazepines, antipsychotics, and cholinesterase inhibitors. The common errors found during the management of delirium are excessive use of antipsychotics or administrating them too late or to overuse benzodiazepines.

Much data is not available for treatment of delirium with available studies showing varying clinical outcomes. Treating the underlying medical condition should be prioritized along with symptomatic treatment.[10]
- *First-generation antipsychotics:* Haloperidol can be given orally (0.5–1 mg) with additional doses every 4 hourly as needed.
- *Second-generation antipsychotics:*
  - Olanzapine can be given orally, (2.5–5 mg) OD and can be hiked up to 20 mg/day.
  - Risperidone (0.5 mg) BD can be used orally, with additional doses, every 4 hourly as needed. Usually given up to 4 mg/day.
  - Quetiapine (12.5–50 mg) BD orally, may be increased to 200 mg/day, if well tolerated.
  - Aripiprazole (5–15 mg/day) orally, maximum up to 30 mg/day.
- *Benzodiazepines:*
  - Lorazepam can be given 0.25–1 mg orally every 2–4 hours as needed, maximum up to 3 mg in 24 hours.
  - Diazepam can be given orally in 5–10 mg dose/day.
- *Cholinesterase inhibitors:*
  - Donepezil can be given 5 mg orally OD.
  - Rivastigmine can be given orally 1.5–6 mg BD
- *Others:*
  - Melatonin, orally 2 mg OD.

In severe cases, injectable haloperidol and lorazepam can be used, but judiciously. **Flowchart 1** describes the pharmacotherapy of agitated patients presenting in psychiatry emergency setting.

Catatonia

It is defined as a clinical syndrome consisting of marked behavioral irregularities which may include motoric excitement or immobility, negativism, stupor, echolalia, or echopraxia. In Diagnostic and Statistical Manual of Mental Disorders, Fifth edition (DSM-5), catatonia is a standalone diagnosis, and also associated with psychotic disorders, schizophrenia, affective disorders, substance use disorder, and underlying medical conditions.

Proper history and clinical assessment should be done before proceeding to treatment. Catatonia should better be treated in indoor setting. The mainstay of pharmacological treatment is benzodiazepine. Most studies have been done using lorazepam. Starting dose is 4 mg/day, 2 mg to be given at baseline, and further 2 mg if there is no effect within 3 hours. If the patient is unable to swallow medications, intramuscular lorazepam can be used. If no improvement occurs within next 1–2 days, higher doses of lorazepam (8–24 mg/24 hours) should be used. One can even consider IV diazepam (10 mg in 500 mL of NS).[7] Antipsychotics should be avoided as they may worsen catatonia and precipitate neuroleptic malignant syndrome (NMS).

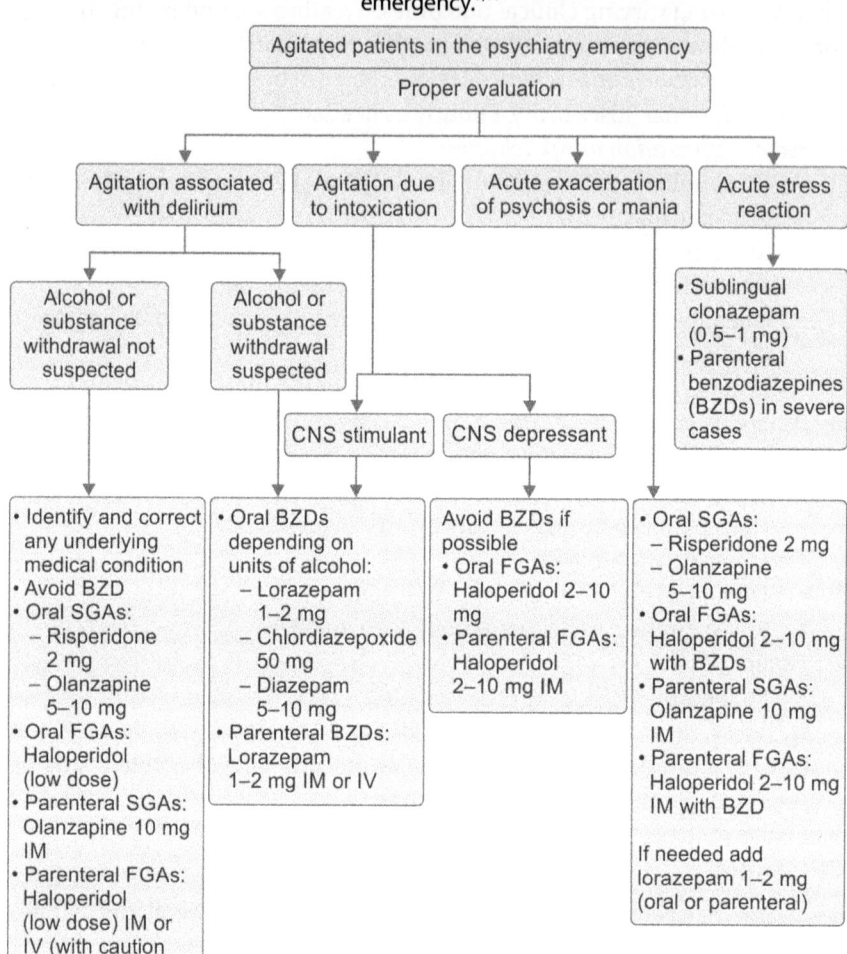

Flowchart 1: Pharmacological intervention of agitated patients in psychiatry emergency.[5,11]

(CNS: central nervous system; FGA: first-generation antipsychotic; IM: intramuscular; IV: intravenous; SGA: second-generation antipsychotic)

In lorazepam nonresponders, next line of treatment should be electroconvulsive therapy (ECT).

Iatrogenic

Few side effects of psychotropic medications can present to psychiatry emergency. Most common among them are following:
- Acute dystonia
- Akathisia
- Neuroleptic malignant syndrome
- Serotonin syndrome.

Acute Dystonia

Acute dystonia is muscle spasm in any part of the body. Most commonly seen are oculogyric crisis (eyes rolling upward) and torticollis (head and neck twisting to one side). Rarely, there is spasm of laryngeal muscles causing acute laryngeal dystonia (ALD) leading to acute respiratory failure which can be life-threatening.[12]

Acute dystonia generally occurs within hours of starting of antipsychotics and within minutes of parenteral administration. First generations are more notorious than second generations.

Treatment of acute dystonia has been described in **Box 1**.

Akathisia

Akathisia is defined as "inability to sit". It is characterized by a subjective feeling of inner restlessness and also objective restlessness, as noted by other people. A sense of dysphoria usually accompanies, and the patient complains of tension when he/she tries to remain still. As observed by others, the patient would appear to have difficulty sitting/standing/lying at one place for a long time.

Treatment of akathisia involves reduction of dose of the offending agent or changing to another antipsychotic with low potency for akathisia. Next option is to add an antiakathisia medication. Beta-blockers are usually considered to be first line for the management of akathisia. Patients who have contraindications to beta-blockers can be treated with mirtazapine. Other drugs that can be used in akathisia are listed in **Box 2**.

Neuroleptic Malignant Syndrome

Neuroleptic malignant syndrome is characterized by muscular rigidity, hyperthermia, altered consciousness, and autonomic dysfunction following exposure to high potency antipsychotics, first-generation antipsychotics, rapid dose increase or rapid dose reduction, antipsychotic polypharmacy, and abrupt withdrawal of anticholinergics.

BOX 1: Pharmacotherapy of acute dystonia.[13]

- Intramuscular or intravenous anticholinergics or antihistaminergic compounds such as promethazine (25 mg)
- Acute dystonia generally relieves within 15–20 minutes of intramuscular and within 5 minutes of intravenous administration
- If dystonia does not relieve after first dose, a second dose of the same drug can be considered after 30 minutes
- Consider an alternate diagnosis after 2–3 failed attempts
- Once the acute dystonia is managed with various agents, one should continue anticholinergic agents for at least 24–48 hours to avoid further recurrence
- However, in routine clinical practice, the anticholinergic agents are generally continued up to 4–7 days

BOX 2: Medications used in akathisia.[13]

Medications doses (in mg/day)
- Beta-blockers:
  - Propranolol 40–80 mg/day
- 5-HT2A receptor antagonists:
  - Mirtazapine 15 mg/day
  - Cyproheptadine 8–16 mg/day
  - Trazodone 100 mg/day
- Anticholinergics:
  - Trihexyphenidyl 2–10 mg/day
- Benzodiazepine:
  - Lorazepam 1–2 mg/day
  - Clonazepam 0.5–1 mg/day
  - Diazepam 5–15 mg/day
- GABA receptor agonists:
  - Pregabalin 50–100 mg/day
  - Gabapentin 300–600 mg/day
- Antihistaminergic agents:
  - Promethazine 25–50 mg/day
- Others:
  - Vitamin B6 (pyridoxine) 200 mg/day
  - N-Acetyl Cysteine 1,000–2,000 mg/day

Clinical findings include fever, diaphoresis, rigidity, fluctuating blood pressure, and tachycardia. Laboratory investigations reveal leukocytosis, increased creatine phosphokinase (CPK), and altered liver function test (LFT). Treatment of NMS should always be a holistic approach in a critical care setup. Withdrawal of the offending drug should be the primary step. No drugs have been approved for the treatment of NMS till date. However, existing literatures are of opinion of parenteral benzodiazepines (in milder cases) and dopamine agonists in severe cases.

- *Benzodiazepines:* Lorazepam intramuscular 1–2 mg can be used as test dose, if effective, one can switch to oral route.
- *Dopamine agonists:*
  - Bromocriptine is started with 2.5 mg twice or thrice a day
  - Amantadine can be given 200–400 mg/day in divided doses. It can be increased to 45 mg/day.
  - Levodopa 50–100 mg/day can be given as continuous IV infusion.

Electroconvulsive therapy can be considered in severe cases not responding to abovementioned drugs.[6]

Serotonin Syndrome

Serotonin syndrome is a life-threatening side effect arising due to serotonin toxicity. It is mainly seen in patients receiving more than one serotonergic agent. If the patient receives CYP3A4 inhibitors along with a selective serotonin reuptake inhibitor (SSRI), then serotonin syndrome can also

precipitate following increased level of serotonin. Clinical features of serotonin syndrome are as follows:
- Mental status changes (confusion and hypomania)
- Agitation
- Myoclonus
- Hyperreflexia
- Diaphoresis
- Shivering
- Tremor
- Diarrhea
- Incoordination
- Fever.

First step in the management of serotonin syndrome includes removal of the offending agent(s). Supportive measures are required to manage the symptoms and prevent the development of complications. These may include measures to reduce the temperature, treat or prevent dehydration, ensure proper nutrition, and avoid organ damage. Moderate and severe cases of serotonin syndrome may require addition of serotonin antagonists like cyproheptadine. A loading dose of 12 mg orally or through a nasogastric tube, followed by 2 mg every 2 hourly until clinical improvement seen, is recommended. Severe cases should always be managed in intensive care unit setup.[13]

CONCLUSION

The demand for psychiatric emergency services has increased in our country. Rising trend in depression, substance abuse and suicide attempts calls for training of almost all clinicians in basic management of these emergencies. Holistic management with other departments is also necessary for improved care level for patients.

TAKE-HOME POINTS

- Lithium is an effective treatment for prevention of suicide in patients with mood disorder, especially depression.
- Clozapine is an approved drug for prevention of suicide in patients with schizophrenia and other nonaffective psychoses.
- Acute management of agitation due to mania/psychosis may be done with oral/injectable antipsychotics along with benzodiazepines in the initial phase.
- Emergency arising out of intoxication of alcohol, sedatives, or opioids may be managed as per existing protocols.
- Delirium may be managed by low dose first- or second-generation antipsychotics along with addition of melatonin in case of sleep issues.
- Patients with catatonia must undergo a lorazepam trial to assess response. ECT is the best option in nonresponders.
- Iatrogenic emergencies such as dystonia, akathisia, NMS, and serotonin syndrome should be dealt with as per available protocol.

REFERENCES

1. Mavrogiorgou P, Brüne M, Juckel G. The management of psychiatric emergencies. Dtsch Arztebl Int. 2011;108(13):222.
2. Jalgaonkar SV, Mapara TI, Parmar UI, Patil ML, Adarkar S, Parkar S. Drug use pattern for emergency psychiatric conditions in a tertiary care hospital: A prospective observational study. Perspect Clin Res. 2021;12(4):203.
3. Schaffer A, Isometsä ET, Tondo L, Moreno DH, Sinyor M, Kessing LV, et al. Epidemiology, neurobiology and pharmacological interventions related to suicide deaths and suicide attempts in bipolar disorder: Part I of a report of the International Society for Bipolar Disorders Task Force on Suicide in Bipolar Disorder. Aust N Z J Psychiatry. 2015;49:785-802.
4. Baldacara L, Grudtner RR, Leite VS, Porto DM, Robis KP, Fidalgo TM, et al. Brazilian Psychiatric Association guidelines for the management of suicidal behavior. Part 2. Screening, intervention, and prevention. Braz J Psychiatry. 2020;43(5):538-49.
5. Raveesh BN, Munoli RN, Gowda GS. Assessment and Management of Agitation in Consultation-Liaison Psychiatry. Indian J Psychiatry. 2022;64(Suppl 2):S484-98.
6. Other psychiatric emergencies. In: Sadock B, Sadock V, Ruiz P (Eds). Kaplan and Sadock's Comprehensive Textbook of Psychiatry. Wolters Kluwer Health; 2017.
7. Schizophrenia and related psychosis. In: Taylor DM, Barnes TR, Young AH (Eds). The Maudsley Prescribing Guidelines in Psychiatry. John Wiley & Sons; 2021.
8. Addictions and substance misuse. In: Taylor DM, Barnes TR, Young AH (Eds). The Maudsley prescribing guidelines in psychiatry. John Wiley & Sons; 2021.
9. An H, Godwin J. Flumazenil in benzodiazepine overdose. CMAJ. 2016;188(17-18):E537.
10. Drug treatment of other psychiatric condition. In: Taylor DM, Barnes TR, Young AH (Eds). The Maudsley prescribing guidelines in psychiatry. John Wiley & Sons; 2021.
11. Keiltyka CA, Nordstrom KD. Agitation. In: Nordstrom KD, Wilson MP (Eds). Quick Guide to Psychiatric Emergencies. Springer; 2018.
12. Collins N, Sager J. Acute laryngeal dystonia: drug-induced respiratory failure related to antipsychotic medications. J Neurol Neuromed. 2018;3(1).
13. Grover S, Sarkar S, Avasthi A. Clinical Practice Guidelines for Management of Medical Emergencies Associated with Psychotropic Medications. Indian J Psychiatry. 2022;64(Suppl 2):S236.

CHAPTER 8

Newer Diagnostic Categories in ICD-11

Adarsh Tripathi, Shivangini Singh

INTRODUCTION

The current diagnostic system, International Statistical Classification of Diseases and Related Health Problems, 10th Edition (ICD-10), uses a categorical approach to diagnose mental disorders. The categorization system uses a set of defining symptoms for a particular illness. To give the appropriate category diagnosis, a certain number of symptoms from this list must be present, which is often predetermined.[1] The categorical system has its own benefits as in most nations, categorical diagnoses are necessary to effectively communicate about mental diseases, justify treatment, and gather epidemiological data.[2] A diagnosis based on categorical approach may also help in determining if the patient is to be treated or not. But categorization of mental diseases has a number of drawbacks, such as significant variations within a specific category, addressing comorbidities, and challenges in defining the subthreshold symptomatology.[3]

The dimensional approach, on the other hand, quantifies the severity of a symptom or the level of a certain psychological function's disruption using a quantitative dimension. Dimensional methods, including subthreshold symptomatology, describe the grades of the intensity of certain symptoms and psychological dysfunctions.[4,5] However, dimensional classification has less clinical use than categorical classification due to its higher complexity and difficulty in defining structured diagnostic criteria. The category system used in ICD-10 was mainly carried over to ICD-11. However, for a certain diagnosis, dimensional expansions in terms of severity, course, and particular symptoms were included. These categorical diagnosis dimensional expansions reflect clinical practice, where dimensional information (such as the severity of the illness) is frequently taken into account when choosing therapies.

Chapter structure was reorganized in ICD-11 with the inclusion of 21 disorder grouping in contrast to the existing 11 disorder grouping in ICD-10 and further new diagnostic categories were identified in ICD-11. Disorders were grouped based on probable common etiological and pathophysiological components as well as shared phenomenology, with neurodevelopmental disorders appearing first and neurocognitive disorders last in the categorization going forward. In the diagnostic criteria, arbitrary cut-offs and duration of symptoms were generally avoided in order to boost the clinical value and ensured the flexible use of clinical judgment.[6] All categories are diagnosed when symptoms are linked to significant distress or functional impairment in vital domains including personal, familial, academic, social, occupational, or other critical domains.

New categories are adopted in order to:
- Make it easier to identify a clinically significant but poorly categorized mental condition in order to give appropriate therapy.
- Enhance the use of morbidity data.
- Encourage research into more potent therapies.[7]

During the early phases of the ICD-11 rollout, it is critical to evaluate the effects of these new categories given the significant consequences for the industry and World Health Organization (WHO) member states. This chapter gives an overview of the new categories added in ICD-11 as per the blocks under which they have been placed under Chapter 06—Mental, behavioral or neurodevelopmental disorders.

BLOCK: OBSESSIVE–COMPULSIVE OR RELATED DISORDERS

Body Dysmorphic Disorder

It is characterized by a persistent fixation and preoccupation with at least one imperfection or defect in one's appearance that is either barely perceptible to others or not at all. Individuals, fixated on the idea of their imperfection, engage in repetitive and excessive behaviors, such as continuously evaluating the appearance or severity of the perceived defect. There is a further subdivision of the category based on the grade of insight of the patient—absent, poor, fair, and good. Body dysmorphic disorder has been categorized as an obsessive-compulsive and related condition due to its specific symptomatology and parallels to the latter [obsessive–compulsive or related disorders (OCRD)] in ICD-11. Earlier the differentials for such symptoms were hypochondriacal disorder, delusional disorder, schizotypal disorder, or other persistent delusional disorder, but it can now be avoided with a more defined category.[8]

Olfactory Reference Syndrome

This disorder is characterized by a constant preoccupation with the idea or belief that one is exuding an allegedly repugnant body odor or filthy breath that is either undetectable to others or only faintly perceptible to them. In response to their excessive preoccupation, people frequently check for body odor or the source of the smell, among other repetitive and excessive behaviors. People are excessively self-consciousness about the odor they perceive. This excessive self-consciousness is frequently accompanied by self-referential thoughts. There is further subdivision of the category based on the grade of insight of the patient—absent, poor, fair, and good. This category was included under OCRD to avoid diagnostic confusion as this phenomenology is seen worldwide and is not just a culture-bound syndrome.[8,9]

Hoarding Disorder

It is characterized by the accumulation of possessions either due to excessive collection of belongings or due to difficulties in getting rid of them, despite their actual worth. Repetitive urges or behaviors that are connected to collecting or purchasing things are the hallmarks of excessive acquisition which is in accordance with Diagnostic and Statistical Manual of Mental Disorders, Fifth edition (DSM-5).[10] People experience distress letting go of belongings and a powerful need to hang onto things with the congestion of their living spaces. There is a further subdivision of the category based on the grade of insight of the patient—absent, poor, fair, and good. Hoarding is distinguishable from OCD by having core symptoms that are distinctive to it (thoughts less intrusive, less insight with acts often leading to pleasure and reward), as well as unique neurological correlations and therapeutic responses.[11]

Body-focused Repetitive Behavior Disorders

The characteristics of this disorder are habitual and recurring actions (such as hair pulling, skin picking, and lip-biting) directed at the integument, which are frequently accompanied by futile attempts to reduce or stop the behavior in question and result in dermatological sequelae. They are further subdivided into four categories—trichotillomania (recurrent pulling of one's hair), excoriation disorder (recurrent picking of one's skin), other specified, and unspecified. Cognitive events such as intrusive thoughts, obsessions, or preoccupations rarely precede sensory sensations; hence, this category was separated from OCD.[12]

BLOCK: DISORDERS SPECIFICALLY ASSOCIATED WITH STRESS

Complex Post-traumatic Stress Disorder

A catastrophic incident or series of traumatic events—often prolonged or recurrent ones from which escape is difficult or impossible—may lead to the development of complex PTSD. The primary symptoms of post-traumatic stress disorder (PTSD) are present, and complex PTSD is additionally defined by:

- Pervasive and severe issues with the regulation of affect
- Persistent views that one is inferior, defeated, or unworthy, coupled with intense and pervasive feelings of failure or humiliation related to the traumatic incident.
- Ongoing persistent issues maintaining connections and feeling close to others.

These points were not taken into account under PTSD (ICD-10); the diagnosis was required to more accurately capture the unique traits and effects of complex trauma. This avoided the multiple diagnoses (comorbid mood, anxiety, or personality disorders) given to patients with PTSD, reducing the stigma. Also, diagnosing complex PTSD as PTSD may lead to treatment needs being underestimated.[7]

Prolonged Grief Disorder

The bereaved may develop extended grief disorder after losing a spouse, parent, child, or another close relative. This condition is characterized by a persistent and pervasive mourning reaction characterized by a longing for the departed or constant concern with the deceased and accompanying great emotional distress. The mourning reaction has persisted for a disproportionately long period of time (more than 6 months, at the very least) following the death, and it clearly exceeds expected societal, religious, or cultural norms for the person's environmental setting and culture. Its inclusion and separation from the culturally typical grief and depression episode are crucial to identifying those in need of support and focusing on appropriate treatment selection and prognoses.[13,14]

BLOCK: FEEDING OR EATING DISORDERS

Binge Eating Disorder

This disease is distinguished from bulimia nervosa by its frequent, repeated bouts of binge eating (e.g., once a week or more over many months), subjective loss of control, sense of anguish, disgust or accompanied guilt, but a lack of frequently occurring improper compensatory behaviors. Putting on weight is not a necessary symptom, although it may be present. The ICD-10 diagnoses of other specified or unspecified eating disorders overlap with the inclusion of binge eating disorder; nonetheless, research throughout time has advocated the creation of this distinct category.[15]

Avoidant/Restrictive Food Intake Disorder

This differs from anorexia nervosa in that it causes weight loss or failure to gain during pregnancy or childhood, is characterized by the consumption of an insufficient quantity or variety of food to meet adequate energy or nutritional requirements. ICD-11 diagnostic guidelines significantly improved accuracy for all feeding and eating disorders and the usage of residual diagnoses was decreased by the addition of binge eating disorder and avoidant/restrictive food intake disorder (ARFID).[16]

Rumination-regurgitation Disorder

Rumination-regurgitation is a condition characterized by the recurrent intentional raising up of previously swallowed food to the mouth for chewing or spitting it out (but not as in vomiting). Regurgitation is a recurring activity that occurs frequently (at least several times each week) and has persisted for a while now (at least several weeks). The patients with this disorder are often undetected and untreated due to a lack of clinician knowledge leading to protracted symptoms in these patients.[17]

BLOCK: DISORDERS OF BODILY DISTRESS OR BODILY EXPERIENCE

Bodily Distress Disorder

Body-related symptoms that cause significant distress to the individual along with excessive attention to the symptoms, for which they frequently contact medical professionals, are the hallmarks of physical distress disorder. The level of focus is obviously out of proportion to the type and course of the ailment. This is in accordance with the "Somatic Symptom and Related Disorders" category of DSM-5 which argues. The fundamental difference is that it drops the terminology of "medically unexplained symptoms" and only focuses on one or more symptoms causing distress to the patient; however, it also increases the chance of overdiagnosis and stigma.[18]

Bodily Integrity Dysphoria

The persistent intense desire to become significantly physically disabled (e.g., paraplegic, major limb amputee, or blind) is the characteristic feature of bodily integrity dysphoria (BID). The onset is usually in the early adolescence and is accompanied by constant discomfort or intense feelings of inappropriateness towards one's current healthy body configuration. In some individuals, the desire or preoccupation might exceed their fantasy, leading them to actually pursue actualization of the desire through surgery (amputation) or self-damaging a limb. It is a unique nosological entity with early experimental research pointing toward a potential neurological component. It is essential to identify this illness early on which may lessen the enormous burden they face.[19,20]

BLOCK: DISORDERS DUE TO ADDICTIVE BEHAVIORS
Gaming Disorder

A pattern of persistent or recurrent gaming activity is what is known as a gaming disorder. It can occur offline or online and is defined by poor control over gaming, prioritizing it more and more over other activities, and using it despite negative effects. Internet gaming addiction is said to be a continuum with risk factors and antecedents leading to "full-blown" addiction, followed by implications in the form of adverse effects and, the need for potential treatment.[21] However, the current diagnostic formulation might still be poor in differentiating it from normal (nonproblematic) gaming behavior.[7]

BLOCK: IMPULSE CONTROL DISORDERS
Compulsive Sexual Behavior Disorder

A continuous pattern of inability to regulate strong, repeated sexual drives or impulses that result in recurrent sexual behavior is the hallmark of this disorder. Its etiology still remains unclear but adding a diagnostic category would provide clinicians a better tool for addressing the unmet clinical requirements of treatment-seeking patients and may even help troubled people feel less ashamed and guilty about asking for help. Its inclusion in the ICD-11 has made it easier to provide appropriate assistance and to create and test therapies with strong empirical backing.[7,22]

Intermittent Explosive Disorder

Recurrent, brief episodes of verbal or physical aggressiveness or property destruction or an inability to control aggressive impulses are characteristics of intermittent explosive disorder. The provocation or the triggering psychosocial stressors are drastically out of proportion to the strength of the outburst or the level of hostility. In ICD-10 it was kept under "other habit and impulse disorders". However, the integrated research criteria's high diagnostic validity suggests it to be sufficient for acceptance and inclusion as a separate diagnostic entity in both DSM-5 and subsequently in ICD-11.[6,23]

CONCLUSION

The creation of the ICD-11 has been by far the most international, bilingual, interdisciplinary, and participatory revision process for the categorization of mental health diseases taking into account the pros and cons of previous classificatory systems (ICD-10 and DSM-V). Its inclusion of the integration of the dimensional methods, the life-span approach, the inclusion of information pertaining to cultures, a tendency toward the biological approach, together with efforts for destigmatization, undoubtedly reinforce its structure, and open it to future possibilities of goal-directed research and newer treatment modalities for all the reformed as well as new categories added in ICD-11.

REFERENCES

1. Parnas J. Differential diagnosis and current polythetic classification. World Psychiatry Off J World Psychiatr Assoc WPA. 2015;14(3):284-7.
2. Kraemer HC, Noda A, O'Hara R. Categorical versus dimensional approaches to diagnosis: methodological challenges. J Psychiatr Res. 2004;38(1):17-25.
3. Krueger RF, Bezdjian S. Enhancing research and treatment of mental disorders with dimensional concepts: toward DSM-V and ICD-11. World Psychiatry Off J World Psychiatr Assoc WPA. 2009;8(1):3-6.
4. Clark LA, Cuthbert B, Lewis-Fernández R, Narrow WE, Reed GM. Three approaches to understanding and classifying mental disorder: ICD-11, DSM-5, and the National Institute of Mental Health's Research Domain Criteria (RDoC). Psychol Sci Public Interest. 2017;18(2):72-145.
5. van Os J, Linscott RJ, Myin-Germeys I, Delespaul P, Krabbendam L. A systematic review and meta-analysis of the psychosis continuum: evidence for a psychosis proneness-persistence-impairment model of psychotic disorder. Psychol Med. 2009;39(2):179-95.
6. Gozi A. Highlights of ICD-11 classification of mental, behavioral, and neurodevelopmental disorders. Indian J Priv Psychiatry. 2019;13(1):11-7.
7. Reed GM, First MB, Billieux J, Cloitre M, Briken P, Achab S, et al. Emerging experience with selected new categories in the ICD-11: complex PTSD, prolonged grief disorder, gaming disorder, and compulsive sexual behaviour disorder. World Psychiatry. 2022;21(2):189-213.
8. Veale D, Matsunaga H. Body dysmorphic disorder and olfactory reference disorder: Proposals for ICD-11. Rev Bras Psiquiatr São Paulo Braz 1999. 2014;36 Suppl 1:14-20.
9. Suzuki K, Takei N, Iwata Y, Sekine Y, Toyoda T, Nakamura K, et al. Do olfactory reference syndrome and jiko-shu-kyofu (a subtype of taijin-kyofu) share a common entity? Acta Psychiatr Scand. 2004;109(2):150-5; discussion 155.
10. Timpano KR, Exner C, Glaesmer H, Rief W, Keshaviah A, Brähler E, et al. The epidemiology of the proposed DSM-5 hoarding disorder: exploration of the acquisition specifier, associated features, and distress. J Clin Psychiatry. 2011;72(6):780-6; quiz 878-9.
11. Fontenelle L, Grant J. Hoarding disorder: a new diagnostic category in ICD-11? Rev Bras Psiquiatr São Paulo Braz 1999. 2014;36 Suppl 1:28-39.
12. Grant JE, Stein DJ. Body-focused repetitive behavior disorders in ICD-11. Rev Bras Psiquiatr Sao Paulo Braz 1999. 2014;36 Suppl 1:59-64.
13. Shear K, Frank E, Houck PR, Reynolds CF. Treatment of complicated grief: a randomized controlled trial. JAMA. 2005;293(21):2601-8.
14. Killikelly C, Maercker A. Prolonged grief disorder for ICD-11: the primacy of clinical utility and international applicability. Eur J Psychotraumatology. 2018;8(Suppl 6):1476441.
15. AlAdawi S, Bax, Bryant-Waugh, Hay P, Rausch Herscovici C, Monteleone P, et al. Revision of ICD: status update on feeding and eating disorders. Adv Eat Disord Theory Res Pract. 2013;1:1-10.
16. Claudino AM, Pike KM, Hay P, Keeley JW, Evans SC, Rebello TJ, et al. The classification of feeding and eating disorders in the ICD-11: results of a field study comparing proposed ICD-11 guidelines with existing ICD-10 guidelines. BMC Med. 2019;17(1):93.

17. Murray HB, Juarascio AS, Lorenzo CD, Drossman DA, Thomas JJ. Diagnosis and treatment of rumination syndrome: a critical review. Am J Gastroenterol. 2019;114(4):562-78.
18. Gureje O, Reed GM. Bodily distress disorder in ICD-11: problems and prospects. World Psychiatry. 2016;15(3):291-2.
19. Blom RM, Hennekam RC, Denys D. Body integrity identity disorder. PLoS ONE. 2012;7(4):e34702.
20. First MB, Fisher CE. Body integrity identity disorder: the persistent desire to acquire a physical disability. Psychopathology. 2012;45(1):3-14.
21. Saunders JB, Hao W, Long J, King DL, Mann K, Fauth-Bühler M, et al. Gaming disorder: Its delineation as an important condition for diagnosis, management, and prevention. J Behav Addict. 2017;6(3):271-9.
22. Kraus SW, Krueger RB, Briken P, First MB, Stein DJ, Kaplan MS, et al. Compulsive sexual behaviour disorder in the ICD-11. World Psychiatry. 2018;17(1):109-10.
23. Coccaro EF. Intermittent explosive disorder as a disorder of impulsive aggression for DSM-5. Am J Psychiatry. 2012;169(6):577-88.

CHAPTER 9

Default Mode Network and Its Role in Various Psychiatric Disorders

Sayanti Ghosh, Malay Kumar Ghosal

INTRODUCTION

Hippocrates postulated that the human brain is responsible for consciousness and intelligence and also conceptualized epilepsy as a brain disorder.[1] But which functions of mind are localized to which specific parts of brain was a comparatively recent and intriguing research question. It dates back to the works of Franz Joseph Gall who in the early part of 19th century gave his theory of cortical localization through the science of phrenology. The phrenology later proved to be pseudoscience, but Gall had laid the foundation of the localization of functions in brain. The first scientific proposition came from the works of Paul Broca and then Carl Wernicke on aphasia. Raymon Cajal gave the theory of neuron doctrine; neurons are structural and functional unit of nervous system. He gave the concept of synapse and flow of information from one neuron to other neuron unidirectionally. Later Edgar Adrian gave the concept of action potential and Dale and Feldberg hypothesized the transmission of action potential from one neuron to other neuron through release of neurotransmitters. However, the theory of cerebral localization came under a strong criticism from the work of Karl Lashley, who gave the hypothesis of law of mass action.[2] According to the proposition, it is the amount of brain tissue damaged that was important and not the area. The dilemma was resolved with the work of Donald Hebb to some extent. His hypothesis about neurons that fire together wire together laid the early foundation of cortical network, where information is processed through interconnected cell groups, and so any function may be represented through widely separated areas together. That also explains diaschisis, where distant neurophysiological changes occur with a focal injury.[3] But the things got clearer with some recent developments, where developments in statistical physics with complex network system, topology and graph theory of mathematical science is being combined with the discoveries on functional imaging such as positron emission tomography (PET) scan and functional magnetic resonance imaging (fMRI).[4] The human brain comprises 2% of the body weight but it consumes 20% of the total oxygen consumption. A part of the brain when active, utilizes more oxygen. This can be measured by blood oxygen level dependent (BOLD) signal in fMRI, or oxygen extraction fraction (OEF) in PET scan. A method of cognitive subtraction is used to find out the areas responsible for a particular action by finding the activity in task and control state. So naturally, one would hypothesize that during some tasks the oxygen utilization of brain will increase in a particular area compared to control subjects. Interestingly, Raichle et al.[4] published an unusual phenomenon in which they found that during task, activity decreases in a particular area of brain, when they measured the OEF data in PET. The areas included posterior cingulate cortex (PCC) and precuneus. They termed medial mystery parietal area (MMPA) for the region.[5] This was later confirmed by fMRI studies and BOLD also. Resting state network was first proposed by Biswal et al.[6] but that was not supported initially by other researchers. Later resting state fMRI showed functional connectivity (FC) between different regions of brain and this was a pathbreaking discovery which actually reveals the functional organization of brain.[7] The unusual phenomenon of decreased activity found by Raichle et al. in brain during task baffled the neuroscientists primarily. This particular network was given the name Default Mode Network (DMN) by Raichle et al.[4] This DMN is now conceptualized as comprising of three areas ventral medial prefrontal cortex (MPFC), dorsal MPFC, and posterior cingulate with precuneus and adjacent parietal cortex.[8] From the regions of DMN it can be surmised that the function includes retrieval of episodic memory and autobiographical memory, emotion regulation, and social cognition. So basically, self-referential mental process is controlled by DMN. It is implicated in different psychiatric disorders, e.g., schizophrenia, depression, Alzheimer's disease, autism, etc. DMN acts in conjunction with two other networks—central executive network (CEN) and salience network (SN). CEN is comprised of dorsolateral prefrontal cortex (DLPFC) and posterior parietal cortex (PPC) and is responsible for attention to external world, working memory, and logical decision making. SN is comprised of dorsal anterior cingulate cortex (ACC) and insular cortex. SN is related to mainly detecting interoceptive signals and emotional regulation. CEN/DMN/SN acts in coordination and SN acts as a switch between DMN and CEN to reorient attention from internal to external world. Aberrant organization and functioning of these three networks are responsible for different psychiatric and neurological problems. This is the triple network model put forward by Menon (2011).[9,10] Here in this short review, we are trying to give very brief outlines of relationships of some important psychiatric disorders and DMN.

DEFAULT MODE NETWORK AND SCHIZOPHRENIA

The concept of schizophrenia and related psychotic disorders was initially conceptualized as disrupted function of a single discrete brain region[11] presenting as positive symptoms, negative symptoms, disorganization, and cognitive deficits. Lately, the concept has advanced with the increased understanding of cognitive brain networks, which suggests a dysfunctional integration of distributed neuronal networks, especially the DMN.[12-15]

Cognitive Deficits in Schizophrenia

Task Suppression and Task Positive Network Reciprocity

There is evidence of abnormal activity and connectivity of the DMN leading to working memory deficits on several task-related fMRI studies in schizophrenia. When working memory demands are parametrically increased, healthy people exhibit greater suppression of the DMN during working memory tasks. But schizophrenia patients fail to show this pattern.[16] It can be thought of as a failure to provide attention to tasks at hand with consequent impairment in task performance. Hence, inattention, working memory deficits, and language problems are noticed.

Task positive networks (TPNs) show an anticorrelation with DMN. When DMN is more active and TPN is less active, there is increased attention to internal feeling states and vice versa. But in schizophrenia, this anticorrelation is seen as being significantly reduced.[17] This occurs specially between MPFC and DLPFC.

Other Psychotic Symptoms in Schizophrenia

Disturbance of the basic sense of self-awareness has been suggested as a core phenotypic marker of schizophrenia spectrum disorders.[18,19] The dysfunctional links between cognitive and emotional dimensions of the human mind comprising of the sense of self, theory of mind, empathy, and hedonia have been thought to underlie schizophrenia phenomenology.[20] This theory of the disturbance of "sense of self" has been supported over the last decade as several studies have suggested that triple network dysfunction specifically the insula/ACC dysfunction, i.e., SN dysfunction is a unified cause of dysfunctions in schizophrenia.[21] Furthermore, structural alteration (grey matter reductions) of hubs of SN such as insula and ACC supports the role of SN.[22-24] These changes precede the occurrence of first psychotic symptoms and transitions to further chronicity are associated with morphological alterations in the adjacent areas of mediofrontal cortex and temporal lobe.[25] Regarding auditory verbal hallucinations (AVHs), studies suggest aberrant FC between DMN and CEN as a denominator of AVH severity.[26] Thus phasic hallucinations could arise from a spontaneous switching off of the dysregulated and unstable DMN secondary to DMN dysfunction.[27] The self-attributional system may thus become dysfunctional resulting in misattribution of internal mental states to external others causing delusions and other positive symptoms. Increased BOLD contrast response in midbrain dopaminergic regions, insula, and other DMN hubs from fMRI studies could underlie the delusions of reference to ambiguous stimuli in schizophrenia subjects compared to control.[9] Internal FC between SN and CEN has also been postulated to underlie the severity of negative symptoms in patients with schizophrenia.[28]

Social Cognition in Schizophrenia

Some social reflection tasks (reflection about oneself and another person) have revealed abnormally increased activation of DMN in the medial PCC and reduced activation of the right ventromedial prefrontal cortex (VMPFC).[29] In schizophrenia though this has not shown correlation with standard scales for social cognition. There is a possibility that these findings might later serve as quantitative neural markers of deficits in social cognition.

DEFAULT MODE NETWORK AND DEPRESSION

There are several research articles that have investigated the role of DMN in major depressive disorders, especially regarding the rumination pattern of thought, which is defined as a recurrent, self-reflective, and uncontrollable focus on depressed mood and its cause and consequences.[30] Rumination intensifies depression, damages social support, and impairs cognitive function.[31] There is increased resting state FC between the DMN and the subgenual prefrontal cortex (PFC) and medial dorsal thalamus, dorsal ACC, and posterior lateral parietal cortex,[32] which suggests an integration of the self-referential processes supported by DMN with the emotionally laden, behaviorally withdrawn process associated with subgenual PFC. This forms the neural substrate for depressive rumination in MDD. Reduced DMN task suppression has been seen during emotional perception and judgement[33] and during passive viewing and reappraisal of negative pictures,[34] which again reinforces the inability of the depressed subject to distract oneself from ruminative thoughts and focus on the task at hand. There is increased FC with the dorsomedial PFC termed "dorsal nexus" due to its widespread hyperconnectivity to seeds in the default, affective, and cognitive networks, which translates clinically to increased self-focus, rumination and distractibility in depressed subjects.[16] Increased levels of DMN dominance compared to TPN is also a feature of MDD, which leads to maladaptive symptoms in MDD.[35]

Both schizophrenia and depression being heterogenous disorders, it will certainly be useful to adopt a dimensional approach based on symptoms to understand the neurobiology. DMN changes in specific areas of the brain are envisioned to be useful in this regard. For example, patients who have auditory hallucinations might recruit the auditory cortex into the cortical midline DMN structures at rest, presumably independent of diagnosis.[36] Similarly people who ruminate will show correlation of DMN activation with limbic structures like subgenual PFC irrespective of their clinical diagnosis.[37] The phenotypic variability could be approached via these dimensional approaches compared to categorical ones as in the Research Domain Criteria (R-DoC). Clinical benefits for those under treatment for these disorders have also been researched by DMN studies. Patients taking antipsychotic medications appear to have more normal DMN activity (more normal task suppression) than patients on atypical antipsychotics.[38] Hence, future drug development could use DMN alterations as a possible outcome measure.

DEFAULT MODE NETWORK IN ALZHEIMER'S DISEASE

The disrupted connectivity of DMN which is one of the important resting state networks in human brain has been implicated in cognitive states such as normal aging and dementia (mostly Alzheimer's disease). Studies have shown that DMN hub regions including the MPFC, PCC, parietal cortex, and precuneus are affected early in Alzheimer's disease and there is high amount of amyloid beta deposition. Due to activity-dependent processing of amyloid precursor protein, it has been hypothesized that the active DMN neurons produce and release large amounts of Amyloid Beta (Aβ). There is increased oligomerization, aggregation of Amyloid Beta (Aβ), and tau hyperphosphorylation due to this. The impaired DMN is consistent with metabolic and structural changes. Memory encoding structures show accumulation of beta amyloid even before symptoms emerge and images of beta-amyloid plaques taken at earliest stage of Alzheimer's disease show a distribution which is remarkably similar to anatomy of DMN.[39] The brainstem long projection fibers (from locus ceruleus, dorsal raphe nucleus) innervate the cortical DMN areas and these show evidence of neurofibrillary degeneration as well. The DMN is coupled with the hippocampus during memory retrieval and not encoding thus confirming the special position of hippocampus between short-term and long-term memory.[40] Studies also provide evidence regarding close links between amyloid deposition, DMN functional changes, and alteration of sleep-awake cycle.[41] Investigation of DMN changes in prodromal or early stages of Alzheimer's disease has been studied by assessment of signal correlation between brain areas and measurement of multi-state entropy (MSE, which measures BOLD signal within a brain area).[42] The latter is thought to show local alterations even before FC is affected or clinical symptoms emerge, hence being envisioned as a putative functional marker for cognitive decline. Disruption in the DMN at the preclinical stage of the disease correlates with the mental status of the patient.

DEFAULT MODE NETWORK IN AUTISM SPECTRUM DISORDER

Deficits in social communication and interaction are the cornerstone of autism spectrum disorder (ASD) diagnosis. The DMN has been found to play a role in specific components of social cognitive dysfunction in ASD, namely self-referential processing which has the ability to process social information relative to oneself and theory of mind or mentalizing which refers to the ability to infer the mental states of others like beliefs, emotions, intentions, and such. Research suggests that aberrations in key nodes of DMN and their dynamic functional interactions underlie the atypical integration and processing of social information. Altered developmental trajectory of structural and functional organization of DMN is a prominent neurobiological feature of ASD.[43] Most task-based fMRI studies in ASD usually reveal hypoactivation of DMN nodes in ASD with decreased recruitment of ventral MPFC (during processing of self-relevant information), dorsal MPFC, and temporoparietal junction (during processing of other relevant information). Resting state fMRI has been used more extensively in several studies of ASD, which reveal increased within-network connectivity between core DMN nodes in children, decreased connectivity in adolescents and adults, and both increase or decrease in mixed age groups.[44] These "inconsistencies" likely reflect the heterogeneity in connectivity profiles as well as changes during brain development.[45] Lynch et al. posited that there may be a "switch" during the period of development in ASD children where connectivity patterns switch from hyperconnectivity to hypoconnectivity.[46] This was further studied in details by Uddin et al. (2013) who identified a particular trend in ASD children related to SN hyperconnectivity, which may assist in identifying specific biomarkers for ASD children.[45] Triple network model of psychopathology suggests that atypical interaction of DMN with SN also contributes to social cognitive dysfunction in ASD. There is evidence of intrinsic functional hyperconnectivity within the SN, CEN, and DMN and other neural systems.[9]

DEFAULT MODE NETWORK IN ATTENTION DEFICIT HYPERACTIVITY DISORDER

In contrast to the mixed FC trends in ASD, studies on attention deficit hyperactivity disorder (ADHD) show a global and widespread trend of increased FC. Increase in FC in the PFC has been noted along with widespread increased FC across whole brain particularly in right inferior frontal gyrus and bilateral MPFC in ADHD children versus typically developing (TD) ones.[47] These can be linked to clinical symptoms of specific attentional deficits such as wandering mind and attentional fluctuations which are again directly linked to DMN FC aberrations between the cerebellar DMN (cer DMN) and regions in visual and dorsal attentional networks in ADHD versus TD individuals.[48]

There has been a growing body of literature which suggests overlap between ASD and ADHD genotypes[49,50] and shared endophenotypes.[51] This has been reflected in high co-occurrence of ASD and ADHD in various studies. This shared prevalence rate necessitates DMN research regarding DMN FC deficits which might be shared in ASD and ADHD. Wang and colleagues

(2019) investigated intrinsic functional connectivity (iFC) in four cohorts (ASD, ASD+ADHD, ADHD, TD) and found increased social impairment and decreased intra-iFC in the bilateral PCC (ASD+ADHD group) and increased inter-iFC between the DMN-somatomotor networks in comparison to ASD group only.[52] Also, the strength of intra-iFC in the DMN was found to be associated with increased autistic trait severity across the ASD groups, especially the ASD+ADHD group. An R-DoC approach is needed to explore these shared connectivity patterns to view the disorders from a dimensional standpoint.

DEFAULT MODE NETWORK AND SUBSTANCE USE DISORDERS

There are several studies which indicate common alterations in resting-state FC across several substance use disorders (SUD) of which hypoconnectivity pattern for the limbic, salience, and frontoparietal network has been found compared to healthy controls. On the other hand, the DMN has shown a complex pattern of hypo- and hyperconnectivity across studies.[53] Association of aberrant patterns of connectivity in DMN has been observed with craving and relapse across different SUD. In addicted individuals, resting state FC of anterior DMN is decreased and that of posterior DMN is increased.[54] The former including ACC and medial orbitofrontal cortex is recognized as the central component of the value system of brain,[55] which participates in emotional processing, decision making,[56] salience attribution,[57] and is associated with dysregulation of reward and motivation circuits in addiction.[58] The posterior DMN has a role in directing attention to internal mental states. The disrupted connectivity between DMN and the cortical areas related to executive function, memory, emotion, and decision making is thought to underlie continued drug-taking behavior despite negative consequences and to stress-triggered relapse. The DMN is prominently engaged during the withdrawal and preoccupation phase of the addiction cycle at the expense of the executive control network and enhanced participation of SN. These lead to problem with disengagement from drug taking and increased salience toward substance use. Acute and chronic drug use-related changes in dopaminergic, glutaminergic, and GABAergic pathways are reflections of altered DMN.[54]

Internet addiction (IA), though not yet recognized as separate disorder, has been studied extensively in last few years regarding functional correlates of IA in resting state DMN and inhibitory control network (ICN) by functional imaging studies.[59] Significant deactivations related to DMN areas (precuneus, posterior cingulate gyrus) has been seen and these were negatively correlated with scales measuring problematic Internet use. Positive correlation with ICN was postulated to be the reason for difficulties in stopping and controlling overuse. A recent study has used resting-state electroencephalography (EEG) source FC within DMN and reward/salience network (RSN) in internet gaming disorder (IGD)[60] and found that hyperconnectivities within the DMN and RSN may be considered potential state markers associated with symptom severity and gaming in IGD.

CONCLUSION

Though the DMN has been classically considered as an "intrinsic" system mostly related to internally oriented cognitive processes such as daydreaming, reminiscing, and future planning, it is also an active and dynamic sense making brain network integrating incoming extrinsic information with prior intrinsic data.[61] It has a role in baseline activation for maintaining steady internal state in rest, mind wandering, autobiographical memory, social cognition, and "knowing oneself". Functional neuroimaging studies allow for systematic study of DMN alterations across various psychiatric disorders. Future putative biomarkers may be helpful for more meaningful diagnostic constructs with dimensional approach in psychiatry and also assist to diagnose the disorders at an early stage. Finally, studies which suggest that DMN changes are plastic and can be changed by treatments offer hope regarding prognosis and management of various psychopathologies.

TAKE-HOME POINTS

- To explain functions of mind with functions of brain is one of the hardest challenges of 21st century.
- The initial effort to understand this by cerebral localization of functions has now given way to circuits in the brain.
- The development of functional neuroimaging with the help of BOLD and OEF have helped a great deal in understanding the large network systems of brain.
- Triple network model is very influential where DMN, CEN and SN acts in tandem to explain different cognitive and emotional functions.
- DMN is comprised of ventral medial prefrontal cortex, dorsal medial prefrontal cortex and posterior cingulate with precuneus and adjacent parietal cortex. The function includes retrieval of episodic memory and autobiographical memory, emotion regulation and social cognition.
- CEN is comprised of dorsolateral prefrontal cortex (DLPFC) and posterior parietal cortex (PPC) and is responsible for attention to external world, working memory, and logical decision making.
- SN is comprised of dorsal anterior cingulate cortex (ACC) and insular cortex. SN is related to mainly detecting interoceptive signals and emotional regulation.
- SN acts as a switch between DMN and CEN to reorient attention from external to internal world.
- The DMN and its connectivity with the other cognitive networks is implicated in various psychiatric disorders such as schizophrenia, depression, ASD, substance use disorders, Alzheimers disorder, etc.
- Psychiatric disorders are lacking in biomarkers currently for diagnosis and classification.
- In future further research in this area may throw light on this area by development of some putative biomarkers.

REFERENCES

1. Britenfeld T, Jurasic MJ, Britenfeld D. Hippocrates: the forefather of neurology. Neurol Sci. 2014;35:1349-52.
2. Milner B, Squire LR, Kandel ER. Cognitive neuroscience and the study of memory. Neuron. 1998;20:445-68.
3. Carrera E, Tononi G. Diaschisis: past present and future. Brain. 2014;137:2408-422.
4. Raichle ME, Macleod AM, Snyder AZ, Powers WJ, Gusnard DA, Shulman GL. A default mode of brain function. PNAS. 2001;98:676-82.
5. Raichle ME. Two views of brain function. In: Gazzaniga MS (Ed). The Cognitive Neurosciences. MIT Press: Cambridge Massachusetts. 2009. pp. 1067-74.
6. Biswal B, Yetkin FZ, Haughton VM, Hyde JS. Functional connectivity of the motor cortex of resting human brain using echo-planar MRI. MRM. 1995;34:537-41.
7. Whitfield-Gabrieli S, Ford JM. Default mode network activity and connectivity in psychopathology. Annu Rev Clin Psychol. 2012;8:49-76.
8. Raichle ME. The brain's default mode network. Annu Rev Neurosci. 2015;38:433-47.
9. Menon V. Large-scale brain networks and psychopathology: a unifying triple network model. Trends Cogn Sci. 2011;15(10):483-506.
10. Bolton TAW, Wotruba D, Buechler R, Theodoridou A, Michels L, Kollias S, et al. Triple network model dynamically revisited: lower salience network state switching in pre-psychosis. Front Physiol. 2020;11:66.
11. Andreasen NC, Nopoulos P, O'Leary DS, Miller DD, Wassink T, Flaum M. Defining the phenotype of schizophrenia: cognitive dysmetria and its neural mechanisms. Biol Psychiatry. 1999;46(7):908-20.
12. Bluhm RL, Miller J, Lanius RA, Osuch EA, Boksman K, Neufeld RWJ, et al. Spontaneous low-frequency fluctuations in the BOLD signal in schizophrenic patients: anomalies in the default network. Schizophr Bull. 2007;33(4):1004-12.
13. Garrity AG, Pearlson GD, McKiernan KA, Lloyd D, Kiehl KA, Calhoun VD. Aberrant "default mode" functional connectivity in schizophrenia. Am J Psychiatry. 2007;164(3):450-7.
14. Whitfield-Gabrieli S, Thermenos HW, Milanovic S, Tsuang MT, Faraone SV, McCarley RW, et al. Hyperactivity and hyperconnectivity of the default network in schizophrenia and in first-degree relatives of persons with schizophrenia. Proc Natl Acad Sci USA. 2009;27;106(4):1279-84.
15. Swanson N, Eichele T, Pearlson G, Kiehl K, Yu Q, Calhoun VD. Lateral differences in the default mode network in healthy controls and patients with schizophrenia. Hum Brain Mapp. 2011;32(4):654-64.
16. Gabrieli SW, Ford JM. Default mode network activity and connectivity in psychopathology. Annu Rev Clin Psychol. 2012;8:49-76.
17. Chai XJ, Whitfield-Gabrieli S, Shinn AK, Gabrieli JD, Nieto Castanon A, McCarthy JM, et al. Abnormal medial prefrontal cortex resting-state connectivity in bipolar disorder and schizophrenia. Neuropsychopharmacology. 2011;36:2009-17.
18. Nelson B, Thompson A, Chanen AM, Amminger GP, Yung AR. Is basic self-disturbance in ultra-high risk for psychosis ('prodromal') patients associated with borderline personality pathology? Early Interv Psychiatry. 2013;7:306-10.
19. Nelson B, Whitford TJ, Lavoie S, Sass LA. What are the neurocognitive correlates of basic self-disturbance in schizophrenia? Integrating phenomenology and neurocognition. Part 1 (Source monitoring deficits). Schizo Phre Res. 2014;152(1):12-9.

20. Nekovarova T, Fajnerova I, Horacek J, Spaniel F. Bridging disparate symptoms of schizophrenia: a triple network dysfunction theory. Front Behav Neurosci. 2014;8:171.
21. Palaniyappan L, White TP, Liddle PF. The concept of salience network dysfunction in schizophrenia: from neuroimaging observations to therapeutic opportunities. Curr Top Med Chem. 2012;12(21):2324-38.
22. Glahn DC, Laird AR, Ellison-Wright I, Thelen SM, Robinson JL, Lancaster JL, et al. Meta-analysis of gray matter anomalies in schizophrenia: application of anatomic likelihood estimation and network analysis. Biol Psychiatry. 2008;64:774-81.
23. Ellison-Wright I, Bullmore E. Anatomy of bipolar disorder and schizophrenia: a meta-analysis. Schizophr Res. 2010;117:1-12.
24. Shepherd AM, Laurens KR, Matheson SL, Carr VJ, Green MJ. Systematic meta-review and quality assessment of the structural brain alterations in schizophrenia. Neurosci Biobehav Rev. 2012;36:1342-56.
25. Chan RC, Di X, McAlonan GM, Gong QY. Brain anatomical abnormalities in high-risk individuals, first-episode and chronic schizophrenia: an activation likelihood estimation meta-analysis of illness progression. Schizophr Bull. 2011;37:177-88.
26. Manoliu A, Riedl V, Zherdin A, Muhlau M, Schwerthoffer D, Scherr M, et al. Aberrant dependence of default mode/central executive network interactions on anterior insular salience network activity in schizophrenia. Schizophr Bull.2014;40:428-37.
27. Northoff G, Qin P. How can the brain's resting state activity generate hallucinations? A 'resting state hypothesis' of auditory verbal hallucinations. Schizophr Res. 2011;127:202-14.
28. Manoliu A, Riedl V, Doll A, Bauml JG, Muhlau M, Schwerthoffer D, et al. Insular dysfunction reflects altered between-network connectivity and severity of negative symptoms in schizophrenia during psychotic remission. Front Hum Neurosci. 2013;7:216.
29. Holt DJ, Cassidy BS, Andrews-Hanna JR, Lee SM, Coombs G, Goff DC, et al. (2011). An anterior-to-posterior shift in midline cortical activity in schizophrenia during self-reflection. Biol Psychiatry. 2011;69(5):415-23.
30. Morrow J, Nolen-Hoeksema S. Effects of responses to depression on the remediation of depressive affect. J Pers Soc Psychol. 19990;58(3):519-27.
31. Nolen-Hoeksema S, Wisco BE, Lyubomirsky S. Rethinking Rumination. Perspecti Psychol Sci. 2008;3(5):400-24.
32. Hamilton PJ, Farmer M, Fogelman P, Gotlib I. Depressive Rumination, the Default-Mode Network, and the Dark Matter of Clinical Neuroscience. Biol Psychiatry. 2015;78(4):224-30.
33. Grimm S, Boesiger P, Beck J, Schuepbach D, Bermpohl F, Walter M, et al. Altered negative BOLD responses in the default-mode network during emotion processing in depressed subjects. Neuropsychopharmacology. 2009;34:932-43.
34. Sheline YI, Barch DM, Price JL, Rundle MM, Vaishnavi SN, Snyder AZ, et al. The default mode network and self-referential processes in depression. Proc Natl Acad Sci USA. 2009;106(6):1942-47.
35. Hamilton JP, Furman DJ, Chang C, Thomason ME, Dennis E, Gotlib IH. Default-mode and task positive network activity in major depressive disorder:

implications for adaptive and maladaptive rumination. Biol Psychiatry. 2011;70:327-33.
36. Northoff G, Qin P, Nakao T. Rest-stimulus interaction in the brain: a review. Trends Neurosci. 2010;33:277-84.
37. Cooney R, Joormann J, Eugène F, Dennis E, Gotlib IH. Neural correlates of rumination in depression. Cogn Affect Behav Neurosci. 2010;10(4):470-8.
38. Surguladze SA, Chu EM, Marshall N, Evans A, Anilkumar AP, Timehin C, et al. Emotion processing in schizophrenia: fMRI study of patients treated with risperidone long-acting injections or conventional depot medication. J Psychopharmacol. 2011;25(6):722-33.
39. Huijbers W, Pennartz CM, Cabeza R, Daselaar SM. The hippocampus is coupled with the default network during memory retrieval but not during memory encoding. PLoS One. 2011;6:e17463.
40. Klunk WE, Engler H, Nordberg A, Wang Y, Blomqvist G, Holt DP, et al. Imaging brain amyloid in Alzheimer's disease with Pittsburgh compound-B. Ann Neurol. 2004;55(3):306-19.
41. Simic G, Babic M, Borovecki F, Hof PR. Early failure of default-mode network and the pathogenesis of Alzheimers disease. CNS Neurosci Ther. 2014;20(7):692-98.
42. Grieder M, Wang DJJ, Dierks T, Wahlund L-O, Jann K. Default mode network complexity and cognitive decline in mild Alzheimer's disease. Front Neurosci. 2018;12:770.
43. Padmanabhan A, Lynch CJ, Schaer M, Menon V. The default mode network in autism. Biol Psychiatry Cogn Neurosci Neuroimaging. 2017;2(6):476-86.
44. Olivito G, Clausi S, Laghi F, Tedesco AM, Baiocco R, Mastropasqua C, et al. Resting-state functional connectivity changes between dentate nucleus and cortical social brain regions in autism spectrum disorders. Cerebellum. 2017;16:283-92.
45. Uddin LQ, Supekar K, Menon V. Reconceptualizing functional brain connectivity in autism from a developmental perspective. Front Hum Neurosci. 2013;7:458.
46. Lynch CJ, Uddin LQ, Supekar K, Khouzam A, Phillips J, Menon V. Default mode network in childhood autism: Posteromedial cortex heterogeneity and relationship with social deficits. Biol Psychiatry. 2013;74:212-9.
47. Bos DJ, Oranje B, Achterberg M, Vlaskamp C, Ambrosino S, de Reus MA, et al. Structural and functional connectivity in children and adolescents with and without attention deficit/hyperactivity disorder. J Child Psychol Psychiatry. 2017;58(7):810-18.
48. Kucyi A, Hove MJ, Biederman J, Van Dijk KR, Valera EM. Disrupted functional connectivity of cerebellar default network areas in attention-deficit/hyperactivity disorder. Hum Brain Mapp. 2015;36:3373-86.
49. Bathelt J, Caan MWA, Geurts HM. More similarities than differences between ADHD and ASD in functional brain connectivity. PsyArXiv. 2020.
50. Chantiluke K, Christakou A, Murphy CM, Giampietro V, Daly EM, Ecker C, et al. Disorder-specific functional abnormalities during temporal discounting in youth with Attention Deficit Hyperactivity Disorder (ADHD), Autism and comorbid ADHD and Autism. Psychiatry Res. 2014;223(2):113-20.
51. Kernbach J, Satterthwaite T, Bassett D, Smallwood J, Margulies D, Krall S, et al. Shared endo-phenotypes of default mode dysfunction in attention deficit/hyperactivity disorder and autism spectrum disorder. Transl Psychiatry. 2018;8(1):133.

52. Wang K, Xu M, Ji Y, Zhang L, Du X, Li J, et al. Altered social cognition and connectivity of default mode networks in the co-occurrence of autistic spectrum disorder and attention deficit hyperactivity disorder. Aust N Z J Psychiatry. 2019;53(8):760-71.
53. Taebi A, Becker B, Brown BK, Roecher E, Biswal B, Zweerings J, et al. Shared network-level functional alterations across substance use disorders: a multi-level kernel density meta-analysis analysis of resting-state functional connectivity studies. Addict Biol. 2022;27(4):e13200.
54. Zhanga R, Volkow ND. Brain default-mode network dysfunction in addiction. Neuroimage. 2019;200:313-31.
55. Bartra O, McGuire JT, Kable JW. The valuation system: a coordinate-based meta-analysis of BOLD fMRI experiments examining neural correlates of subjective value. Neuroimage. 2013;76:412-27.
56. Fuster JM. Prefrontal cortex. In: Adelman (Ed). Comparative neuroscience and neurobiology (Readings from the Encyclopedia of Neuroscience). Boston, MA: Birkhäuser; 1988. pp. 107-9.
57. Goldstein RZ, Volkow ND. Dysfunction of the prefrontal cortex in addiction: neuroimaging findings and clinical implications. Nat Rev Neurosci. 2011;12:652-69.
58. Volkow ND, Fowler JS, Wang GJ. The addicted human brain: insights from imaging studies. J Clin Investig. 2003;111:1444-51.
59. Darnai G, Perlaki G, Zsidó AN, Inhóf O, Orsi G, Horváth R, et al. Internet addiction and functional brain networks: task-related fMRI study. Sci Rep. 2019;9:15777.
60. Lee JY, Choi CH, Park M, Park S, Choi JS. Enhanced resting-state EEG source functional connectivity within the default mode and reward-salience networks in internet gaming disorder. Psychol Med. 2022;52(11):2189-97.
61. Yeshurun Y, Nguyen M, Hasson U. The default mode network: where the idiosyncratic self meets the shared social world. Nat Rev Neurosci. 2021;22(3):181-92.

CHAPTER 10

Role of Stem Cells and Nutraceuticals in Psychiatry

Kartik Singhai, Biju Viswanath, Krishna Prasad Muliyala

STEM CELLS IN PSYCHIATRY

Introduction

The concept of personalized medicine entails providing tailored treatment to the individual. It aims to provide an accurate diagnosis, predict disease susceptibility, and thereby help to arrive at the most efficient therapeutic option. This often involves using genetic or other biomarker information catering to the nuances of each patient.

The etiological or neurobiological basis of many psychiatric conditions remains elusive, which translates into limited biological interventions being available. There are no consistently proven biomarkers or objective markers of prognostication in psychiatry. Patients are often exposed to treatment partially on a trial and error basis, thus enhancing the associated morbidity. Hence, there is an increasing focus on personalized or precision-based medicine. Newer modalities such as stem cell (SC) research are a step forward in this direction.

Stem cells are the units of biological organization with exclusive self-renewal capability and differentiation potential to give rise to multiple cell lineages.[1,2] These traits render them useful for the development and regeneration of organ and tissue systems.

In the present chapter, we shall discuss the application of SCs in various psychiatric disorders. The second part of the chapter shall entail a brief discussion on nutraceuticals and their application to psychiatric disorders.

It is worthwhile to mention at the outset itself that while SCs hold immense promise for a wide variety of applications, their understanding and applicability at present in the field of psychiatry are more restricted to eliciting the neurobiology and disease models of psychiatric disorders. Their therapeutic role currently for the same is not well elucidated.

Basic Concepts

Induced Pluripotent Stem Cells

Hierarchically, based on the kind of tissue they give rise to, SCs can be totipotent SCs (body of an embryo and tissues of the placenta), pluripotent (all three germ layers) or multipotent SCs (one of the germ layers), and omnipotent or tissue committed SCs (tissue-specific cells which give rise to one line of cells).[1,3,4]

The last decade or so of research has seen the expansion of the utility of induced pluripotent stem cells (iPSCs) in understanding patient-specific disease models and pathophysiology.[5] iPSCs are cells derived from the skin or blood after being reprogrammed into an embryonic-like pluripotent state, using various transcription factors. Kobayashi and Yamanaka, in their landmark paper in 2006, reported about pluripotent SCs induced from mouse embryonic or adult fibroblasts.[6] These cells, the iPSCs, displayed properties of embryonic SCs and expressed those marker genes. The neural stem cells (NSCs) that can be formed from iPSCs have the potential to be differentiated into other cell types such as astrocytes and functionally active neurons and glia.[6,7] While human iPSCs were initially obtained from skin biopsy-derived fibroblasts, getting iPSCs from peripheral blood mononuclear cells and cells in the urine has also become feasible.[8,9]

Further, the technique of gene editing has expanded our usage of iPSCs. Gene editing aims to modify living organisms' genes, understand gene function, and possibly utilize it to treat diseases.[10] The CRISPR-Cas9 approach (clustered regularly interspaced short palindromic repeats and CRISPR-associated protein 9) is relevant here. The CRISPR/Cas9 system is constituted by two important molecules (guide RNA and Cas nuclease) that can be used to insert one or more DNA sections into the genome to hijack the DNA repair machinery.[11,12] CNS disorders which have a defined genetic alteration have been studied using these iPSCs model. CNS disorders having a defined genetic alteration can be well studied using this system. Furthermore, through insertion, deletion, or by replacing nucleotides, or by modulation of gene expression the identified pathogenic mutation can be corrected.[11,12]

Brain Organoids

Brain organoids (BO) are SC-derived 3D suspension cultures that self-assemble into an organized structure with cell types and cytoarchitectures recapitulating the developing brain.[13,14] Neurodevelopmental and neuropsychiatric disorders that do not present with observable neuroanatomical phenotypes can be studied using this BO, which help to learn the alterations in neuronal migration, cortical layering, and axon guidance which characterize these disorders.[13,14]

Role of Induced Pluripotent Stem Cells

Induced pluripotent stem cells are attractive candidates for future developments in personalized psychiatry since. Modelling the iPSC-disease model reproduces a pathologic condition in vitro by reprogramming the patient's somatic cells into iPSCs, then redifferentiating the patient-specific iPSCs into disease-specific cells.

The potential and goal of iPSC models are to create an approximation of aspects of illness or risk in the context of a particular human cell, with a particular human genome. This can then be studied to elucidate pathogenic mechanisms and identify remediation or rescue targets. The relative immaturity of iPSC-derived neural cells creates a barrier in creating accurate in vitro models of neuropsychiatric disorders. The similarity of 2D and 3D models to early fetal neurons is supported by gene expression and electrophysiological studies.[15-17] This fetal-like identity of iPSCs is often considered as a limitation, but it could work to an advantage. They may provide the much needed insight into otherwise difficult to access biological processes if they are able to recapitulate aspects of human neurodevelopment. Therefore, iPSC-based models provide a system to study cause and effect relationships for disorders with a proposed neurodevelopmental origin, such as schizophrenia (SZ) and autism.

Individual Disorders

The studies described below are examples of some of the significant studies performed using iPSCs in psychiatry. The field is ever-growing, and interested readers can also go through Alciati et al. (2022), Dixon and Muotri (2022), and Kalin (2022). A simplified summary of findings is presented in **Table 1**.

Schizophrenia

Schizophrenia is a type of severe mental illness characterized by positive, negative, disorganization, cognitive, and affective symptoms. It is associated with subtle cortical brain changes. Neurogenesis being a neuroprotective factor, its dysfunction can lead to the progression of SZ. SC studies mainly attempt to understand the pathogenesis of the illness.

Brennand et al. in 2011 published the first human study using human iPSCs. Compared to controls, iPSC-derived neurons from patients with SZ showed lesser neuronal connectivity, lower neurite numbers, and lesser PSD95 synaptic protein levels, besides altered gene expression profiles of the cAMP, wingless-related integration site (Wnt) signaling pathways, and glutamate receptors.[18] Regulation of cell proliferation and differentiation during embryonic development is the key function of the Wnt.[5,18] Similar findings have been noted in postmortem brain of patients with SZ as well as animal models of SZ. Loxapine was shown to ameliorate these changes in further experiments.[18]

TABLE 1: Summary of findings from selected studies utilizing stem cell models for various psychiatric disorders.

S. no.	Disorder	Cell model	Findings/implications	Authors/References
1.	Schizophrenia	• iPSC-derived dentate gyrus • iPSC differentiated into NCCs • SZ-iPSC and HC-iPSC derived BO	• Depleted neuronal programming factors • Reduced PSD95 synaptic protein levels • Wnt signaling pathways' expression is altered • Downregulation of genes involved in cell adhesion	Notaras et al. (2022); Kathuria et al. (2020); Ahmed et al. (2018)
2.	Major depressive disorder	• iPSCs from SSRI remitters and SSRI nonremitters differentiated to serotonergic neurons • iPSC-derived dopaminergic neurons • MDD responders and nonresponders to bupropion; their LCLs reprogrammed to iPSCs and differentiated to mature prefrontal cortex neurons	• Enhanced colocalization of synaptic markers in bupropion responders • Exposure to ketamine promotes synaptic plasticity • Differences in serotonergic neuron morphology probably lead to differential response to SSRIs	Avior et al. (2021); Cavalleri et al. (2018); Vadodoria et al. (2020)
3.	Bipolar disorder	• iPSC-derived neural progenitor cells • CXCR expressing NPCs	• Abnormalities in WNT/GSK3 signaling • BD iPSC-derived neurons show significantly different gene expression, especially transcripts involved in calcium signaling • Neuronal activity functionally less supported by BD astrocytes	Vadodoria et al. (2021); Bame et al. (2020); Truve et al. (2020); Chen et al. (2014)
4.	Autism spectrum disorder	• 2D and 3D FXS models based on isogenic FMR1 knock-out mutant and wild-type human iPSC lines • iPSC 3D models of FXS	• Excitation/inhibition ratio and glial cell proliferation need essential support from FMRP	Brighi et al. (2021); Mariani et al. (2016)

(BD: bipolar disorder; BO: brain organoids; FXS: fragile X syndrome; HC: healthy controls; iPSC: induced pluripotent stem cells; LCLs: lymphoblastoid cell lines; MDD: major depressive disorder; NCC: neuron committed cell; NPCs: neural progenitor cells; SSRI: selective serotonin reuptake inhibitor; SZ: schizophrenia)

Another study by Narla et al. showed impaired migration capacity in induced NSCs in patients with SZ vis-a-vis healthy and high-risk genetic controls. This was further studied to identify the nFGFR1 signaling as a potential therapeutic target.[19]

Another brain process under study is hippocampal neurogenesis and its aberrations in SZ. Yu et al. in their study found that hippocampal neural precursor cells (NPCs) derived from SZ-iPSC showed decreased neuronal activity and decreased release of spontaneous neurotransmitters.[20]

It has also been postulated that mitochondrial dysfunction could have a putative role in SZ pathogenesis. Studies investigating the same using iPSC-NPC and neurons of patients of SZ have shown signs of increased oxidative species damage and disturbed mitochondrial respiration and morphology among patients as compared to controls.[5,21]

Phenotypes associated with early neurodevelopmental defects have been implicated in another set of studies using BO to study SZ. Some of the findings elicited from RNA sequencing in BOs include aberrant gene expression pathways involved in synaptic biology, nervous system development, mitochondrial function, and excitatory and inhibitory neurotransmission modulation.[22]

In another study on BO derived from SZ patients, progenitor survival was altered and neurogenesis was disrupted, resulting in fewer neurons within developing cortical areas.[23] Depletion of neuronal programming factors were seen in SZ progenitors when studied using single-cell sequencing. This study indicates that the risk of developing SZ is contributed by multiple mechanisms involving SZ-derived BO converging upon neurodevelopmental pathways.[23]

Overall, these studies in patients with SZ indicate early genetic dysregulation leading to alteration in development of neurons and the brain.

Major Depressive Disorder

Decreased neurogenesis and volume in the hippocampus, along with reduced levels of brain-derived growth factor, is a known etiopathological factor in patients with major depressive disorder (MDD). It is implicated that this suppression in neurogenesis is due to elevated steroids induced by chronic stress, and antidepressants may work to stimulate neurogenesis to exert their therapeutic effects.

Most of the evidence of SC models and their usage in MDD is derived from studying mechanisms of antidepressants. Further, the majority of the studies have focused on treatment-resistant depression.[5]

A study was conducted in patients with MDD by generating iPSCs from both remitters and nonremitters.[24] Patients, who after treatment with selective serotonin reuptake inhibitor (SSRI) did not reach remission, showed serotonin-induced hyperactivity downstream of upregulated excitatory serotonergic receptors (5-HT2A and 5-HT7). This was in contrast to what was seen in iPSCs derived from patients who remitted on SSRIs and in healthy controls.[24]

In another study, the effects of bupropion were studied using rapidly generated cortical neurons from patient-derived lymphoblastoid cell lines from a set of patients with MDD.[25] Changes in dendritic spine morphology and gene expression were seen in cells of patients who responded to bupropion.

Ketamine, a glutamate N-methyl-D-aspartate (NMDA) receptor antagonist, is a novel treatment for treatment-resistant depression and suicidality. An iPSC-based study has explored the mechanism of action for the antidepressant effects of ketamine. The findings indicate that ketamine elicits structural plasticity by recruitment of AMPAR (α-amino-3-hydroxy-5-methyl-4-isoxazolepropionic acid), mammalian target of rapamycin (mTOR), and brain-derived neurotrophic factor (BDNF) signaling in both mouse mesencephalic and human-iPSCs-derived dopaminergic (DA) neurons.[26]

Achour et al. (2021) assessed the effect of luteolin on human NSC fate determination and the lipopolysaccharide (LPS)-induced neuroinflammation in a mouse model of depression with astrocyte genesis defect.[27] Findings reveal that luteolin upregulated the expressions of genes related to neurotrophin, DA, hippo, and Wnt signaling pathways, and downregulated the genes involved in p53, TNF, FOXO, and Notch signaling pathways. Luteolin treatment also significantly increased mature BDNF, dopamine, and noradrenaline levels in the hypothalamus of LPS-induced depression mice. While findings do not retain statistical significance, possible therapeutic benefits of luteolin and thus also giving a clue onto underlying molecular mechanisms in depression were important gains from this study.

Bipolar Disorder

The focus of iPSC-based studies for bipolar disorder (BD) has been on understanding the pathogenic mechanisms, additionally taking the help of examination of effects of lithium and/or other BD medication exposure on the various signaling pathways.

Chen et al. studied the changes in gene expression in iPSCs from patients with BD and compared with healthy controls.[28] The expression of transcripts for membrane bound receptors and ion channels was significantly increased in BD-derived neurons compared with controls. Also, lithium pretreatment of BD neurons significantly altered their calcium transient and wave amplitude. Further, there have been studies on microRNAs (miRNAs) in BD iPSC-derived cells. MiRNAs regulate the expression of multiple BD-linked genes that are implicated in the development and differentiation of neurons and neuroplasticity; miR-34a has been implicated to play a role in the pathogenesis of BD. This miRNA has also been found to be reduced by in vitro application of lithium and valproic acid.[29]

A study explored expression differences in CXCR4 expressing central nervous system NPCs between a pair of BD-affected brothers and their parents.[30] The CXCR4 is a G protein-coupled chemokine receptor that on binding to its ligands orchestrates multiple signaling pathways involved in cell migration, hematopoiesis, and cell homing. The BD affected siblings had many phenotypic differences in neurogenesis and gene expression necessary for neural plasticity quite unlike the parents.

Inflammatory responses in patients with BD have been another area of study with upcoming evidence. Available evidence suggests a role of astrocytes, which have shown to be transcriptionally different in BD patients compared to controls. Attili et al. (2020) studied cell lines from BD patients and controls and found that exosomes from astrocyte cell lines were more concentrated in the BD group than the controls.[31]

Another set of studies have proposed that electrophysiological activity of iPSC-derived neuronal cells may help in predicting response to lithium.[5,32] Lithium treatment reversed selectively the hyperexcitability phenotype in BD. This was seen only in neurons that were derived from patients who responded to lithium treatment. This supports the possible utility of this model of iPSCs in helping design new drugs.

Truve et al. (2020) performed a study aimed at finding the genes, proteins, and genetic variants that are possibly involved in the development of BD.[33] Methods employed were generation of human iPSC, human iPSC-NSC, and human iPSC-neuron/glial cultures; quantitative proteomics; whole genome sequencing; and genotyping and comparison with a former data set. The protein within the NSCs and mature cells obtained from BD-patient cell samples with the most significant up-regulation was NLRP2. Another set of proteins that were differentially expressed in BD compared to control-derived cells were the FEZ2 and CADM2 proteins. Novel candidate mutations were identified in the *ANK3, NEK3, NEK7, TUBB, ANKRD1*, and *BRD2* genes. Review of literature on the candidate variants and deregulated proteins inform that the molecules putatively involved are connected to microtubule function. Axon structure and axonal transport are highly dependent on microtubule function. A functional dynamic microtubule has a role in response to cellular and environmental stress. Compromise in microtubule function can lead to deregulated expressions, which can possibly explain the inherited vulnerability to stressful life events that can precipitate mood episodes in BD. If mutations compromise microtubule dynamics, it could lead to deregulated expression. This forms a possible explanation for the inherited vulnerability to stressful life events that have been proposed to trigger mood episodes in BD patients.

Bame et al. (2020) utilized iPSCs to study differential expressions of miRNAs in a group of BD patients compared to healthy controls. 58 miRNAs were identified, which were differentially expressed between the two groups.[34]

Quantitative polymerase chain reactions validated six miRNAs that were elevated and two miRNAs that were expressed at lower levels in BD-derived neurons. The targets of these miRNAs are putatively involved in regulating a number of cellular pathways, which include axon guidance, mitogen-activated protein kinase pathway, Ras protein signaling pathway (proteins serve as transducers that couple cell surface receptors to intracellular effector pathways), Hippo pathway (regulates cell number by modulating cell proliferation, cell death, and cell differentiation), neurotrophin-modulated signaling pathways, and the Wnt signal transduction pathway.

Sukumaran et al. (2022) in their study aimed to study migration patterns of iPSC-derived NPCs from individuals with familial BD with a healthy control group as comparison.[35] Migrating cells were studied through time-lapse analysis. Findings revealed abnormal parameters in cell migration, including speed and directionality of NPCs. Further, transcriptomic analysis showed downregulation of a network of genes, centering on EGF/ERBB proteins.

Autism Spectrum Disorder

The potential of iPSCs to recapitulate early neurodevelopmental conditions makes them a suitable material to study a neurodevelopmental disorder such as autism spectrum disorder (ASD).

Mariani et al. studied gene expression in ASD iPSC-derived BO.[36] They found that an overexpression of the gene *FOXG1* lead downstream to an increase in brain volume and an imbalance in the excitation/inhibition systems of the developing cortex was observed. However, some studies have shown conflicting results in terms of the proportion of GABAergic inhibitory precursors compared to glutamatergic precursors.[36]

An essential gene linked with ASD is the one for fragile X syndrome (FXS). This syndrome is caused due to the transcriptional *FMR1* gene being silenced on the X-chromosome during development of the embryo. The silencing causes aberrant differentiation in the neural progenitor cells derived from human iPSC.

Bright et al. generated iPSC 3D models of FXS. These models revealed cortical neuron gene expression was altered and differentiation was impaired when compared to the wild-type human iPSCs.[37] Cortical BO models have demonstrated higher number of glial cells (astrocytes) and bigger organoid size. These findings support that FMRP is essential for correct excitation/inhibition ratio and to correctly support proliferation of neurons and glial cells in human brain development.

NUTRACEUTICALS IN PSYCHIATRY

The word nutraceutical is a combination of the words "nutrition" and "pharmaceuticals" and is defined as food components or active principles present in aliments that have positive effects for health and quality of life, including for prevention or treating disorders.[38]

Similarly, the field of Nutritional Psychiatry as a paradigm entails clinical consideration (where appropriate) of prescriptive dietary modification/improvement and/or the select judicious use of nutrient-based supplementation to prevent or manage psychiatric disorders.[39] The field is still in its nascent stages; however, intervention studies provide good promise for preventing and treating conditions such as depression.

The International Society for Nutritional Psychiatry Research published an index paper in 2015[40] in which one of the critical articulations was—

"... we advocate that evidence-based nutritional change should be regarded as an efficacious and cost-effective means to improve mental health. In addition to dietary modification, we recognise that nutrient-based (nutraceutical) prescription has the potential to assist in the management of mental disorders at the individual and population level. Many of these nutrients have a clear link to brain health, including: omega-3s, B vitamins (particularly folate and B12), choline, iron, zinc, magnesium, S-adenosyl methionine (SAMe), vitamin D, and amino acids. While we advocate for these to be consumed in the diet where possible, additional select prescription of these as nutraceuticals may also be justified".

A recent review depicted that probiotics and prebiotics might improve mental function via several mechanisms.[41] Clinical studies have shown beneficial effects of their application in depression, anxiety, Alzheimer's disease, and ASDs. However, further evidence is needed to establish the clinical significance and their equivalence or superiority to current treatments.

In MDD, evidence suggests that St. John's wort (Hypericum Perform) may have antidepressant properties via its serotonin-reuptake blocking mechanism. A Cochrane review revealed hypericum seems somewhat effective when less strict diagnostic criteria are used, but tends to be nonsuperior to placebo in major depression.[42] Saffron and curcumin are the other phytochemicals with some evidence in the positive direction.[43] Within nutraceuticals, omega-3 fatty acid, followed by adjunctive probiotics, and zinc have shown some evidence in the positive direction for unipolar depression.

For SZ, N-acetyl cysteine and methyl-folate have varying degrees of evidence support and recommendations for treating negative symptoms.[43]

Similarly, the role of omega-3 fatty acids as an augmentation or adjacent treatment strategy in SZ or prevention of conversion into psychosis in individuals at ultra-high risk for the same has been suggested by certain clinical studies.[44] The proposed mechanism is that omega-3 fatty acids correct the reduced synthesis and uptake of polyunsaturated fatty acids and abnormal fatty acid-binding protein levels in patients of SZ.[45] However, the evidence base and hence the strength of recommendation remains low.

TABLE 2: Summary of evidence (supporting Grade A evidence) and strength of recommendation as per clinician guidelines for the treatment of psychiatric disorders with nutraceuticals and phytoceuticals: The World Federation of Societies of Biological Psychiatry (WFSBP) and Canadian Network for Mood and Anxiety Treatments (CANMAT) Taskforce.

S. no.	Nutraceuticals/Phytoceuticals	Schizophrenia	Unipolar depression	Bipolar depression
1.	Adjunctive omega-3 fatty acid	Inconclusive	+++	+
2.	Adjunctive N-acetyl cysteine	++	NA	+/–
3.	Vitamin D	+	+	NA
4.	Methylfolate	++	+	NA
5.	St. John's wort	NA	+++	NA
6.	Curcumin	NA	++	NA
7.	Saffron	NA	++	NA

(NA: not applicable)

Proposed benefits but with inconclusive evidence are present for a variety of other interventions such as folate, vitamin B_{12} and D_3, alfa-lactalbumin and S-adenosylmethionine for depression, and kava, valerian, and passionflower for anxiety and insomnia.[46]

A meta-analysis on dietary interventions for ASDs revealed that dietary supplementation, omega-3 supplementation and vitamin supplementation, was more effective than placebo for certain cluster of symptoms such as anxiety, general autistic psychopathology, core symptoms, or the associated symptoms.[47] However, the effect sizes of such interventions were relatively small and hence bear limited clinical utility.

This field is currently limited by a lack of data and methodological issues such as heterogeneity, residual confounding, measurement error, and challenges in measuring and ensuring dietary adherence in intervention studies. Future directions will be to elucidate clear biological pathways and targets that link the benefit of nutraceuticals to mental disorders, to replicate and scale up promising strategies via more scientifically rigorous interventions, and to advocate for policy changes aimed at improving the food environment at the population level **(Table 2)**.[48]

CONCLUSION

In the past decade, stem cell research in psychiatry has gained much needed pace. It gives the field a direction in its search for the etiology of mental disorders. Their remain significant challenges in this field of research such as difficulty in access to the organ of origin, i.e., the brain, coupled with the heterogeneity of findings and complexities in synthesizing the same. Research findings at their current level are far from conclusive and causal, however, continual work in the same is likely to lead towards clinically translational results.

TAKE-HOME POINTS

- iPSC-based models provide a basis to understand disorders of possible neurodevelopmental origin, such as schizophrenia and autism.
- Depleted neuronal programming factors, altered Wnt signaling expression, down regulation of cell adhesion molecules are some of the findings found associated with schizophrenia.
- Enhanced colocalization of synaptic markers in bupropion responders and better synaptic plasticity in patients receiving ketamine was seen in patients with major depressive disorder.
- Research pertaining to iPSC and BD has shown abnormalities in WNT/GSK3 signaling and neuronal activity being less supported by astrocytes derived from a population with BD.
- Apart from omega-3-fatty acid and N-acetylcysteine, evidence base is highly limited for the use of nutraceuticals in mental disorders.

REFERENCES

1. Ratajczak MZ, Zuba-Surma E, Kucia M, Poniewierska A, Suszynska M, Ratajczak J, et al. Pluripotent and multipotent stem cells in adult tissues. Adv Med Sci. 2012;57(1):1-17.
2. Morrison SJ, Kimble J. Asymmetric and symmetric stem-cell divisions in development and cancer. Nature. 2006;441:1068-74.
3. Thomson JA, Itskovitz-Eldor J, Shapiro SS, Waknitz MA, Swiergiel JJ, Marshall VS, et al. Embryonic stem cell lines derived from human blastocysts. Science. 1998;282:1145-7.
4. Brons IG, Smithers LE, Trotter MW, Rugg-Gunn P, Sun B, Chuva de Sousa Lopes SM, et al. Derivation of pluripotent epiblast stem cells from mammalian embryos. Nature. 2007;448(7150):191-5.
5. Alciati A, Reggiani A, Caldirola D, Perna G. Human-Induced Pluripotent Stem Cell Technology: Toward the Future of Personalized Psychiatry. J Pers Med. 2022;12(8):1340.
6. Takahashi K, Yamanaka S. Induction of Pluripotent Stem Cells from Mouse Embryonic and Adult Fibroblast Cultures by Defined Factors. Cell. 2006;126:663-76.
7. Abdullah AI, Pollock A, Sun T. The path from skin to brain: Generation of functional neurons from fibroblasts. Mol Neurobiol. 2012;45:586-95.
8. Park B, Yoo KH, Kim C. Hematopoietic Stem Cell Expansion and Generation: The Ways to Make a Breakthrough. Blood Res. 2015;50:194-203.
9. Liu G, David BT, Trawczynski M, Fessler RG. Advances in Pluripotent Stem Cells: History, Mechanisms, Technologies, and Applications. Stem Cell Rev. Rep. 2020;16:3-32.
10. De Masi C, Spitalieri P, Murdocca M, Novelli G, Sangiuolo F. Application of CRISPR/Cas9 to Human-Induced Pluripotent Stem Cells: From Gene Editing to Drug Discovery. Hum Genom. 2020;14:25.

11. Duarte F, Déglon N. Genome Editing for CNS Disorders. Front Neurosci. 2020;14:10-22.
12. Bassett AR. Editing the Genome of HiPSC with CRISPR/Cas9: Disease Models. Mamm Genome. 2017;28:348-64.
13. Lancaster MA, Renner M, Martin CA, Wenzel D, Bicknell LS, Hurles ME, et al. Cerebral Organoids Model Human Brain Development and Microcephaly. Nature. 2013;501:373-9.
14. Eglen RM, Reisine T. Human IPS Cell-Derived Patient Tissues and 3D Cell Culture Part 1: Target Identification and Lead Optimization. SLAS Technol. 2019;24:3-17.
15. De Los Angeles A, Fernando MB, Hall NAL, Brennand KJ, Harrison PJ, Maher BJ, et al. Induced Pluripotent Stem Cells in Psychiatry: An Overview and Critical Perspective. Biol Psychiatry. 2021;90(6):362-72.
16. Gunhanlar N, Shpak G, van der Kroeg M, Gouty-Colomer LA, Munshi ST, Lendemeijer B. A simplified protocol for differentiation of electrophysiologically mature neuronal networks from human induced pluripotent stem cells. Mol Psychiatry. 2018;23:1336-44.
17. Burke EE, Chenoweth JG, Shin JH, Collado-Torres L, Kim SK, Micali N. Dissecting transcriptomic signatures of neuronal differentiation and maturation using iPSCs. Nat Commun. 2020;11:462.
18. Brennand KJ, Simone A, Jou J, Gelboin-Burkhart C, Tran N, Sangar S, et al. Modelling Schizophrenia Using Human Induced Pluripotent Stem Cells. Nature. 2011;473:221-5.
19. Narla ST, Lee YW, Benson CA, Sarder P, Brennand KJ, Stachowiak EK, et al. Common Developmental Genome Deprogramming in Schizophrenia—Role of Integrative Nuclear FGFR1 Signaling (INFS). Schizophr Res. 2017;185:17-32.
20. Yu DX, Di Giorgio FP, Yao J, Marchetto MC, Brennand K, Wright R, et al. Modeling Hippocampal Neurogenesis Using Human Pluripotent Stem Cells. Stem Cell Rep. 2014;2:295-310.
21. Ahmad R, Sportelli V, Ziller M, Spengler D, Hoffmann A. Tracing Early Neurodevelopment in Schizophrenia with Induced Pluripotent Stem Cells. Cells. 2018;7:140.
22. Kathuria A, Lopez-Lengowski K, Jagtap SS, McPhie D, Perlis RH, Cohen BM, et al. Transcriptomic Landscape and Functional Characterization of Induced Stem Cell–Derived Cerebral Organoids In. JAMA Psychiatry. 2020;77:745.
23. Notaras M, Lodhi A, Dündar F, Collier P, Sayles NM, Tilgner H, et al. Schizophrenia is defined by cell-specific neuropathology and multiple neurodevelopmental mechanisms in patient-derived cerebral organoids. Mol Psychiatry. 2022;27:1416-34.
24. Vadodaria KC, Ji Y, Skime M, Paquola A, Nelson T, Hall-Flavin D, et al. Serotonin-Induced Hyperactivity in SSRI-Resistant Major Depressive Disorder Patient-Derived Neurons. Mol Psychiatry. 2019;24:795-807.
25. Avior Y, Ron S, Kroitorou D, Albeldas C, Lerner V, Corneo B, et al. Depression patient-derived cortical neurons reveal potential biomarkers for antidepressant response. Transl Psychiatry. 2021;11:201.
26. Cavalleri L, Merlo Pich E, Millan MJ, Chiamulera C, Kunath T, Spano PF, et al. Ketamine Enhances Structural Plasticity in Mouse Mesencephalic and Human IPSC-Derived Dopaminergic Neurons via AMPAR-Driven BDNF and MTOR Signaling. Mol Psychiatry. 2018;23:812-23.

27. Achour M, Ferdousi F, Sasaki K, Isoda H. Luteolin Modulates Neural Stem Cells Fate Determination: In vitro Study on Human Neural Stem Cells, and in vivo Study on LPS-Induced Depression Mice Model. Front Cell Dev Biol. 2021;9:753279.
28. Chen HM, DeLong CJ, Bame M, Rajapakse I, Herron TJ, McInnis MG, et al. Transcripts Involved in Calcium Signaling and Telencephalic Neuronal Fate Are Altered in Induced Pluripotent Stem Cells from Bipolar Disorder Patients. Transl Psychiatry. 2014;4:e375.
29. Hunsberger JG, Fessler EB, Chibane FL, Leng Y, Maric D, Elkahloun AG, et al. Mood Stabilizer-Regulated MiRNAs in Neuropsychiatric and Neurodegenerative Diseases: Identifying Associations and Functions. Am J Transl Res. 2013;5:450-64.
30. Madison JM, Zhou F, Nigam A, Hussain A, Barker DD, Nehme R, et al. Characterization of Bipolar Disorder Patient-Specific Induced Pluripotent Stem Cells from a Family Reveals Neurodevelopmental and MRNA Expression Abnormalities. Mol Psychiatry. 2015;20:703-17.
31. Attili D, Schill DJ, DeLong CJ, Lim KC, Jiang G, Campbell KF, et al. Astrocyte-Derived Exosomes in an iPSC Model of Bipolar Disorder. Adv Neurobiol. 2020;25:219-35.
32. Mertens J, Wang QW, Kim Y, Yu DX, Pham S, Yang B, et al. Differential Responses to Lithium in Hyperexcitable Neurons from Patients with Bipolar Disorder. Nature. 2015;527:95-9.
33. Truvé K, Parris TZ, Vizlin-Hodzic D, Salmela S, Berger E, Ågren H, et al. Identification of candidate genetic variants and altered protein expression in neural stem and mature neural cells support altered microtubule function to be an essential component in bipolar disorder. Transl Psychiatry. 2020;10(1):390.
34. Bame M, McInnis MG, O'Shea KS. MicroRNA Alterations in Induced Pluripotent Stem Cell-Derived Neurons from Bipolar Disorder Patients: Pathways Involved in Neuronal Differentiation, Axon Guidance, and Plasticity. Stem Cells Dev. 2020;29(17):1145-59.
35. Sukumaran SK, Paul P, Guttal V, Holla B, Vemula A, Bhatt H, et al. Abnormalities in migration of neural precursor cells in familial bipolar disorder. Dis Model Mech. 2022;15(10):dmm049526.
36. Mariani J, Coppola G, Zhang P, Abyzov A, Tomasini L, Amenduni M, et al. FOXG1-Dependent Dysregulation of GABA/Glutamate Neuron Differentiation in Autism Spectrum Disorders. Cell. 2016;162:375-90.
37. Brighi C, Salaris F, Soloperto A, Cordella F, Ghirga S, de Turris V, et al. Novel Fragile X Syndrome 2D and 3D Brain Models Based on Human Isogenic FMRP-KO IPSCs. Cell Death Dis. 2021;12:498.
38. Brower V. Nutraceuticals: poised for a healthy slice of the healthcare market? Nat Biotechnol. 1998;16:728-31.
39. Sarris J. Nutritional psychiatry: from concept to the clinic. Drugs. 2019;79(9):929-34.
40. Sarris J, Logan AC, Akbaraly TN, Paul Amminger G, Balanza-Martinez V, Freeman MP, et al. International Society for Nutritional Psychiatry Research consensus position statement: nutritional medicine in modern psychiatry. World Psychiatry. 2015;14(3):370-1.
41. Ansari F, Pourjafar H, Tabrizi A, Homayouni A. The effects of probiotics and prebiotics on mental disorders: a review on depression, anxiety, Alzheimer, and autism spectrum disorders. Curr Pharma Biotechnol. 2020;21(7):555-65.

42. Linde K, Berner MM, Kriston L. St John's wort for major depression. Cochrane Database Syst Rev. 2008;(4):CD000448.
43. Sarris J, Ravindran A, Yatham LN, Marx W, Rucklidge JJ, McIntyre RS, et al. Clinician guidelines for the treatment of psychiatric disorders with nutraceuticals and phytoceuticals: The World Federation of Societies of Biological Psychiatry (WFSBP) and Canadian Network for Mood and Anxiety Treatments (CANMAT) Taskforce. World J Biol Psychiatry. 2022;23(6):424-55.
44. Goh KK, Chen CY, Chen CH, Lu ML. Effects of omega-3 polyunsaturated fatty acids supplements on psychopathology and metabolic parameters in schizophrenia: A meta-analysis of randomized controlled trials. J Psychopharmacol. 2021;35(3):221-35.
45. Hsu MC, Huang YS, Ouyang WC. Beneficial effects of omega-3 fatty acid supplementation in schizophrenia: possible mechanisms. Lipids Health Dis. 2020;19(1):159.
46. Chiappedi M, de Vincenzi S, Bejor M. Nutraceuticals in psychiatric practice. Recent Patents on CNS Drug Discovery (Discontinued). 2012;7(2):163-72.
47. Fraguas D, Díaz-Caneja CM, Pina-Camacho L, Moreno C, Duran-Cutilla M, Ayora M, et al. Dietary interventions for autism spectrum disorder: a meta-analysis. Pediatrics. 2019;144(5):e20183218.
48. Jacka FN. Nutritional Psychiatry: Where to Next? EBioMedicine. 2017;17:24-9.

CHAPTER 11

Treatment-resistant Bipolar Disorder: Approach to Management

Alka A Subramanyam, Mansi P Somaiya, Prerna B Khar, Swati B Shelke

INTRODUCTION

Bipolar disorder is a chronic mental illness characterized by periods of elevated or irritable mood (mania or hypomania) alternating with periods of depression. Treatment for bipolar disorder typically involves mood stabilizers, antipsychotics, and psychotherapy. However, some patients with bipolar disorder do not respond to these treatments or experience only partial improvement in their symptoms. These patients are said to have treatment-resistant bipolar disorder. This article will discuss the current understanding of treatment-resistant bipolar disorder and the available treatment options.

The concept of "treatment resistance" itself is a matter of much debate in neuroscience. For operational purposes, however, we will go by the definition outlined below.

Most studies have considered treatment-resistant bipolar disorder (TRBD) as a failure in two or more interventions, i.e., "failure to reach sustained symptomatic remission for 8 consecutive weeks after two different treatment trials, at adequate therapeutic doses, with at least two recommended monotherapy treatments or at least one monotherapy treatment and another combination treatment".[1]

CRITERIA ON TREATMENT-RESISTANT BIPOLAR DISORDER

Various definitions are proposed for treatment resistance; however, there is no uniform and consensual definition. Various considerations are to be taken while terming resistance, such as:[2,3]

- *Phase*—manic, depressive, hypomanic, mixed, breakthrough episodes during maintenance treatment, and functional outcome.
- *Treatment*—adequate trial, which includes dose and duration of the medication.

While considering calling it treatment resistance, the clinician needs to take into account if the therapeutic approaches were administered—to achieve response with an optimum dose, duration and frequency of administration. Hence, a minimum threshold dose of treatment needs to be administered. Poor adherence to medication is often a reason for relapse, which needs to be ruled out. Also, exclude patients who are intolerant to treatment or experience side effects.

Treatment: Resistant bipolar disorder is marked by recurring mood episodes that can take various forms (manic, depressive, hypomanic, or mixed) over a span of 12 months. These episodes can occur in any order and be separated by remission periods of up to 2 months.

Rapid cycling BD can be viewed as a special form of TRBD. This variant of the illness is defined by 4 or more episodes of illness within a 12-month period.[3]

TREATMENT RESISTANCE

Resistance can be seen in the acute phase or maintenance phase:
- *Acute:* Failure of response to a specified number of treatments that are generally considered effective.
- *Maintenance:* Continued cycling despite adequate trials of previously demonstrated effective treatments.

Factors Responsible in Treatment-resistant Bipolar Disorder

Dysregulation in the immune system, including microglial alterations, inflammation, oxidative damage, cytokines, and brain-derived neurotrophic factor changes, are factors resulting in treatment resistance. This predisposes amygdala hyperreactivity to emotional stimuli. Additionally, white matter abnormalities, and cognitive deficits predispose to mood episodes.[3] This is also very personalized, and hence, at times becomes difficult to treat for the very same reason.

Review the following before terming resistance:[3]
- Diagnosis
- Compliance on medications
- Medical conditions
- Substance triggered
- Endocrinological, neurological, and autoimmune diseases
- Neurodegenerative disorders
- Psychosocial factors.

Duration of trial: Duration must be at least a minimum of 3 weeks and should be provided at an adequate dose, excluding titration period in mania.

CASE VIGNETTE

XYZ is a 42-year-old married lady with a history of first episode characterized by mania, followed by depressive episodes. Currently presenting with depressive symptoms; claims to be adherent on medications. Despite an adequate trial of lithium with lamotrigine, continues to report depressive symptoms. The clinician optimized the doses of medications and got the lithium levels done, which were well within range. Thereafter, two courses of antidepressants were tried in optimum doses but she continued to report depressive symptoms. How does the clinician proceed?

Approach to Treatment Resistance

It is important to rule out pseudoresistance before the true treatment resistance can be established. **Table 1** illustrates the difference between treatment resistance and pseudoresistance in a case of bipolar disorder.

Resistant Bipolar Mania

When all first-/second-line agents have failed, the next step involves add-on/switch therapy. As per the Canadian Network for Mood and Anxiety Treatments (CANMAT) and International Society for Bipolar Disorders (ISBD) 2018 guidelines, the following agents can be tried as the third line of management **(Table 2)** (Molecules are mentioned in alphabetical order and not order of preference, as overall evidence is limited).[4]

Tamoxifen is recommended further down in the list due to the risk of uterine cancer and the lack of clinical experience, despite evidence for efficacy.

TABLE 1: Difference between true resistance and pseudoresistance.

True resistance	*Pseudoresistance*
Diagnosis has been established	Diagnosis is not clear
Adherence to treatment has been established	There is erratic adherence to medication/unsupervised medication
Adequate doses and duration have been tried	Inadequate medication doses/for suboptimal duration
There is an absence of comorbidities/substance abuse	There is presence of nonpsychiatric medical/psychiatric comorbidities (e.g., thyroid disorders, substance abuse)
Trial of psychotherapy has been employed	Psychotherapy has not been employed
Expressed emotions of family members and other psychosocial factors have been addressed to	There are high expressed emotions in family members/caregivers—clouding the perception of improvement. Other psychosocial factors affecting the prognosis

TABLE 2: Level of evidence for molecule/modality for resistant bipolar depression (CANMAT).[4]

Agent	Level of evidence
Carbamazepine/oxcarbazepine lithium/divalproate	Level 3
Chlorpromazine	Level 2
Clonazepam	Level 2
Clozapine	Level 4
Haloperidol + lithium/divalproate	Level 2
rTMS	Level 3
Tamoxifen	Level 2
Tamoxifen + lithium/divalproate	Level 2

(CANMAT: Canadian Network for Mood and Anxiety Treatment; rTMS: repetitive transcranial magnetic stimulation)

International College of Neuropsychopharmacology (CINP) Guidelines[5]

In patients resistant (principally) to lithium, valproate, or carbamazepine, the following can be considered as described in **Table 3**.

Step 1: Add aripiprazole (30 mg), asenapine (20 mg), folic acid, quetiapine (800 mg), or valnoctamide (1,200 mg) to lithium/valproate/carbamazepine.

Step 2: Lithium/valproate/carbamazepine + haloperidol (12 mg)/olanzapine (40 mg).

Step 3: Lithium/valproate/carbamazepine + phenytoin (400 mg).

Step 4: Lithium/valproate/carbamazepine + clozapine (500 mg)/electroconvulsive therapy (ECT)/allopurinol (600 mg)/oxcarbazepine (1,200 mg)/folic acid (3 mg)/levetiracetam (2,000–3,000 mg)/pregabalin (75–150 mg)/L-thyroxine (till free T4 is high than upper limit).

Maximum dosages are mentioned in the bracket.

Role of Clozapine

Just as it has a role in treatment-resistant schizophrenia, clozapine has an important role in TRBD. The benefits of using it are as follows:[6]
- Decreasing the number of hospitalizations
- Symptomatic and functional improvement
- Reduces aggressive behavior in young patients with TRBD
- Reduces suicidality and overdose/self-harm
- Effective in rapid cycling disorder (considered a type of treatment resistance).[7]

TABLE 3: Bipolar mania (acute) with molecules and guidelines (for treatment resistance).

Molecule/Modality	CANMAT[4]	CINP[5]
Carbamazepine/oxcarbazepine + Li/DVP	Level 3	Step 4
Chlorpromazine	Level 2	Not recommended
Clonazepam	Level 2	Not recommended
Clozapine	Level 4	Step 4 (Addition to Li/Val/CBZ)
Haloperidol + Li/DVP	Level 2	Step 2 (Add to Li/Val/CBZ
rTMS	Level 3	Not recommended
Tamoxifen	Level 2	Not recommended
Tamoxifen + Li/DVP	Level 2	Not recommended
Aripiprazole	Not recommended	Step 1 (Add to Li/Val/CBZ)
Olanzapine	Not mentioned	Step 2 (Add to Li/Val/CBZ)
Quetiapine	Not mentioned	Step 1 (Add to Li/Val/CBZ)
Valnoctamide	Not recommended (Level 1 negative)	Step 1 (Add to Li/Val/CBZ)
Folic acid	Not mentioned	Step 1 (Add to Li/Val/CBZ)
Asenapine	Not mentioned	Step 1 (Add to Li/Val/CBZ)
Phenytoin	Not mentioned	Step 3 (Add to Li/Val/CBZ)
ECT	Not mentioned	Step 4 (Add to Li/Val/CBZ)
Allopurinol	Not recommended (Level 1 negative)	Step 4 (Add to Li/Val/CBZ)
Levetiracetam	Not mentioned	Step 4 (Add to Li/Val/CBZ)
Pregabalin	Not mentioned	Step 4 (Add to Li/Val/CBZ)
L-thyroxine	Not mentioned	Step 4 (Add to Li/Val/CBZ)

(CANMAT: Canadian Network for Mood and Anxiety Treatments; CBZ: carbamazepine; CINP: International College of Neuropsychopharmacology; DVP: divalproex; ECT: electroconvulsive therapy; Li: lithium; rTMS: repetitive transcranial magnetic stimulation; Val: valproate)

Role of Novel Agents

The use of nutraceuticals such as branched chain amino acids, folic acid, and l-tryptophan is anecdotal. The use of other agents such as medroxyprogesterone, memantine, mexiletine, levetiracetam, phenytoin, and verapamil has largely been experimental and mainly in adjunct with other antimanic agents. There have also been few case reports of using glasses that block blue light. Larger controlled trials are needed, however, before a recommendation for their use in mania can be made.[4]

Other Strategies for Treatment Refractory Bipolar Disorder

Risperidone/aripiprazole is injectable once in 15 days and can be considered as a part of relapse prevention.[4] Few case reports have mentioned the use of eslicarbazepine in resistant mania cases, but more trials need to be conducted for conclusive evidence.[8] Cariprazine has also received recent approval by the Food and Drug Administration (FDA) for treating mania and mixed episodes.[7]

Maintenance Treatments

As per the National Institute for Health and Care Excellence (NICE)/the British Association for Psychopharmacology (BAP) guidelines,[7] prophylaxis for bipolar disorder can be carried out as follows:
- *First line:* Lithium monotherapy
- *Second line:* Olanzapine, aripiprazole, risperidone, or quetiapine in combination with valproate or lithium
- *Third line:* Alternative antipsychotic (lurasidone, asenapine, ziprasidone) or alternative mood stabilizer (carbamazepine, lamotrigine) in combination
- *Fourth line:* Antipsychotic with two mood stabilizers.

As per the CANMAT guidelines,[4] in case first-/second-line agents are not effective, the following can be considered as third line:
- Aripiprazole + lamotrigine (Level 2)
- Clozapine (adjunctive) (Level 4)
- Gabapentin (adjunctive) (Level 4)
- Olanzapine + fluoxetine (Level 2).

Resistant Bipolar Depression

As per the CANMAT and ISBD guidelines in resistant depression:[3,4] **Table 4** illustrates the different modalities.
- Lithium along with carbamazepine, pramipexole, monoamine oxidase inhibitors, tricyclic antidepressants (TCAs), venlafaxine, selective serotonin reuptake inhibitors (SSRIs) (except paroxetine) or lamotrigine
- Divalproex with venlafaxine, TCAs, SSRIs (except paroxetine) or lamotrigine
- Quetiapine with lamotrigine.

The clinician must bear in mind that treating a unipolar depression versus bipolar depression—the difference lies in using a mood stabilizer and concerns of potential mood destabilizing effects on antidepressants.

Acute Episode of Resistant Depression

Potential drugs and combinations once the first-line modalities fail are as follow, additionally described in **Table 5**:

TABLE 4: Level of evidence with modality for resistant bipolar depression.[5]

Agent	Level of evidence
Lamotrigine	Level 1 (Efficacy)
	Level 2 (Recommendation)
Pramipexole	Level 2
Ketamine	Level 1 (Efficacy)
	Level 4 (Recommendation)
Modafinil	Level 2
Haloperidol + Li/DVP	Level 2
Light therapy	Level 1
ECT	Level 2

(DVP: divalproex; ECT: electroconvulsive therapy; Li: lithium)

- *Lamotrigine:* It may be added in those who continue to experience depressive symptoms on Lithium.[5] A combination of lamotrigine and lithium resulted in 50–70% response in various studies.[9,10]
- *Pramipexole:* It is a D2/D3 agonist with an antidepressant effect. In patients with resistant bipolar depression, addition of pramipexole to mood stabilizers led to improvement in the depressive symptoms. Additionally, it is a safe and tolerable option along with mood stabilizers.[2,11]
- *Modafinil:* It has been tried as an adjuvant agent in resistant bipolar depression. It has been shown to be effective in reducing depressive symptoms without a manic/hypomanic switch. There is limited evidence, and hence, more studies are required to corroborate the evidence.[2,5,12,13]

Antiepileptic drugs:
- *Levetiracetam:* Tried as an add-on, with 30% response.[5,13]
- *Gabapentin:* Reports of use as an adjuvant, in acute bipolar depression is noted.[5]
- *Valproate:* Divalproex was seen to be effective in patients with bipolar depression, in a few controlled studies. Substituting lithium with valproate is another modality tried.[2,3]
- *Carbamazepine:* It has been used in randomized placebo-controlled trials and has shown efficacy. However, large-scale studies are necessary to conclude the evidence.[2]
- *Ketamine:* Along with lithium or valproate, ketamine, when added to treatment regime, improves both depressive and anxiety symptoms. It has also reported a decrease in suicidality, anhedonia, and fatigue.[5]
- *Modafinil:* Adjuvant modafinil, added to a mood stabilizer, showed positive response without a switch. There is limited evidence, and hence, more studies are required to corroborate the evidence.[5,13]

TABLE 5: Acute bipolar depression with molecules and guidelines.

Treatment	CINP[5]	CANMAT[4]
Lithium and lamotrigine	First step in TR	
Pramipexole (adjunct)	First step in TR	Third line (Level 3)
Modafinil (adjunct)	First step in TR	Third line (Level 2)
Levetiracetam	Not recommended	
Valproate		Second line (Level 2)
Carbamazepine		Third line (Level 2)
Ketamine (IV)	Third step in TR	Third line (Level 3)
Lurasidone	Third step in TR	
Cariprazine		Second line (Level 2)
Olanzapine		Third line (Level 1)
Olanzapine and fluoxetine combination		Second line (Level 2)
Aripiprazole (adjunct)		Level 4
Armodafinil (adjunct)		Level 4
Asenapine (adjunct)		Level 4
Amitriptyline (adjunct)	Third step in TR	
Bupropion (adjunct)	Third step in TR	
Paroxetine (adjunct)	Third step in TR	
Clozapine	Third step in TR	
Deep rTMS	First step in TR	Third line (Level 2)
Deep brain stimulation	Not recommended	
Electroconvulsive therapy	First step in TR	Second line (Level 3)
Sleep deprivation therapy	Third step in TR	Third line (Level 3)
Light therapy	First step in TR	Third line (Level 3)
Group psychoeducation	Add-on to all modalities	Insufficient evidence
Cognitive behavior therapy	Add-on to first in TR	Second line (Level 2)
Family focused therapy	Limited data	Second line (Level 2)
Interpersonal and social rhythm therapy	Limited data	Third line (Level 2)

(CANMAT: Canadian Network for Mood and Anxiety Treatments; CINP: International College of Neuropsychopharmacology; IV: intravenous; TR: treatment resistance)

Atypical antipsychotics:
- *Lurasidone, aripiprazole:* There is an evidence of use as add-on therapy; however, data is still inconclusive.[5]
- *Other drugs:* Pioglitazone, celecoxib, levothyroxine, pregnanolone, and N-acetyl cysteine have been tried in small studies and have shown some benefit when used as an add-on modality of treatment.

- *Systematic treatment enhancement program for bipolar disorder (STEP BD):* Lamotrigine, inositol, and risperidone, when used as adjuvant agents, showed no intergroup significant differences in recovery in treatment-resistant depression. Remission was noted in 23%, 17%, and 4.6%, respectively.[1]
- *Other therapies:* Sleep deprivation and light therapies have been tried as add-on and shown some benefit when used as an adjuvant.[5]

Brain stimulation techniques:
Electroconvulsive therapy: ECT has been an efficacious modality of treatment of bipolar depression. A randomized controlled trial comparing efficacy of ECT with pharmacologic treatment revealed a significant response to ECT, with remission in both groups.[3]

Deep transcranial magnetic stimulation: Very few studies have been carried out using deep transcranial magnetic stimulation (TMS). Deep TMS on the prefrontal cortex has shown efficacy in treatment of acute bipolar depression, when over weekdays for 4 consecutive weeks. It has preliminary evidence and large-scale studies need to be carried out for its efficacy in patients with bipolar depression. Its relative safety, faster recovery, and less likelihood toward memory impairment make it a promising modality in treatment.[3]

Deep brain stimulation: Not much evidence in efficacy is reported.

Bipolar Depression Resistant to Maintenance Treatment

Modalities recommended: See also **Table 6** for the different modalities.

Risperidone—a long-acting injectable: Studies showed significant improvement with prolonging time to relapse. It is also suggested to add cognitive behavior therapy (CBT) or psychoeducation with the above modality.[5]

Atypical antipsychotics: The next choice of intervention can include, adding aripiprazole and ziprasidone to the given treatment. It has been tried in resistant bipolar disorder patients, with Level 2 evidence.[5]

Anticonvulsants: Phenytoin and gabapentin also have been tried with no conclusive evidence.[5]

Psychotherapies: Any structured therapy, when added to a medication, offers additional benefit in treatment which is evident in outcome, lesser relapse rates, reduction in symptoms, better adherence, fewer mood episodes, better social functioning, and lesser rates of hospitalization.

A variety of psychotherapies have been evaluated, which include:
- *Family-focused treatment:* This encompasses psychoeducation, communication skills training, problem-solving skills, skills to address

TABLE 6: Bipolar depression (maintenance) with molecules and guidelines.

Treatment	CINP[5]	CANMAT[4]
Risperidone long-acting injectable	First step	
Aripiprazole	Second step	Aripiprazole with lamotrigine (Level 2)
Ziprasidone	Second step	
Gabapentin (adjunct)	Third step	Level 4
Phenytoin	Third step	
Clozapine (adjunct)	Fourth step	Level 4
ECT	Fourth step	
Lithium plus lamotrigine	Fourth step	
Lithium plus valproate	Fourth step	
Olanzapine	Fourth step	
Olanzapine plus fluoxetine		Level 2

(CANMAT: Canadian Network for Mood and Anxiety Treatments; CINP: International College of Neuropsychopharmacology; ECT: electroconvulsive therapy)

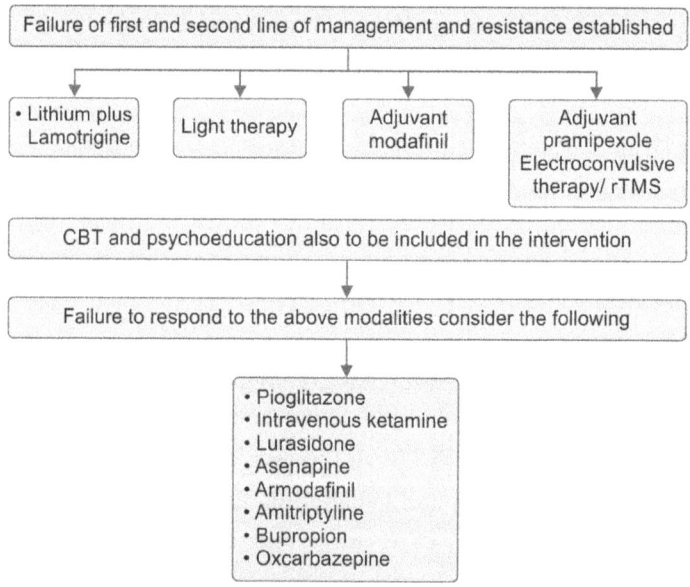

Flowchart 1: Treatment-resistant acute bipolar depression.

Failure of first and second line of management and resistance established

- Lithium plus Lamotrigine
- Light therapy
- Adjuvant modafinil
- Adjuvant pramipexole Electroconvulsive therapy/ rTMS

CBT and psychoeducation also to be included in the intervention

Failure to respond to the above modalities consider the following

- Pioglitazone
- Intravenous ketamine
- Lurasidone
- Asenapine
- Armodafinil
- Amitriptyline
- Bupropion
- Oxcarbazepine

(CBT: cognitive behavior therapy; rTMS: repetitive transcranial magnetic stimulation)

stress within the family, fewer relapses, better adherence, and greater reduction in symptoms.[2]

- *Cognitive therapy:* Adjuvant to medications, it has been associated with fewer relapses, better compliance, reduced symptoms, better social functioning, and reduced hospitalization duration.[2]

Treatment-resistant Bipolar Disorder: Approach to Management

Flowchart 2: Treatment-resistant acute bipolar mania (CINP guidelines).

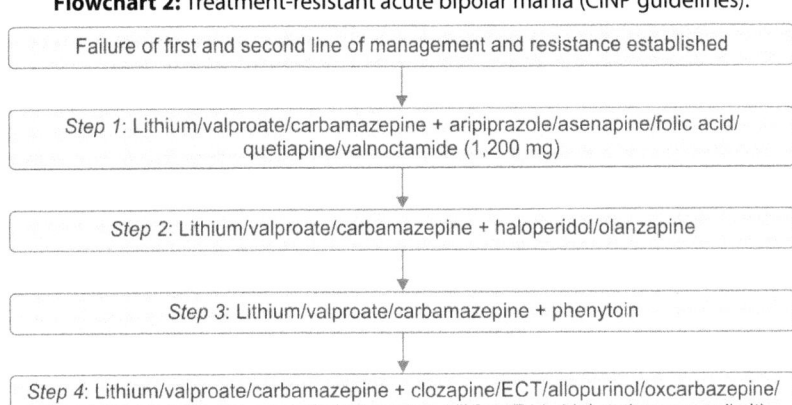

(CINP: International College of Neuropsychopharmacology)

Flowchart 3: Treatment-resistant maintenance bipolar disorder.[4,5]

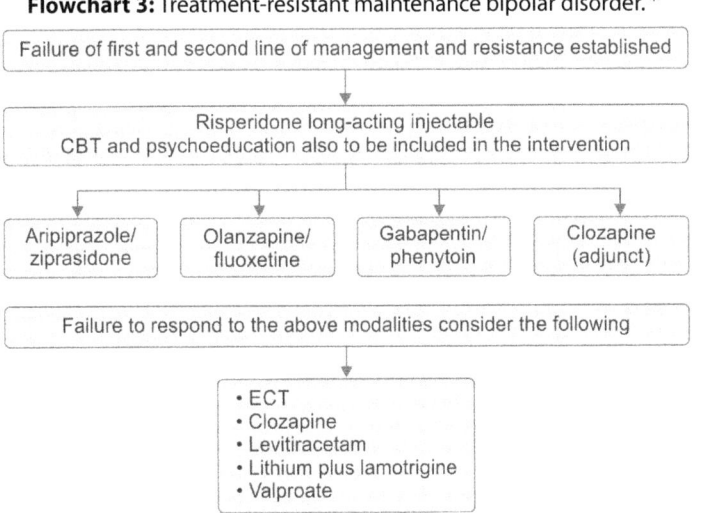

(CBT: cognitive behavior therapy; ECT: electroconvulsive therapy)

- *Group psychoeducation:* It reduced the frequency of episodes and duration of hospitalizations.[2]
- *Interpersonal and social rhythm therapy:* It includes interpersonal therapy, which includes addressing interpersonal problems, setting and regulating a routine, and associating the link between mood symptoms and social roles.[2]

OVERVIEW

For the readers benefit, we have tried to summarize the treatment protocol for resistant bipolar disorders into three algorithms **(Flowcharts 1 to 3)**.

Please note: Flowcharts have been created with whatever small evidence database we have. They are likely to evolve as evidence gets more robust.

CONCLUSION

Treatment resistance is truly a challenge for most clinicians. Though the concept and the criteria are yet under evolution, this is a small attempt to try to collate the available knowledge and approach to make it easier for clinicians to manage these cases.

> **TAKE-HOME POINTS**
>
> Treatment-resistant bipolar disorder (TRBD) is a challenging scenario in clinical practice due to variability in consensus in definition, various contributing factors and management. It is considered a failure in two or more interventions, i.e., "failure to reach sustained symptomatic remission for 8 consecutive weeks after two different treatment trials, at adequate therapeutic doses, with at least two recommended monotherapy treatments or at least one monotherapy treatment and another combination treatment". Resistance can be seen in the acute phase which is failure of response to a specified number of treatments that are generally considered effective. Maintenance phase which is continued cycling despite adequate trials of previously demonstrated effective treatments. The factors contributing to treatment resistance are dysregulation in the immune system, including microglial alterations, inflammation, oxidative damage, cytokines, and brain-derived neurotrophic factor changes are factors resulting in treatment resistance.
>
> *Bipolar mania*
> - Once treatment resistance has been established and 1st/2nd line of treatment have failed, a combination of Lithium/ Valproate/Carbamazepine + Aripiprazole/ Asenapine /Folic acid/Quetiapine/Valnoctamide (1200 mg) can be considered.
> - Lithium/Valproate/Carbamazepine + Haloperidol/Olanzapine can be considered as the next line of management.
> - A combination of Lithium/Valproate/Carbamazepine + Phenytoin can also be considered.
> - Other combinations that be tried are: Lithium/Valproate/Carbamazepine + Clozapine ECT/Allopurinol/Oxcarbazepine/Folic acid/Levetiracetam)/Pregabalin/L-Thyroxine (till free T4 is higher than upper limit).
> - Clozapine has a special role in treatment resistance as it reduces the aggression, the need for hospitalization, leads to overall functional improvement, reduced suicidality and is effective in rapid cycling bipolar disorder.
>
> *Bipolar depression:*
> - In the acute phase of bipolar depression, once the first and second line of management and resistance is established, a combination of Lithium and Lamotrigine can be considered.
> - Light therapy, adjuvant Modafinil or Pramipexole can be considered.
> - ECT and rTMS are neuromodulation techniques which can be used in treatment resistance.

Contd...

Contd...
- Failure to respond to above modalities, intravenous Ketamine, Asenapine, Armodafinil, Amitriptyline, Bupropion can be considered.
- CBT and psychoeducation can also be used in treatment resistance.

Bipolar disorder-maintenance phase:
- For treatment resistance, consider Risperidone long-acting injectable. CBT and psychoeducation can also be included in the intervention.
- Aripiprazole, Ziprasidone can be used as adjuvants. Olanzapine with Fluoxetine can also be used as a combination. Gabapentin and phenytoin are other options. Adjunct Clozapine is another option in management. Failure to respond to the above modalities ECT, Clozapine, Levetiracetam, Lithium and Lamotrigine or Valproate are other lines of interventions.

REFERENCES

1. Diaz AP, Fernandes BS, Quevedo J, Sanches M, Soares JC. Treatment-resistant bipolar depression: concepts and challenges for novel interventions. Braz J Psychiatry. 2022;44(2):178-86.
2. Gitlin M. Treatment-resistant bipolar disorder. Mol Psychiatry. 2006;11(3): 227-40.
3. Bauer IE, Soares JC, Selek S, Meyer TD. The Link between Refractoriness and Neuroprogression in Treatment-Resistant Bipolar Disorder. Mod Trends Pharmacopsychiatry. 2017;31:10-26.
4. Yatham LN, Kennedy SH, Parikh SV, Schaffer A, Bond DJ, Frey BN, et al. Canadian Network for Mood and Anxiety Treatments (CANMAT) and International Society for Bipolar Disorders (ISBD) 2018 guidelines for the management of patients with bipolar disorder. Bipolar Disord. 2018;20(2):97-170.
5. Yatham LN, Kennedy SH, Parikh SV, Schaffer A, Bond DJ, Frey BN, et al. Canadian Network for Mood and Anxiety Treatments (CANMAT) and International Society for Bipolar Disorders (ISBD) 2018 guidelines for the management of patients with bipolar disorder. Bipolar Disord. 2018;20(2):97-170.
6. Wilkowska A, Wiglusz MS, Cubała WJ. Clozapine in treatment-resistant bipolar disorder with suicidality. Three case reports. Front Psychiatry. 2019;10:520.
7. Taylor D (Ed). The Maudsley Prescribing Guidelines in Psychiatry, 14th edition. Hoboken, NJ: Wiley-Blackwell; 2021.
8. Hui Poon S, Sim K, J Baldessarini R. Pharmacological approaches for treatment-resistant bipolar disorder. Curr Neuropharmacol. 2015;13(5):592-604.
9. Nierenberg AA, Ostacher MJ, Calabrese JR, Ketter TA, Marangell LB, Miklowitz DJ, et al. Treatment-resistant bipolar depression: a STEP-BD equipoise randomized effectiveness trial of antidepressant augmentation with lamotrigine, inositol, or risperidone. Am J Psychiatry. 2006;163(2):210-6.
10. Kagawa S, Mihara K, Nakamura A, Nemoto K, Suzuki T, Nagai G, et al. Relationship between plasma concentrations of lamotrigine and its early therapeutic effect of lamotrigine augmentation therapy in treatment-resistant depressive disorder. Ther Drug Monit. 2014;36(6):730-3.

11. Goldberg JF, Burdick KE, Endick CJ. Preliminary randomized, double-blind, placebo-controlled trial of pramipexole added to mood stabilizers for treatment-resistant bipolar depression. Am J Psychiatry. 2004;161(3):564-6.
12. Frye MA, Grunze H, Suppes T, McElroy SL, Keck Jr PE, Walden J, et al. A placebo-controlled evaluation of adjunctive modafinil in the treatment of bipolar depression. Am J Psychiatry. 2007;164(8):1242-9.
13. Post RM, Altshuler LL, Frye MA, Suppes T, McElroy SL, Keck Jr PE, et al. Preliminary observations on the effectiveness of levetiracetam in the open adjunctive treatment of refractory bipolar disorder. J Clin Psychiatry. 2005;66(3):370-4.

CHAPTER 12

Ketamine and Psychiatry

Rajesh Nagpal, Malvika Nagpal

INTRODUCTION

(S)- and (R)-Ketamine are the two optical enantiomers of (R,S)-Ketamine, a phenylcyclohexylamine.[1] Ketamine was derived from phencyclidine (PCP) minus the psychomimetic effects but still has induced dissociative effects and has abuse potential, albeit less than PCP. Harold V. Maddox created PCP, on March 26, 1956. Animal effects of PCP have been researched by Domino. Greifenstein conducted the first PCP human trials in 1958 under the trade name Sernyl. Sernyl evoked that there is considerable excitation with a protracted postoperative recovery, but did not produce depression in cardiovascular and respiratory systems. Because of its psychedelic effects, it was added to Schedule II of the Federal Controlled Substance Act (CSA) in 1978 and was sold as "angel dust" on the streets. PCP had serious psychotomimetic side effects and an abuse potential. It was removed from the market in 1978.[2] Ketamine was created in 1962 by the scientist Calvin Stevens, a consultant for Parke-Davis Laboratories in Detroit, Michigan.

In 1964, Domino and Corssen investigated the drug's effects on people. These writers explained the phenomenon of dissociative anesthesia. Ketamine was given to soldiers during the Vietnam War after it was granted a patent in 1966 under the name Ketalar for human use.

In 1970, it was first used commercially as a rapid-acting intravenous (IV) anesthetic.[3] Ketamine was included in the CSA's class III list of drugs in 1999 due to abuse. The withdrawal of ketamine was brought on by its hallucinogenic effects and the introduction of propofol. The pathophysiology of hyperalgesia and mental performance, however, underwent a revolutionary change with the identification of the N-methyl-D-aspartate receptor (NMDAR) and ketamine's noncompetitive suppression of it.

Remifentanil was introduced in the early 1990s before opioid-induced hyperalgesia was identified. This led to a paradigm shift in the treatment of pain and the resurgence of ketamine as an antihyperalgesic medication. In the field of treatment-resistant depression (TRD), ketamine is currently receiving attention, and it has been suggested as a potential rapid antidepressant in individuals with a high risk of suicide.

Due to its brief half-life and lack of clinically significant respiratory depression, ketamine is a beneficial medication as an anesthetic agent. It is interesting to note that in addition to its analgesic,[4] anti-inflammatory,[5] and anesthetic effect in multiple subsets such as children, adults, and pregnant females, it also has shown antidepressant activity.[6]

Ketamine has been an uncompetitive NMDAR antagonist and dissociative anesthetic for the past 20 years, but it has just made a breakthrough as a unique and potent rapid-acting antidepressant. Individuals with severe depressive illness received a single subanesthetic dose of IV ketamine (0.5 mg/kg over 40 minutes) in a landmark randomized controlled trial (RCT) conducted by Berman et al. Within hours of the injection, ketamine had a noticeable antidepressant effect that grew gradually over the next three days. Since then, this result has been confirmed in several studies of both unipolar and bipolar depression (including treatment-resistant individuals).[6-9,10]

CLINICAL EFFECTS

Dissociative Anesthesia

Individuals can experience dissociative anesthesia, which is characterized by catatonia, catalepsy, and amnesia but does not result in total unconsciousness, at ketamine doses of 1-2 mg/kg given intravenously (bolus) or 4-11 mg/kg given orally.[11] For the induction of dissociative anesthesia, peak ketamine plasma concentrations of roughly 1,200-2,400 ng/mL, or 5-10 mM, are required.[12]

Ketamine was found to produce anesthesia at an average steady-state plasma concentration of 2,200 ng/mL or 9.3 mM.[13]

It can be administered orally (500 mg)[14] or intrarectally (8-15 mg/kg)[15] to cause drowsiness and/or general anesthesia in people.

When delivered at a dose of 3-9 mg/kg, intranasal (S)-ketamine causes drowsiness in the patients.[16] According to reports, (S)-ketamine is two to three times more potent as an anesthetic for humans than (R)-ketamine and the racemic combination.[17]

Analgesic

Ketamine has been used in pediatric patients for treating fractures,[18] burns,[19] or cases of traumatic amputation as an analgesic agent both quantitatively and qualitatively similar to opioids, but with a reduced amount of respiratory depressive effects. IV ketamine has been used to treat both acute and chronic postoperative pain.[20]

The different dosages used are:
- *Orally:* If given as an adjuvant along with morphine, dose is 0.5 mg/kg, twice daily or can be given independently as a single dose of 2 mg/kg[21]
- *Intranasally:* Dose ranging from 10 to 50 mg, twice daily[22]
- *Transdermally:* Dose of 25 mg, released over the course

It may be appropriate to utilize intranasal route of (S)-ketamine as an analgesic in prehospital settings where IV administration is challenging and also in situations when immediate delivery is necessary for injuries since it lowers pain scores in just 5 minutes of administration.[23] (S)-ketamine is a more potent analgesic medication than racemic ketamine, despite (S)-ketamine having greater adverse effects, similar to their distinct anesthetic effects.

Antidepressant

The 1970s witnessed the initial indications of ketamine's antidepressant properties. The earliest reports of ketamine's potential antidepressant effects in humans date back to 1973, when Khorramzadeh and Lotfy (1973) reported that IV administration of ketamine at subanesthetic doses ranging from 0.2 to 1.0 mg/kg (IV bolus) caused an abreaction and facilitated psychotherapy in a cohort of 100 psychiatric patients admitted in hospital. Unfortunately, modern diagnostic criteria and therapeutic guidelines could not clearly define the precise symptoms of depression, which ketamine helped to relieve. Ketamine was denoted to as a generic abreactive agent in this investigation.[24]

In 2000, the first placebo-controlled study that suggested ketamine has antidepressant properties was published. According to the findings of that study, a 40-minute IV infusion of 0.5 mg/kg ketamine produced a more potent and quick antidepressant response in depressed patients than a placebo did.[10] This result was later confirmed in a double-blind, placebo-controlled, RCT that included individuals with treatment-resistant major depressive disorder.[6] This study showed that in patients who have not responded to at least two prior conventional antidepressants, ketamine has an antidepressant effect that manifests within 2 hours of infusion and lasts on an average for about 7 days.

These results have been duplicated in numerous further clinical studies in patients with TRD.[8,25] A study used a psychoactive placebo (i.e., midazolam) to create the functional unblinding of treatment brought on by the dissociative effects of ketamine, which happen even at low subanesthetic doses. They found that patients who received ketamine had a higher response rate when compared to those who received midazolam. Moreover, ketamine is said to have antidepressant effects in those with bipolar disorder.[7,26] Both IV and intranasal administration of (S)-ketamine has been demonstrated to help treat depression.[27]

Further research has demonstrated that ketamine is effective in treating major depressive disorder by lowering anhedonia[28] and suicidal ideation.[29]

In a small pilot study, there is evidence for antidepressant responses in treatment-resistant individuals achieved at doses as low as 0.1 mg/kg (5-minute IV infusion or intramuscular injection).[30] Although this study showed that ketamine at lower dosages has fewer negative effects, it may be useful in the treatment of depression. This conclusion is yet to be replicated in a larger study.

There is proof that ketamine given in subanesthetic doses repeatedly could have positive long-term benefits. For instance, the clinical outcomes for TRD improved after repeated subanesthetic ketamine administration.[30-32]

Anti-inflammatory

The body uses inflammation as a vital homeostatic process to combat infections and mend tissue damage. When cells of the innate immune system are stimulated, whether by invasive pathogens or by tissue damage, inflammatory processes are set off. These cells release proinflammatory cytokines, which then trigger the adaptive immune system's components to start an inflammatory response.[33] Administering ketamine during or before surgical procedures has been utilized to achieve a better postoperative result, principally because of its actions to decrease the formation of excess proinflammatory cytokines.

In a study, individuals were exposed to preoperative subanesthetic dosages of ketamine, which had anti-inflammatory effects (i.e., reduced proinflammatory cytokines).[34] Given that increased interleukin 6 (IL-6) levels have been linked to poor postoperative outcomes, the potential of ketamine to lower proinflammatory cytokine levels may be therapeutically significant. More research is underway on this topic currently. Ketamine is also beneficial in treating major depressive disorder-related aberrant inflammatory bone markers. Particularly, in individuals with major depressive disorder, a 40-minute IV infusion of ketamine (0.5 mg/kg) elevated levels of osteoprotegerin receptor activator of nuclear factor kB ligand and osteopontin—but was ineffective in healthy controls.[35]

Given that this was seen after saline infusion as well, it is possible that the infusion itself caused a transient stress-related rise in IL-6 levels.[36] These findings collectively show that ketamine's anti-inflammatory benefits occur primarily in the presence of immunological stimulation, but the drug has no effect on the balance of cytokines in the absence of an inflammatory response.[37] As ketamine is typically taken during the induction of anesthesia, which occurs prior to surgery, it may therefore serve as an immunomodulator rather than an immunosuppressive drug.

SIDE EFFECTS

Psychoactive Effects

They primarily involve psychotomimetic and dissociative effects. During recovering from ketamine-induced anesthesia, some patients have reported dissociative and out-of-body experiences, which are effects of ketamine that depend on dose.[38]

Both randomized controlled studies[39] and nonrandomized studies reported these effects.[40] For example, a study demonstrated that a 40-minute

IV infusion of the subanesthetic dose of 0.5 mg/kg ketamine causes distortion in perception which are consistent with dissociative states as well as positive and negative psychotomimetic symptoms. Around 10 minutes of the ketamine infusion beginning, these effects began to show up, and by 40 minutes of the treatment's end, they started to fade.[41]

Memory and Cognitive Impairment

Many research studies have discovered detrimental effects of subanesthetic ketamine treatment on cognition. Several investigations have found that ketamine tends to reduce memory functions in both the explicit (episodic and semantic) and implicit (procedural) forms either during or shortly after treatment.[42] A 40-minute IV infusion of 0.5 mg/kg of ketamine also impairs alertness, verbal fluency, and delayed recall; these effects fade quickly after the infusion is finished. By receiving ketamine infusions, instantaneous recollection and general cognitive function appear to be unaffected.[41]

Abuse

Although some people may find ketamine's initial psychotropic effects to be uncomfortable, the drug's dissociative characteristics have made it popular for recreational usage. Yet some users may become more agitated or have anxiety/panic attacks.[43] Despite the dearth of controlled studies examining ketamine's misuse potential, reports of recreational usage provide important information regarding the drug's short- and long-term consequences.[44] For recreational ketamine usage, the dosage typically ranges from 1 to 2 mg/kg for IV route, 50–150 mg for intramuscular route, 100–500 mg orally, or 30–400 mg for intranasal insufflation.[45]

Users report that the lesser dosage causes mild stimulatory, dissociative, and hallucinogenic effects, while the higher dosage results in psychotomimetic symptoms and a dissociation from reality, even though the exact effects of these specific doses used recreationally cannot be directly ascertained due to a dearth of controlled studies. Nasal insufflation is the most popular method of recreational delivery, with an average "high" onset time of 5–10 minutes and a duration of 40–75 minutes. Users claim that ketamine causes a profoundly dissociative experience at the highest doses, which is further characterized by an altered state of consciousness and sensory detachment (often known as the k-hole), which some people compare to a near-death experience.[46]

Ketamine dosage, dependent on plasma concentrations between 50 and 200 ng/mL,[47] may be linked to visual hallucinations, altered perceptions of self and time, and floating sensation.[48] Unwanted side effects that illegal users have described include palpitations, chest pain, vomiting, blurred vision, and slurred speech.[49] Ketamine-induced reduced tactile and musculoskeletal sensations have been theorized to generate experiences of weightlessness or detachment from one's own body, which may be a factor in the extracorporeal sensations.[38]

Moreover, prolonged ketamine usage may cause flashbacks and cognitive problems, and reduced sociability; nonetheless, the other psychotropic effects support ongoing use.[50] Although having reinforcing qualities, ketamine dependence is not common but has been documented.[49,51]

Direct and Indirect Peripheral Effects

Ketamine could cause issues including vestibular disturbances, including dizziness and nausea/vomiting at the subanesthetic dosage.[41,52]

In both clinical (0.5–1.0 mg/kg IV)[8] and recreational settings, ketamine's effects on the sympathetic nervous system are associated with wide cardiovascular consequences (e.g., tachycardia, hypertension, and palpitations).

Additionally, (S)-, (R)-, and (R, S)-ketamine are not found to have significantly different hemodynamic effects (blood pressure and pulse rate).[53] (S)-ketamine specifically contributes to (R, S)-ketamine's cardiovascular effects, like hypertension suggested by a study.[54] In general, a recent study of IV ketamine infusions in patients found that the blood pressure variations are mild and clinically insignificant.[55] Although modest respiratory side effects are reported at doses of 0.3–3 mg/kg,[11,56] this is generally regarded as clinically not significant.

Nystagmus, diplopia, and dilatation of the eyes have all been noted as side effects of ketamine in both therapeutic settings and recreational settings.[41,57] The main substance associated with several ocular side effects, like impaired vision, is (S)-ketamine.[58] Moreover, ketamine abuse has been linked to musculoskeletal side effects such as myoclonus, twitching, spasms, ataxia, and fasciculation.[45,46]

Ketamine use for recreational purposes for an extended period is connected to urological issues such as ulcerative cystitis, hematuria, discomfort, incontinence, and dysuria.[59] Given that long-term ketamine users exhibit erythema, edema, and epithelial inflammation during cystoscopy, it is hypothesized that ketamine may directly harm the interstitial cells of the bladder.[60] Moreover, computed tomography showed perivesical inflammation, mucosal augmentation, and a noticeable thickening of the bladder wall associated with ketamine usage for recreational purposes.[61] At least one case report has been documented with subanesthetic ketamine, associated with urine urgency and incontinency.[62]

Long-term Effects

Since therapeutic efficacy of ketamine mostly needs repeated drug administration,[63] it is crucial to take into account any potential side effects that may be specifically associated to chronic ketamine administration. The effects following a protracted ketamine therapy are either vaguely described or rarely documented. The persistent memory problems are most frequently associated with ketamine misuse on a regular basis.[50] In the absence of multimodal intoxication, deaths from ketamine overdoses are extremely rare (Jansen, 2001); nonetheless, accidents involving people who have used ketamine, such as those involving falls from great heights, intense hypothermia, and car accidents, have reported to cause accidental deaths.[64]

The immediate dissociation, derealization, and dizziness that ketamine causes are also known to lessen with repeated dosing.[65] Yet, in randomized controlled trials that look at the effects of repeated IV subanesthetic ketamine exposure, dissociative and psychotomimetic effects are seen.[66] The majority, if not all, of ketamine's side effects are dose-dependent, momentary, and self-correcting.[30]

Neurotoxicity

As a result of newer indications (such as antidepressant effects) requiring recurring ketamine administration, there are concerns regarding more severe adverse treatment effects, such as the development of Olney's lesions. Olney's lesions are characterized by vacuoles that form in the cytoplasm of certain populations of neuronal cells. They were first identified in 1989.[67,68] These neuronal vacuolation events primarily occur in the posterior cingulate and retrosplenial cortices in rats following treatment with NMDAR antagonists (such as PCP, MK-801, and ketamine)[67,69] Modest doses of competitive [CPP (3-(2-carboxypiperazin-4-yl)propyl-l-phosphonoic acid), CGS-19755, and CGP-37849] or noncompetitive medicines (PCP, MK-801, ketamine, and dextrorphan) do not seem to induce long-term cell damage because vacuolation seems to return within 24 hours after treatment. Nonetheless, there is a slight possibility that using NMDAR antagonists like ketamine repeatedly at low doses (or in large doses) might result in particular permanent damage. Determining whether Olney's lesions are related to long-term ketamine use in humans is controversial and difficult. One magnetic resonance imaging research discovered that recreational ketamine users had cortical atrophy in the frontal, parietal, and occipital lobes (total ketamine usage: 0.5–12 years), and that considerable shrinkage was connected to the beginning of drug use happening 2-4 years earlier.[70]

Another research of recreational users (total time of ketamine use: 1–10.5 years) likewise found a loss of frontal cortical white matter microstructure integrity, and this loss was connected to overall lifetime ketamine use.[71]

PHARMACOKINETICS
Metabolism

Ketamine is subjected to extensive metabolism, first converting to norketamine through nitrogen demethylation, which is largely performed by the cytochrome (CYP) P450 liver enzymes CYP3A4 and CYP2B6.[72] Ketamine is demethylated in a stereospecific way, with CYP3A4 demethylating the (S) enantiomer more quickly than the (R) enantiomer while CYP2B6 demethylates both enantiomers of ketamine equally efficiently. The individual variation in ketamine metabolism is partly related to variations in P450 enzyme expression.[73] Shortly after the dosing, it was shown that (2R,6R;2S,6S)-HNK also accumulates in brain tissue.[74,75] Within 10 minutes of ketamine treatment, the brain showed signs of ketamine, norketamine, and (2R,6R;2S,6S)-HNK. The maximum level of ketamine in the brain was 51.66%, which is greater than the equivalent plasma level. In contrast, the maximum levels of norketamine and (2R,6R;2S,6S)-HNK in the brain tissue were 58.96 and 26.13% lower, respectively, than the corresponding maximum plasma levels.[76]

The observation that DHNK levels in brain tissue were below the limits of quantification is consistent with the fact that DHNK divides into red blood cells and has minimal blood–brain barrier penetration.[77]

Absorption

There are several ways to give ketamine to people, including IV, intramuscular, oral, intranasal, epidural, and intrarectal.[14,78] IV infusion is the most common method of administration since it quickly reaches maximal plasma concentrations.[79] With a high bioavailability of 93%, intramuscular administration of ketamine is used in emergency situations involving uncooperative patients, neonates, and children. It reaches peak plasma concentration within 5–30 minutes of administration. However, a population pharmacokinetic analysis discovered that the bioavailability following intramuscular administration of ketamine in children was significantly lower (41%).[80]

Ketamine's oral bioavailability is limited to 16–29% due to substantial first-pass hepatic metabolism, with peak drug concentrations reaching in 20–120 minutes. The estimated 8–11% oral bioavailability of (S)-ketamine[81] is consistent with (S)-ketamine having a higher first-pass metabolism than (R,S)-ketamine. Ketamine bioavailability in the nasal and intrarectal regions is 45–50% and 25–30%, respectively.[14,79,82,83]

Ketamine can be administered intranasally rather than intravenously since it is less intrusive, quickly absorbed into the body, and does not undergo first-pass hepatic metabolism.[14]

Distribution

Ketamine is rapidly distributed into highly perfused organs, such as the brain, and has a significant steady-state volume of distribution. Plasma protein binding ranges from 10 to 50%. One IV (bolus) dose of 1 mg/kg (S)-ketamine was administered, and one minute later, the plasma concentration of the drug increased [calculated from Geisslinger et al; maximum concentration (C_{max}) = 2,600 ng/mL: 11 mM]. These results are particularly important when comparing the effects of (S)-ketamine with those of racemic ketamine or (R)-ketamine as (S)-ketamine needs fewer doses to reach equivalent or greater plasma ketamine concentrations.[58]

Elimination

Although plasma levels of ketamine fell below detectable limits within 1 day of an IV antidepressant dose of ketamine (0.5 mg/kg administered over a 40-minute infusion), circulating levels of DHNK and (2R,6R; 2S,6S)-HNK were detected for up to 3 days after ketamine infusion in patients with bipolar depression or treatment-resistant major depression.[84,85] Norketamine and ketamine levels were found in children who received anesthetic doses of ketamine for up to 14 and 11 days, respectively, with reported concentrations of 0.1-1,442 ng/mL for norketamine and 2-1204 ng/mL for ketamine. In adult humans, ketamine has a rapid rate of clearance and a short elimination half-life (2-4 hours).[86]

Ketamine is predominantly eliminated by the kidneys, where it is excreted in small amounts as ketamine (2%), norketamine (2%), and DHNK (16%).[87] According to Dinis-Oliveira (2017), the majority of the medicine is excreted as the glucuronic acid-labile conjugates of HK and HNK, which are excreted in the bile and urine. Whether administered intravenously (half-life: 186 minutes; whole body clearance: 19.1 mL/min/kg) or intramuscularly (half-life: 155 minutes; total body clearance: 23.2 mL/min/kg), ketamine's terminal plasma half-life and clearance rates do not differ appreciably in adult adults.[79]

Despite this, there is evidence that repeated administration of ketamine lengthens its elimination time. For instance, a research found that following three single IV infusions of ketamine over a 2-year period (doses varied from 0.75 to 1.59 mg/kg), the clearance of the drug decreased from 2 days after the first infusion to 5 days after the second and 11 days after the third.[86] Norketamine continues to be regularly removed (i.e., 5 days after each infusion). In children, ketamine is eliminated nearly twice as fast as in adults. There are considerable differences across species in ketamine's half-life values, areas under the curve (AUCs), C_{max}, and clearance rates.[88]

When evaluating the behavioral effects of various dosage schedules of ketamine and its different metabolites in rats, mice, and humans, this is a crucial problem to consider. Direct comparisons are difficult, since it is unknown how much ketamine and its metabolites are present in the brain after ketamine injection in humans.

PHARMACODYNAMICS

As ketamine is an NMDAR antagonist, NMDAR inhibition is principally responsible for its well-recognized analgesia and anesthetic effects. NMDARs are just one of ketamine's pharmacological targets, though. Many additional receptors and ion channels, such as dopamine, serotonin, sigma, opioid, and cholinergic receptors, as well as hyperpolarization-activated cyclic nucleotide-gated (HCN) channels, have been observed to interact with ketamine. In multiple animal testing, it was discovered that (2R,6R)-HNK is a more potent antidepressant than (2S,6S)-HNK, which is consistent with the (R)-ketamine enantiomer's stronger antidepressant effects when compared to the (S)-ketamine enantiomer.[76]

Mechanism of Action: N-Methyl-D-Aspartate Receptors

Historically, the NMDAR has been the most widely acknowledged receptor target for ketamine, acting as a noncompetitive open-channel blocker.[89] *GluN1*, *GluN2A-D*, and *GluN3A-B* are three of the seven genes that encode the glutamatergic ion channels known as NMDARs. Calcium ions can activate a variety of intracellular pathways in neurons and glial cells because NMDARs are very permeable to them. Magnesium (Mg^{2+}) tonically blocks NMDAR channels when they are in their resting state. Effective receptor activation requires the following: (1) membrane depolarization, which shifts the Mg^{2+} block, and (2) glutamate binding and the coactivator D-serine or glycine.

Clinical Effects

David Lodge and colleagues first identified ketamine as an NMDAR antagonist,[90] and other researchers later corroborated their findings.[91] By binding to the allosteric PCP site that is located within the channel pore of the receptor, ketamine inhibits the NMDAR noncompetitively.[2] Ketamine has a moderately strong (86%) trapping capability (binding within the ion channel pore following closure of the channel) to inhibit NMDARs. It binds to the same site as PCP (98% trapping) and MK-801 (100% trapping).

Ketamine's dissociative anesthetic and amnesic effects, as well as its antidepressant, analgesic, and altered psychotomimetic effects are all assumed to be caused by NMDAR blockage. Another proposed as a cause of the cognitive abnormalities brought on by ketamine is NMDAR inhibition.[92] When external Mg^{2+} is present, (S)-ketamine has a potency/affinity for the NMDAR's PCP site that is roughly four times more than that of (R)-ketamine and double that of the racemic combination.[93]

Ketamine's immediate antidepressant effects, which start to take action hours after administration, have sparked extensive research efforts to understand this phenomena. This discovery and the elucidation of the relevant mechanisms involved have the potential to revolutionize the treatment of depression given that currently approved antidepressants take weeks or even months to fully exert their antidepressant effects,[94] and that many patients with major depressive disorders are resistant to traditional antidepressant pharmacotherapies. A 40-minute IV infusion of (S)-ketamine has immediate antidepressant effects (within 2 hours of treatment) according to clinical human studies on depressed individuals.[65]

Also, people with depression who are resistant to treatment and using oral traditional antidepressants have mentioned treatment-dependent antidepressant benefits of (S)-ketamine administered intranasally.[95]

Esketamine nasal spray (Spravato™) has been developed and is currently approved for use in TRD in both Europe and the United States when used in conjunction with an oral antidepressant, despite the fact that ketamine is still regarded as an off-label treatment for TRD.

Although glutamate release from glutamatergic neurons is generally suppressed by gamma-aminobutyric acid (GABA)-ergic interneurons, it has been hypothesized that the fast antidepressant action of ketamine and esketamine are mediated by blocking NMDARs on these interneurons. Seven acute cortical glutamate surge, activation of postsynaptic α-amino-3-hydroxy-5-methyl-4-isoxazolepropionic acid (AMPA) receptors, and subsequent impacts on synaptogenesis and neuroplastic pathways are the outcomes of this disinhibition. Because other NMDAR antagonists, like memantine, lack antidepressant effects, this may be a red herring in and of itself.

Drug Therapy Use of Ketamine's Metabolites

An article claims that the capacity of ketamine to be metabolized determines the extent of its antidepressant effects in mice.[76] Even though certain ketamine HNK metabolites, such as (2S,6S)-HNK and (2R,6R)-HNK, which are produced by the metabolism of (S)-ketamine and (R)-ketamine, respectively, do not bind to or functionally inhibit the NMDAR at antidepressant-relevant concentrations,[96,97] they do have an antidepressant effect. These findings cast more doubt on the NMDAR inhibition theory underlying ketamine's antidepressant properties. Moreover, (2R,6R)-HNK has antidepressant properties in animal studies without the sensory disorientation, ataxia, or misuse potential of ketamine.

Ketamine's psychotropic side effects, such as dissociation and alterations in sensory perception, as well as its misuse potential have been connected to its NMDAR-inhibiting capabilities.[92]

FUTURE

The recent findings that ketamine metabolites contribute to ketamine's antidepressant effects offer new research directions and raise the prospect of employing these metabolites to treat depression. HNK metabolites may contribute to the clinical effects of subanesthetic doses of ketamine because of their direct or indirect actions on nicotinic acetylcholine receptors (nAChRs), D-serine, or other targets.[98] This research might serve as a foundation for a novel ketamine metabolite paradigm that postulates therapeutically applicable effects associated with ketamine's metabolic conversion but excludes NMDAR inhibition.[99] Future preclinical studies are needed to support the contention that NMDAR inhibition is not required for the effectiveness of ketamine's metabolites as fast-acting antidepressants and to identify the underlying mechanism of action of these metabolites. It also remains to be investigated whether ketamine metabolites have a role in the anti-inflammatory or analgesic actions of ketamine.

CONCLUSION

Ketamine is a promising treatment option for several psychiatric disorders, including major depressive disorder, treatment-resistant depression and bipolar disorder. Its rapid onset of action makes it an attractive alternative to traditional antidepressant medications. While ketamine's exact mechanisms of action are not fully understood, it is thought to modulate glutamate neurotransmission and enhance synaptic plasticity in key brain regions involved in mood regulation and emotional processing.

Although ketamine has been shown to be effective in several clinical trials, there are still some limitations to its use. These include concerns over its potential for abuse and addiction, as well as its potential to cause dissociative and other side effects. As such, the use of ketamine in clinical settings is closely monitored and regulated.

Despite these limitations, the use of ketamine in psychiatry holds great promise. Ongoing research is focused on further elucidating its mechanisms of action, identifying biomarkers to predict treatment response, and developing new formulations and delivery methods to enhance its efficacy and safety. In addition, there is growing interest in combining ketamine with other treatments, such as psychotherapy and other medications, to optimize outcomes and improve the overall treatment of psychiatric disorders.

In summary, ketamine represents a novel and exciting addition to the psychiatric treatment armamentarium. While there is still much to learn about this drug, the current evidence suggests that it may play a crucial role in the future of psychiatric treatment, offering hope to millions of patients who have not found relief from traditional treatments.

TAKE-HOME POINTS

- Ketamine is a promising treatment option for major depressive disorder, treatment-resistant depression and bipolar disorder.
- Ketamine has a rapid onset of action and lasting effects, making it an attractive alternative to traditional antidepressant medications.
- Ketamine has a relatively safe profile when administered in a clinical setting.
- While the mechanisms of action of ketamine are not fully understood, it is thought to modulate glutamate neurotransmission and enhance synaptic plasticity.
- Future research is needed to fully understand the long-term effects and mechanisms of action of ketamine in psychiatric treatment.

REFERENCES

1. Adams JD, Castagnoli N, Trevor AJ. Quantitative analysis of ketamine enantiomers. Proc West Pharmacol Soc. 1978;21:471-2.
2. Mion G, Villevieille T. Ketamine Pharmacology: An Update (Pharmacodynamics and Molecular Aspects, Recent Findings). CNS Neurosci Ther. 2013;19(6):370-80.
3. Dundee JW, Knox JW, Black GW, Moore J, Pandit SK, Bovill J, et al. Ketamine as an induction agent in anaesthetics. Lancet. 1970;1(7661):1370-1.
4. Weisman H. Anesthesia for pediatric ophthalmology. Ann Ophthalmol. 1971;3(3):229-32.
5. Roytblat L, Talmor D, Rachinsky M, Greemberg L, Pekar A, Appelbaum A, et al. Ketamine attenuates the interleukin-6 response after cardiopulmonary bypass. Anesth Analg. 1998;87(2):266-71.
6. Zarate CA, Singh JB, Carlson PJ, Brutsche NE, Ameli R, Luckenbaugh DA, et al. A Randomized Trial of an N-methyl-D-aspartate Antagonist in Treatment-Resistant Major Depression. Arch Gen Psychiatry. 2006;63(8):856-64.
7. Diazgranados N, Ibrahim L, Brutsche NE, Newberg A, Kronstein P, Khalife S, et al. A Randomized Add-on Trial of an N-methyl-D-aspartate Antagonist in Treatment-Resistant Bipolar Depression. Arch Gen Psychiatry. 2010;67(8):793-802.
8. Murrough JW, Iosifescu DV, Chang LC, Al Jurdi RK, Green CE, Perez AM, et al. Antidepressant Efficacy of Ketamine in Treatment-Resistant Major Depression: A Two-Site Randomized Controlled Trial. Am J Psychiatry. 2013;170(10):1134-42.
9. Singh JB, Fedgchin M, Daly E, Xi L, Melman C, De Bruecker G, et al. Intravenous Esketamine in Adult Treatment-Resistant Depression: A Double-Blind, Double-Randomization, Placebo-Controlled Study. Biol Psychiatry. 2016;80(6):424-31.
10. Berman RM, Cappiello A, Anand A, Oren DA, Heninger GR, Charney DS, et al. Antidepressant effects of ketamine in depressed patients. Biol Psychiatry. 2000;47(4):351-4.
11. Gao M, Rejaei D, Liu H. Ketamine use in current clinical practice. Acta Pharmacol Sin. 2016;37(7):865-72.
12. Grant IS, Nimmo WS, McNicol LR, Clements JA. Ketamine disposition in children and adults. Br J Anaesth. 1983;55(11):1107-11. doi: 10.1093/bja/55.11.1107. PMID: 6639827.
13. Idvall J, Ahlgren I, Aronsen KF, Stenberg P. Ketamine infusions: pharmacokinetics and clinical effects. Br J Anaesth. 1979;51(12):1167-73.
14. Craven R. Ketamine. Anaesthesia. 2007;62(Suppl 1):48-53.

15. Malinovsky JM, Servin F, Cozian A, Lepage JY, Pinaud M. Ketamine and norketamine plasma concentrations after i.v., nasal and rectal administration in children. Br J Anaesth. 1996;77(2):203-7.
16. Tsze DS, Steele DW, Machan JT, Akhlaghi F, Linakis JG. Intranasal ketamine for procedural sedation in pediatric laceration repair: a preliminary report. Pediatr Emerg Care. 2012;28(8):767-70.
17. Himmelseher S, Pfenninger E. Die klinische Anwendung von S-(+)-Ketamin-eine Standortbestimmung. Anasthesiol Intensivmed Notfallmed Schmerzther. 1998;33(12):764-70.
18. Kennedy RM, Porter FL, Miller JP, Jaffe DM. Comparison of fentanyl/midazolam with ketamine/midazolam for pediatric orthopedic emergencies. Pediatrics. 1998;102(4 Pt 1):956-63.
19. McGuinness SK, Wasiak J, Cleland H, Symons J, Hogan L, Hucker T, et al. A systematic review of ketamine as an analgesic agent in adult burn injuries. Pain Med. 2011;12(10):1551-8.
20. Laskowski K, Stirling A, McKay WP, Lim HJ. A systematic review of intravenous ketamine for postoperative analgesia. Can J Anaesth. 2011;58(10):911-23.
21. Marchetti F, Coutaux A, Bellanger A, Magneux C, Bourgeois P, Mion G. Efficacy and safety of oral ketamine for the relief of intractable chronic pain: A retrospective 5-year study of 51 patients. Eur J Pain. 2015;19(7):984-93.
22. Carr DB, Goudas LC, Denman WT, Brookoff D, Staats PS, Brennen L, et al. Safety and efficacy of intranasal ketamine for the treatment of breakthrough pain in patients with chronic pain: a randomized, double-blind, placebo-controlled, crossover study. Pain. 2004;108(1):17-27.
23. Johansson J, Sjöberg J, Nordgren M, Sandström E, Sjöberg F, Zetterström H. Prehospital analgesia using nasal administration of S-ketamine—a case series. Scand J Trauma Resusc Emerg Med. 2013;21(1):38.
24. Khorramzadeh E, Lotfy AO. The use of ketamine in psychiatry. Psychosomatics. 1973;14(6):344-6.
25. Lapidus KAB, Levitch CF, Perez AM, Brallier JW, Parides MK, Soleimani L, et al. A randomized controlled trial of intranasal ketamine in major depressive disorder. Biol Psychiatry. 2014;76(12):970-6.
26. Ibrahim L, Diazgranados N, Franco-Chaves J, Brutsche N, Henter ID, Kronstein P, et al. Course of Improvement in Depressive Symptoms to a Single Intravenous Infusion of Ketamine vs Add-on Riluzole: Results from a 4-Week, Double-Blind, Placebo-Controlled Study. Neuropsychopharmacology. 2012;37(6):1526-33.
27. Canuso CM, Singh JB, Fedgchin M, Alphs L, Lane R, Lim P, et al. Efficacy and Safety of Intranasal Esketamine for the Rapid Reduction of Symptoms of Depression and Suicidality in Patients at Imminent Risk for Suicide: Results of a Double-Blind, Randomized, Placebo-Controlled Study. Am J Psychiatry. 2018;175(7):620-30.
28. Ballard ED, Wills K, Lally N, Richards EM, Luckenbaugh DA, Walls T, et al. Anhedonia as a clinical correlate of suicidal thoughts in clinical ketamine trials. J Affect Disord. 2017;218:195-200.
29. Ballard ED, Ionescu DF, Vande Voort JL, Niciu MJ, Richards EM, Luckenbaugh DA, et al. Improvement in suicidal ideation after ketamine infusion: Relationship to reductions in depression and anxiety. J Psychiatr Res. 2014;58:161-6.

30. Loo CK, Gálvez V, O'Keefe E, Mitchell PB, Hadzi-Pavlovic D, Leyden J, et al. Placebo-controlled pilot trial testing dose titration and intravenous, intramuscular and subcutaneous routes for ketamine in depression. Acta Psychiatr Scand. 2016;134(1):48-56.
31. Rasmussen KG, Lineberry TW, Galardy CW, Kung S, Lapid MI, Palmer BA, et al. Serial infusions of low-dose ketamine for major depression. J Psychopharmacol. 2013;27(5):444-50.
32. Fava M, Freeman MP, Flynn M, Judge H, Hoeppner BB, Cusin C, et al. Double-blind, placebo-controlled, dose-ranging trial of intravenous ketamine as adjunctive therapy in treatment-resistant depression (TRD). Mol Psychiatry. 2020;25(7):1592-603.
33. Newton K, Dixit VM. Signaling in innate immunity and inflammation. Cold Spring Harb Perspect Biol. 2012;4(3):a006049.
34. Roussabrov E, Davies JM, Bessler H, Greemberg L, Roytblat L, Yardeni IZ, et al. Effect of ketamine on inflammatory and immune responses after short-duration surgery in obese patients. Open Anesth J. 2008;2(1):40-5.
35. Kadriu B, Gold PW, Luckenbaugh DA, Lener MS, Ballard ED, Niciu MJ, et al. Acute ketamine administration corrects abnormal inflammatory bone markers in major depressive disorder. Mol Psychiatry. 2018;23(7):1626-31.
36. Cho JE, Shim JK, Choi YS, Kim DH, Hong SW, Kwak YL. Effect of low-dose ketamine on inflammatory response in off-pump coronary artery bypass graft surgery. Br J Anaesth. 2009;102(1):23-8.
37. Loix S, De Kock M, Henin P. The anti-inflammatory effects of ketamine: state of the art. Acta Anaesthesiol Belg. 2011;62(1):47-58.
38. White PF, Way WL, Trevor AJ. Ketamine—its pharmacology and therapeutic uses. Anesthesiology. 1982;56(2):119-36.
39. Li CT, Chen MH, Lin WC, Hong CJ, Yang BH, Liu RS, et al. The effects of low-dose ketamine on the prefrontal cortex and amygdala in treatment-resistant depression: A randomized controlled study. Hum Brain Mapp. 2016;37(3):1080-90.
40. Ionescu DF, Rosenbaum JF, Alpert JE. Pharmacological approaches to the challenge of treatment-resistant depression. Dialogues Clin Neurosci. 2015;17(2):111-26.
41. Krystal JH, Karper LP, Seibyl JP, Freeman GK, Delaney R, Bremner JD, et al. Subanesthetic effects of the noncompetitive NMDA antagonist, ketamine, in humans. Psychotomimetic, perceptual, cognitive, and neuroendocrine responses. Arch Gen Psychiatry. 1994;51(3):199-214.
42. Mathew KL, Whitford HS, Kenny MA, Denson LA. The long-term effects of mindfulness-based cognitive therapy as a relapse prevention treatment for major depressive disorder. Behav Cogn Psychother. 2010;38(5):561-76.
43. Arditti J, Spadari M, de Haro L, Brun A, Bourdon JH, Valli M. Ketamine-reves et realites. Acta Clin Belg. 2002;57(Suppl 1):31-3.
44. Corazza O, Assi S, Schifano F. From "Special K" to "Special M": the evolution of the recreational use of ketamine and methoxetamine. CNS Neurosci Ther. 2013;19(6):454-60.
45. Bokor G, Anderson PD. Ketamine: an update on its abuse. J Pharm Pract. 2014;27(6):582-6.

46. Wolff K, Winstock AR. Ketamine: from medicine to misuse. CNS Drugs. 2006;20(3):199-218.
47. Bowdle A, Radant A, Cowley DS, Kharasch ED, Strassman RJ, Roy-Byrne PP. Psychedelic Effects of Ketamine in Healthy Volunteers: Relationship to Steady-state Plasma Concentrations. Anesthesiology. 1998;88(1):82-8.
48. Wilkins LK, Girard TA, Cheyne JA. Anomalous bodily-self experiences among recreational ketamine users. Cogn Neuropsychiatry. 2012;17(5):415-30.
49. Muetzelfeldt L, Kamboj SK, Rees H, Taylor J, Morgan CJA, Curran HV. Journey through the K-hole: phenomenological aspects of ketamine use. Drug Alcohol Depend. 2008;95(3):219-29.
50. Ke X, Ding Y, Xu K, He H, Wang D, Deng X, et al. The profile of cognitive impairments in chronic ketamine users. Psychiatry Res. 2018;266:124-31.
51. Blier P, Zigman D, Blier J. On the safety and benefits of repeated intravenous injections of ketamine for depression. Biol Psychiatry. 2012;72(4):e11-2.
52. Ghoneim MM, Hinrichs JV, Mewaldt SP, Petersen RC. Ketamine: behavioral effects of subanesthetic doses. J Clin Psychopharmacol. 1985;5(2):70-7.
53. White PF, Schüttler J, Shafer A, Stanski DR, Horai Y, Trevor AJ. Comparative pharmacology of the ketamine isomers. Studies in volunteers. Br J Anaesth. 1985;57(2):197-203.
54. Geisslinger G, Hering W, Thomann P, Knoll R, Kamp HD, Brune K. Pharmacokinetics and pharmacodynamics of ketamine enantiomers in surgical patients using a stereoselective analytical method. Br J Anaesth. 1993;70(6):666-71.
55. Riva-Posse P, Choi KS, Holtzheimer PE, Crowell AL, Garlow SJ, Rajendra JK, et al. A connectomic approach for subcallosal cingulate deep brain stimulation surgery: prospective targeting in treatment-resistant depression. Mol Psychiatry. 2018;23(4):843-9.
56. Corssen G, Domino EF. Dissociative anesthesia: further pharmacologic studies and first clinical experience with the phencyclidine derivative CI-581. Anesth Analg. 1966;45(1):29-40.
57. Backonja M, Arndt G, Gombar KA, Check B, Zimmermann M. Response of chronic neuropathic pain syndromes to ketamine: a preliminary study. Pain. 1994;56(1):51-7.
58. Mathisen LC, Skjelbred P, Skoglund LA, Øye I. Effect of ketamine, an NMDA receptor inhibitor, in acute and chronic orofacial pain. Pain. 1995;61(2):215-20.
59. Nahapiet J, Ghoshal S. Social capital, intellectual capital, and the organizational advantage. Acad Manage Rev. 2009;119-58.
60. Shahani R, Streutker C, Dickson B, Stewart RJ. Ketamine-associated ulcerative cystitis: a new clinical entity. Urology. 2007;69(5):810-2.
61. Mason K, Cottrell AM, Corrigan AG, Gillatt DA, Mitchelmore AE. Ketamine-associated lower urinary tract destruction: a new radiological challenge. Clin Radiol. 2010;65(10):795-800.
62. Vickers BA, Lee W, Hunsberger J. A case report: subanesthetic ketamine infusion for treatment of cancer-related pain produces urinary urge incontinence. A A Case Rep. 2017;8(9):219-21.
63. Segmiller F, Rüther T, Linhardt A, Padberg F, Berger M, Pogarell O, et al. Repeated S-ketamine infusions in therapy resistant depression: a case series. J Clin Pharmacol. 2013;53(9):996-8.

64. Jansen KL, Darracot-Cankovic R. The nonmedical use of ketamine, part two: a review of problem use and dependence. J Psychoactive Drugs. 2001;33(2):151-8.
65. Singh JB, Fedgchin M, Daly EJ, De Boer P, Cooper K, Lim P, et al. A Double-Blind, Randomized, Placebo-Controlled, Dose-Frequency Study of Intravenous Ketamine in Patients With Treatment-Resistant Depression. Am J Psychiatry. 2016;173(8):816-26.
66. George D, Gálvez V, Martin D, Kumar D, Leyden J, Hadzi-Pavlovic D, et al. Pilot Randomized Controlled Trial of Titrated Subcutaneous Ketamine in Older Patients with Treatment-Resistant Depression. Am J Geriatr Psychiatry. 2017;25(11):1199-209.
67. Olney JW, Labruyere J, Price MT. Pathological changes induced in cerebrocortical neurons by phencyclidine and related drugs. Science. 1989;244(4910):1360-2.
68. Olney JW, Labruyere J, Wang G, Wozniak DF, Price MT, Sesma MA. NMDA antagonist neurotoxicity: mechanism and prevention. Science. 1991;254(5037):1515-8.
69. Carliss RD, Radovsky A, Chengelis CP, O'Neill TP, Shuey DL. Oral administration of dextromethorphan does not produce neuronal vacuolation in the rat brain. Neurotoxicology. 2007;28(4):813-8.
70. Wang C, Zheng D, Xu J, Lam W, Yew DT. Brain damages in ketamine addicts as revealed by magnetic resonance imaging. Front Neuroanat. 2013;7:23.
71. Liao Y, Tang J, Ma M, Wu Z, Yang M, Wang X, et al. Frontal white matter abnormalities following chronic ketamine use: a diffusion tensor imaging study. Brain. 2010;133(Pt 7):2115-22.
72. Rao LK, Flaker AM, Friedel CC, Kharasch ED. Role of Cytochrome P4502B6 Polymorphisms in Ketamine Metabolism and Clearance. Anesthesiology. 2016;125(6):1103-12.
73. Hijazi Y, Boulieu R. Contribution of CYP3A4, CYP2B6, and CYP2C9 isoforms to N-demethylation of ketamine in human liver microsomes. Drug Metab Dispos. 2002;30(7):853-8.
74. Leung LY, Baillie TA. Comparative pharmacology in the rat of ketamine and its two principal metabolites, norketamine and (Z)-6-hydroxynorketamine. J Med Chem. 1986;29(11):2396-9.
75. Paul RK, Singh NS, Khadeer M, Moaddel R, Sanghvi M, Green CE, et al. (R,S)-Ketamine metabolites (R,S)-norketamine and (2S,6S)-hydroxynorketamine increase the mammalian target of rapamycin function. Anesthesiology. 2014;121(1):149-59.
76. Zanos P, Moaddel R, Morris PJ, Georgiou P, Fischell J, Elmer GI, et al. NMDAR inhibition-independent antidepressant actions of ketamine metabolites. Nature. 2016;533(7604):481-6.
77. Can A, Zanos P, Moaddel R, Kang HJ, Dossou KSS, Wainer IW, et al. Effects of Ketamine and Ketamine Metabolites on Evoked Striatal Dopamine Release, Dopamine Receptors, and Monoamine Transporters. J Pharmacol Exp Ther. 2016;359(1):159-70.
78. Andrade C. Ketamine for Depression, 3: Does Chirality Matter? J Clin Psychiatry. 2017;78(6):e674-7.
79. Clements JA, Nimmo WS, Grant IS. Bioavailability, Pharmacokinetics, and Analgesic Activity of Ketamine in Humans. J Pharm Sci. 1982;71(5):539-42.

80. Hornik C, Gonzalez D, van den Anker J, Atz AM, Yogev R, Poindexter BB, et al. Population Pharmacokinetics of Intramuscular and Intravenous Ketamine in Children. J Clin Pharmacol. 2018;58:1092-104.
81. Peltoniemi MA, Saari TI, Hagelberg NM, Laine K, Neuvonen PJ, Olkkola KT. S-ketamine concentrations are greatly increased by grapefruit juice. Eur J Clin Pharmacol. 2012;68:979-86.
82. Grant IS, Nimmo WS, Clements JA. Pharmacokinetics and analgesic effects of i.m. and oral ketamine. Br J Anaesth. 1981;53(8):805-10.
83. Kharasch ED, Labroo R. Metabolism of ketamine stereoisomers by human liver microsomes. Anesthesiology. 1992;77(6):1201-7.
84. Zhao G, Guo Y, Bao S, Meng L, Zhang L. Prevention of propofol-induced pain in children: pretreatment with small doses of ketamine. J Clin Anesth. 2012;24(4):284-8.
85. Zarate CA Jr, Brutsche NE, Ibrahim L, Franco-Chaves J, Diazgranados N, Cravchik A, et al. Replication of ketamine's antidepressant efficacy in bipolar depression: a randomized controlled add-on trial. Biol Psychiatry. 2012;71(11):939-46.
86. Adamowicz P, Kala M. Urinary Excretion Rates of Ketamine and Norketamine Following Therapeutic Ketamine Administration: Method and Detection Window Considerations. J Anal Toxicol. 2005;29(5):376-82.
87. Dinis-Oliveira RJ. Metabolism and metabolomics of ketamine: a toxicological approach. Forensic Sci Res. 2017;2(1):2-10.
88. Haas DA, Harper DG. Ketamine: A review of its pharmacologic properties and use in ambulatory anesthesia. Anesth Prog. 1992;39(3):61-8.
89. MacDonald JF, Miljkovic Z, Pennefather P. Use-dependent block of excitatory amino acid currents in cultured neurons by ketamine. J Neurophysiol. 1987;58(2):251-66.
90. Anis NA, Berry SC, Burton NR, Lodge D. The dissociative anaesthetics, ketamine and phencyclidine, selectively reduce excitation of central mammalian neurones by N-methyl-aspartate. Br J Pharmacol. 1983;79(2):565-75.
91. Harrison NL, Simmonds MA. Quantitative studies on some antagonists of N-methyl D-aspartate in slices of rat cerebral cortex. Br J Pharmacol. 1985;84(2):381-91.
92. Shaffer CL, Osgood SM, Smith DL, Liu J, Trapa PE. Enhancing ketamine translational pharmacology via receptor occupancy normalization. Neuropharmacology. 2014;86:174-80.
93. Temme L, Schepmann D, Schreiber JA, Frehland B, Wünsch B. Comparative pharmacological study of common NMDA receptor open channel blockers regarding their affinity and functional activity toward GluN2A and GluN2B NMDA receptors. ChemMedChem. 2018;13(5):446-52.
94. Rush AJ, Trivedi MH, Wisniewski SR, Nierenberg AA, Stewart JW, Warden D, et al. Acute and Longer-Term Outcomes in Depressed Outpatients Requiring One or Several Treatment Steps: a STAR*D Report. Am J Psychiatry. 2006;163(11):1905-17.
95. Daly EJ, Singh JB, Fedgchin M, Cooper K, Lim P, Shelton RC, et al. Efficacy and Safety of Intranasal Esketamine Adjunctive to Oral Antidepressant Therapy in Treatment-Resistant Depression: A Randomized Clinical Trial. JAMA Psychiatry. 2018 Feb;75(2):139-48.

96. Zanos P, Moaddel R, Morris PJ, Riggs LM, Highland JN, Georgiou P, et al. Ketamine and ketamine metabolite pharmacology: Insights into therapeutic mechanisms. Pharmacol Rev. 2018;70(3):621-60.
97. Zanos P, Gould TD. Mechanisms of ketamine action as an antidepressant. Mol Psychiatry. 2018;23(4):801-11.
98. Moaddel R, Luckenbaugh DA, Xie Y, Villaseñor A, Brutsche NE, Machado-Vieira R, et al. D-serine plasma concentration is a potential biomarker of (R,S)-ketamine antidepressant response in subjects with treatment-resistant depression. Psychopharmacology (Berl). 2014;232(2):399-409.
99. Singh NS, Zarate CA, Moaddel R, Bernier M, Wainer IW. What is hydroxynorketamine and what can it bring to neurotherapeutics? Expert Rev Neurother.2014;14(11):1239-42.

CHAPTER 13

Newer Noninvasive Neuromodulatory Techniques in Psychiatry

Samir Kumar Praharaj, Nishant Goyal

INTRODUCTION

Neuromodulation techniques include use of *electrical, magnetic, photic,* or *ultrasonic* stimulation to excite or inhibit specific brain targets. They can be classified as *invasive* [e.g., deep brain stimulation, (DBS)] or *noninvasive* [e.g., transcranial magnetic stimulation (TMS)], and *seizural* [e.g., electroconvulsive therapy (ECT)] or *nonseizural* [e.g., transcranial electrical stimulation (tES)]. These techniques not only affect the neurotransmitter systems, but also have other effects such as altering the brain circuitry, neuroplasticity, changing the rhythms or oscillations in the brain, and functional connectivity. These brain effects could now be studied using functional imaging such as functional magnetic resonance imaging (fMRI), positron emission tomography (PET), or electrophysiological imaging such as electroencephalography (EEG) and event-related potentials (ERP). Noninvasive brain stimulation (NIBS) techniques have various clinical applications including investigation of psychiatric disorders (e.g., *virtual lesions* to study brain function), as well as therapeutic uses, specifically when they are resistant or intolerant to conventional pharmacotherapy.

Localization techniques are used to target the brain areas while using more focal forms of NIBS. These includes using 10-20 EEG system based on scalp measurements, or using individualized localization with structural or functional MRI, PET, or single-photon emission computed tomography (SPECT) scan and/or near infrared spectroscopy (NIRS) (e.g., *neuronavigation*). Furthermore, the use of robotic arm helps to deliver NIBS precisely (e.g., *robotic TMS*). There is an explosion of literature on neuromodulation since the last two decades. We review the current NIBS methods (excluding ECT) that have potential application in the field of psychiatry. Of these, magnetic and electrical neuromodulation have been well studied, whereas, photic and ultrasonic neuromodulation are still in nascent stages of development.

MAGNETIC NEUROMODULATION

Magnetic stimulation includes repetitive TMS (rTMS) and magnetic seizure therapy (MST). There are other magnetic stimulation techniques, such as low frequency magnetic stimulation (LFMS), which are less well studied than TMS.

Transcranial Magnetic Stimulation

Transcranial magnetic stimulation involves the use of time-varying high field magnetic stimulation to produce electrical currents in the brain based on *Faraday's principle of electromagnetic induction*, thus bypassing the scalp impedance that is a concern in ECT. Also, the stimulation is much more focal, which results in either excitation or inhibition of the underlying cortex depending on the frequency of stimulation. *High-frequency* (HF) stimulation (>5 Hz) is considered excitatory, whereas, *low-frequency* (LF) stimulation (<1 Hz) is inhibitory. There are widespread effects of rTMS beyond the point of stimulation, because of white matter projections to other brain areas, which may contribute to the therapeutic benefits. The brain areas stimulated or inhibited depend on the coil types used. Different coil types are used for more focal stimulation (e.g., *figure-of-eight* coil) or double-cone coil, or to target deeper cortical and subcortical structures [e.g., *Hessed* (H)-coil] for therapeutic effect. Recently, *priming* rTMS is also found to show promising results in the treatment of obsessive–compulsive disorder (OCD) and late life depression.

Several studies have demonstrated efficacy of HF-rTMS to left dorsolateral prefrontal cortex (DLPFC) and LF-rTMS to right DLPFC in depression.[1] Clinical application of TMS in bipolar disorder is mostly for depression, which shows similar effect as unipolar depression, and few studies have demonstrated efficacy in mania.[2] In schizophrenia, 1-Hz TMS over left temporoparietal junction (TPJ) has been consistently shown to improve persistent auditory hallucinations in short term, with medium effect sizes.[3] Other TMS techniques that have been used for auditory hallucinations are HF-TMS over right temporoparietal cortex, HF-primed 1-Hz TMS, neuronavigational TMS, but with mixed results. There is small and inconsistent effect of HF-TMS to the left DLPFC in negative and cognitive symptoms in schizophrenia.[3] In OCD, stimulation of supplementary motor area (SMA) or pre-SMA, and orbitofrontal cortex (OFC) target has been found to be effective.[4,5] TMS over DLPFC has been used to reduce craving and improve abstinence rates in patients with addiction with alcohol, tobacco, and cocaine.[6] The other applications for TMS include generalized anxiety disorder, post-traumatic stress disorder, eating disorders, and obesity.[7,8]

Patterned/Theta Burst Stimulation

To improve upon conventional rTMS, bursts of three stimuli at 50-Hz every 200 ms, at 5-Hz frequency, called *theta burst stimulation* (TBS), have been developed which mimics the intrinsic properties of neuronal firing (Chung et al. 2015). Depending on continuous pulses without interruption (*continuous TBS* or cTBS) or intermittent 2-second train of bursts every 10 seconds (*intermittent TBS* or iTBS) stimulation, it can either inhibit or excite the underlying cortex, respectively. This *patterned TMS* has reduced the treatment duration markedly (e.g., from 45 minutes with slow rTMS to 3 minutes with iTBS in the treatment of depression), and induces plasticity changes more effectively.[9] Studies have demonstrated that iTBS has equal efficacy as HF-rTMS in the treatment of depression not responding to pharmacotherapy.[10,11] *Prolonged iTBS* (piTBS) which is three times of standard protocol using 600 pulses (i.e., 1,800 pulses per session) is suggested to be more effective, as TMS after effects are more prominent with total number of pulses.[12] TBS with adjusted burst frequency (20 Hz, instead of standard 50 Hz) has been investigated in depression, and may have distinct effects.[12] Inhibitory protocol using cTBS over TPJ is being used for the treatment of auditory hallucinations in schizophrenia.

Accelerated Transcranial Magnetic Stimulation

To reduce treatment duration from standard 4–6 weeks, accelerated forms of TMS protocols have been developed. For example, Stanford neuromodulation therapy (SNT), which was previously known as Stanford accelerated intelligent neuromodulation therapy (SAINT), uses high dose, resting-state fMRI-guided iTBS protocol (10 daily sessions for 5 days) for depression.[13] Spaced iTBS protocol uses piTBS (i.e., 1,800 pulses per session), 10 sessions/day over 5 days (i.e., 90,000 pulses), and reported dramatic improvement in depression;[12] however, these protocols require replication. Accelerated TMS is also being for the treatment of other conditions such as schizophrenia and OCD.

Deep Transcranial Magnetic Stimulation

One of the major limitations of conventional TMS is the depth of penetration (1.5–2.5 cm). This has been overcome by use of specially designed coils (e.g., H-coils) to target deeper structures, up to 6 cm.[14] The H7 coil is designed to target the medial prefrontal cortex and anterior cingulate cortex, and is found to be effective in the treatment of OCD.[15] H1 coil targeting DLPFC, which has broader and deeper targets than figure-of-8 coil, has been used to treat depression, and appears promising.[16]

Synchronized Transcranial Magnetic Stimulation

Synchronized TMS (sTMS) uses rotating spherical neodymium magnets over midline of the scalp to deliver low-field sinusoidal waveform stimulation, which is synchronized to the alpha EEG frequency of the individual. Antidepressant effects are achieved at lower energy levels than conventional TMS using brain's natural resonance.[12]

Quadripulse Stimulation

Another form of patterned TMS includes *quadripulse stimulation* (QPS), which includes repeated trains of four pulse bursts. QPS can be excitatory or inhibitory depending on the interstimulus interval (ISI), i.e., short ISI facilitates and long ISI suppresses. Putatively, QPS is being explored for the treatment of Parkinson's disease, depression, and epilepsy.[17]

Magnetic Seizure Therapy

Magnetic seizure therapy involves the use of magnetic stimulation to induce a seizure, which is considered to have more focal effects than ECT, with lesser cognitive adverse effects.[18] Conventionally, MST uses 100 Hz stimulation over vertex to induce seizure, and has been found to be effective in depression, with less cognitive adverse effects. Newer MST protocols with lower frequencies (e.g., 50 or 25 Hz), and different sites (e.g. prefrontal cortex) are being explored in depression.

NONINVASIVE ELECTRICAL NEUROMODULATION

Among noninvasive electrical neuromodulation, transcranial direct current stimulation (tDCS) is the most studied technique, besides ECT. Other less commonly used techniques are transcranial alternating current stimulation (tACS), transcranial random noise stimulation (tRNS), and transcranial pulsed current stimulation (tPCS). There are several noninvasive cranial electrical neuromodulation techniques including transcutaneous auricular vagus nerve stimulation (taVNS), transcutaneous cervical VNS (tcVNS), and auricular neuromodulation (AN).

Transcranial Electrical Stimulation

Transcranial electrical stimulation involves stimulation using *direct current*, i.e., tDCS, and *alternating current*, i.e., tACS. It is a low-cost noninvasive neuromodulation technique that is being explored in the treatment of psychiatric disorders. The mechanism of action is very different from TMS, as the small current is not sufficient to induce action potentials, but can change the neuronal excitability in a polarity-specific manner, i.e., *cathodal* stimulation is inhibitory, whereas, *anodal* stimulation is excitatory.

Transcranial Direct Current Stimulation

In tDCS, low amplitude current (usually 1-2 mA) is used to stimulate brain areas using anode and cathode applied over specific areas, to excite or inhibit underlying neurons. It has a modulatory effect on the neurons, through changes in the postsynaptic potentials. It has shown promise in the treatment of auditory hallucinations, negative and cognitive symptoms in schizophrenia, in alleviating symptoms of depression, OCD, anxiety disorders, and reducing craving in substance use disorders.[19] In a randomized trial, tDCS showed almost similar efficacy as escitalopram, when continued for sufficiently longer periods.[20] Although some studies have reported improvement in persistent auditory hallucinations with cathodal tDCS over TPJ, the results are mixed.[21] *High-definition tDCS* (HD-tDCS) is a more focal form of electrical stimulation that has been explored in the treatment of psychiatric disorders.[22]

Transcranial Alternating Current Stimulation

Transcranial alternating current stimulation involves use of alternating current to modulate the brain oscillations identified through electroencephalography (EEG) or magnetoencephalography (MEG). It can be used to couple or decouple the connection between two neural circuits by synchronizing or desynchronizing their oscillations. The stimulation frequency is set to the EEG frequency that is targeted. It produces lasting changes in brain through entrainment of brain oscillations and neuroplasticity. It has shown promising roles in schizophrenia (frontal alpha tACS, frontal theta tACS), depression (bifrontal alpha tACS), and OCD (frontal gamma tACS).[23]

Cranial Nerve Neuromodulation

Vagus nerve stimulation is an invasive technique that has been demonstrated to have antidepressant effect in treatment-resistant conditions. In contrast, taVNS involves transcutaneous stimulation of auricular branch of vagus nerve, and has been studied in the treatment of depression, putatively through its anti-inflammatory effects and modulation of neural circuits.[24] Similarly, external trigeminal nerve stimulation (e-TNS) has shown efficacy for the management of ADHD in children and adolescents,[25] and migraine.[26]

PHOTIC NEUROMODULATION

Light in near-infrared region (810 nm wavelength) using laser or light-emitting diodes (LEDs) has been demonstrated to penetrate skull and has biologic effects, specifically when used in pulsed mode (e.g., at 10 Hz). Transcranial photobiomodulation (tPBM) is possible using wavelengths in the range of 808-835 nm, laser devices, higher power densities, and pulsed parameters. Most of the physiological effects of tPBM are related to its effects on mitochondrial energy production and increasing regional blood flow. Several studies have demonstrated efficacy of tPBM over prefrontal cortex in depression; however, the optimum parameters (e.g., LED vs. laser, continuous vs. pulsed wave) are yet to be known.[27] Other approaches of PBM include intranasal, intraoral, and intra-aural applications, though these approaches are less well studied.[28]

ULTRASONIC NEUROMODULATION

Ultrasounds at lower intensities (0.5-100 W/cm^2) when delivered in pulsed mode, do not produce thermal effects, but induce mechanical effects on tissues, and opens up the field of ultrasonic neuromodulation. In contrast, high-intensity ultrasound at intensities >500 W/cm^2 is used for focal tissue ablation for the treatment of movement disorders [e.g., transcranial magnetic resonance (MR)-guided HIFU], and has been extended to produce bilateral capsulotomies in the treatment of treatment-resistant OCD. Transcranial focused ultrasound stimulation (tFUS) has been demonstrated to differentially modulate (i.e., excite and inhibit) brain circuit and neural activity across a broad range of acoustic stimulus parameters. The advantages of tFUS over TMS includes: (1) It is not affected by the tissue shapes (e.g., gyral curvature) thus reducing variability in responses; (2) Compatibility with EEG and MRI, and can be used along with these modalities; and (3) targeting deeper brain structures (i.e., DBS target sites).[29]

CONCLUSION

Among the neuromodulation techniques, TMS and tDCS are the most well studied. Newer protocols and techniques are being developed, which provide higher efficacy, lesser time, and wider applicability.[30] More research is needed in these newer techniques for establishing the optimal parameters and protocols. There are guidelines being developed for further research in specific areas of neuromodulation (e.g., Ekhtiari et al.[31] for neuromodulation in addiction research). With the recent advances in neuromodulation techniques involving large-scale clinical trials pave the way for the field of *interventional psychiatry*.[32]

ACKNOWLEDGMENTS

Dr Samir Kumar Praharaj and Dr Nishant Goyal acknowledge the support of Department of Biotechnology (DBT), Wellcome Trust India Alliance (IA/CRC/19/1/610005).

TAKE-HOME POINTS

- Noninvasive neuromodulation techniques are being used for investigational as well as therapeutic applications.
- Patterned TMS (theta burst stimulation), which is more physiological, and accelerated TMS has reduced treatment time and treatment days.
- Use of H-coils has facilitated targeting deeper cortical and subcortical structures.
- Newer TES techniques such as the use of alternating current to modulate brain oscillations could produce lasting changes in neural plasticity.
- Neuronavigation techniques have been helpful to improve localization of brain areas in focal forms of NIBS.
- Photic and ultrasonic neuromodulation are other emerging techniques of NIBS.

REFERENCES

1. Fitzgerald PB, Gill S, Breakspear M, Kulkarni J, Chen L, Pridmore S, et al. Revisiting the effectiveness of repetitive transcranial magnetic stimulation treatment in depression, again. Aust N Z J Psychiatry. 2022;56:905-9.
2. Gold AK, Ornelas AC, Cirillo P, Caldieraro MA, Nardi AE, Nierenberg AA, et al. Clinical applications of transcranial magnetic stimulation in bipolar disorder. Brain Behav. 2019;9:e01419.
3. Mehta UM, Naik SS, Thanki MV, Thirthalli J. Investigational and therapeutic applications of transcranial magnetic stimulation in schizophrenia. Curr Psychiatry Rep. 2019;21:89.
4. Lusicic A, Schruers KR, Pallanti S, Castle DJ. Transcranial magnetic stimulation in the treatment of obsessive-compulsive disorder: current perspectives. Neuropsychiatr Dis Treat. 2018;14:1721-36.
5. Acevedo N, Bosanac P, Pikoos T, Rossell S, Castle D. Therapeutic neurostimulation in obsessive-compulsive and related disorders: a systematic review. Brain Sci. 2021;11:948.
6. Antonelli M, Fattore L, Sestito L, Di Giuda D, Diana M, Addolorato G. Transcranial magnetic stimulation: a review about its efficacy in the treatment of alcohol, tobacco and cocaine addiction. Addict Behav. 2021;114:106760.
7. Kozel FA. Clinical repetitive transcranial magnetic stimulation for posttraumatic stress disorder, generalized anxiety disorder, and bipolar disorder. Psychiatr Clin North Am. 2018;41:433-46.
8. Jáuregui-Lobera I, Martínez-Quiñones JV. Neuromodulation in eating disorders and obesity: a promising way of treatment? Neuropsychiatr Dis Treat. 2018;14:2817-35.
9. Chung SW, Hoy KE, Fitzgerald PB. Theta-burst stimulation: a new form of TMS treatment for depression? Depress Anxiety. 2015;32:182-92.
10. Blumberger DM, Vila-Rodriguez F, Thorpe KE, Feffer K, Noda Y, Giacobbe P, et al. Effectiveness of theta burst versus high-frequency repetitive transcranial magnetic stimulation in patients with depression (THREE-D): a randomised non-inferiority trial. Lancet. 2018;391:1683-92.
11. Bulteau S, Laurin A, Pere M, Fayet G, Thomas-Ollivier V, Deschamps T, et al. Intermittent theta burst stimulation (iTBS) versus 10 Hz high-frequency repetitive transcranial magnetic stimulation (rTMS) to alleviate treatment-resistant

unipolar depression: a randomized controlled trial (THETA-DEP). Brain Stimul. 2022;15:870-80.
12. Cheng CM, Li CT, Tsai SJ. Current updates on newer forms of transcranial magnetic stimulation in major depression. Adv Exp Med Biol. 2021;1305:333-49.
13. Cole EJ, Phillips AL, Bentzley BS, Stimpson KH, Nejad R, Barmak F, et al. Stanford neuromodulation therapy (SNT): a double-blind randomized controlled trial. Am J Psychiatry. 2022;179:132-41.
14. Bersani FS, Minichino A, Enticott PG, Mazzarini L, Khan N, Antonacci G, et al. Deep transcranial magnetic stimulation as a treatment for psychiatric disorders: a comprehensive review. Eur Psychiatry. 2013;28:30-9.
15. Harmelech T, Roth Y, Tendler A. Deep TMS H7 coil: features, applications & future. Expert Rev Med Devices. 2021;18:1133-44.
16. Zibman S, Pell GS, Barnea-Ygael N, Roth Y, Zangen A. Application of transcranial magnetic stimulation for major depression: Coil design and neuroanatomical variability considerations. Eur Neuropsychopharmacol. 2021;45:73-88.
17. Matsumoto H, Ugawa Y. Quadripulse stimulation (QPS). Exp Brain Res. 2020;238:1619-25.
18. Chen M, Yang X, Liu C, Li J, Wang X, Yang C, et al. Comparative efficacy and cognitive function of magnetic seizure therapy vs. electroconvulsive therapy for major depressive disorder: a systematic review and meta-analysis. Transl Psychiatry. 2021;11:437.
19. Chase HW, Boudewyn MA, Carter CS, Phillips ML. Transcranial direct current stimulation: a roadmap for research, from mechanism of action to clinical implementation. Mol Psychiatry. 2020;25:397-407.
20. Brunoni AR, Moffa AH, Sampaio-Junior B, Borrione L, Moreno ML, Fernandes RA, et al.; ELECT-TDCS Investigators. Trial of Electrical Direct-Current Therapy versus Escitalopram for Depression. N Engl J Med. 2017;376:2523-33.
21. Guttesen LL, Albert N, Nordentoft M, Hjorthøj C. Repetitive transcranial magnetic stimulation and transcranial direct current stimulation for auditory hallucinations in schizophrenia: Systematic review and meta-analysis. J Psychiatr Res. 2021;143:163-75.
22. Parlikar R, Vanteemar SS, Shivakumar V, Narayanaswamy CJ, Rao PN, Ganesan V. High definition transcranial direct current stimulation (HD-tDCS): a systematic review on the treatment of neuropsychiatric disorders. Asian J Psychiatr. 2021;56:102542.
23. Elyamany O, Leicht G, Herrmann CS, Mulert C. Transcranial alternating current stimulation (tACS): from basic mechanisms towards first applications in psychiatry. Eur Arch Psychiatry Clin Neurosci. 2021;271:135-56.
24. Liu CH, Yang MH, Zhang GZ, Wang XX, Li B, Li M, et al. Neural networks and the anti-inflammatory effect of transcutaneous auricular vagus nerve stimulation in depression. J Neuroinflammation. 2020;17:54.
25. McGough JJ, Sturm A, Cowen J, Tung K, Salgari GC, Leuchter AF, et al. Double-blind, sham-controlled, pilot study of trigeminal nerve stimulation for attention-deficit/hyperactivity disorder. J Am Acad Child Adolesc Psychiatry. 2019;58:403-11.e3.
26. Stanak M, Wolf S, Jagoš H, Zebenholzer K. The impact of external trigeminal nerve stimulator (e-TNS) on prevention and acute treatment of episodic and chronic migraine: a systematic review. J Neurol Sci. 2020;412:116725.

27. Askalsky P, Iosifescu DV. Transcranial photobiomodulation for the management of depression: current perspectives. Neuropsychiatr Dis Treat. 2019;15:3255-72.
28. Salehpour F, Gholipour-Khalili S, Farajdokht F, Kamari F, Walski T, Hamblin MR, et al. Therapeutic potential of intranasal photobiomodulation therapy for neurological and neuropsychiatric disorders: a narrative review. Rev Neurosci. 2020;31:269-86.
29. Fini M, Tyler WJ. Transcranial focused ultrasound: a new tool for non-invasive neuromodulation. Int Rev Psychiatry. 2017;29:168-77.
30. Hyde J, Carr H, Kelley N, Seneviratne R, Reed C, Parlatini V, et al. Efficacy of neurostimulation across mental disorders: systematic review and meta-analysis of 208 randomized controlled trials. Mol Psychiatry. 2022;27:2709-19.
31. Ekhtiari H, Tavakoli H, Addolorato G, Baeken C, Bonci A, Campanella S, et al. Transcranial electrical and magnetic stimulation (tES and TMS) for addiction medicine: a consensus paper on the present state of the science and the road ahead. Neurosci Biobehav Rev. 2019;104:118-40.
32. Venkatasubramanian G, Mehta UM, Goyal N, Praharaj SK, Umesh S, Muralidharan K, et al. Clinical research center for neuromodulation in psychiatry: a multi-center initiative to advance interventional psychiatry in India. Indian J Psychiatry. 2021;63:503-5.

CHAPTER 14

Mental Health Services for Homeless Populations

Nimesh G Desai

INTRODUCTION

The scientific advances in treatment methods for mental disorders, have had significant impact in the situation of millions of persons with mental illnesses (PMIs), and the larger scenario is unquestionably more positive. The judicially driven deinstitutionalization movement and the possibility of PMIs, with severe mental disorders (SMDs) living in the community has been a remarkable achievements. This has also helped social attitudes and some development of social care models, and family-based rehabilitation of those PMIs, with SMDs, who require some support. Mental healthcare systems have also undergone transformation, and continue to evolve. Amongst the few unintended negative social impact of this overall positive trend has been, the phenomenal increase in the number of PMIs with SMDs on the streets of major cities, towns and even smaller places. The nuclearization of families and other changing socioeconomic realities has further contributed to the problem of homeless populations in general, including the homeless PMIs. The service needs for these populations, the large gaps therein, and the pockets of interest from different quarters have led to some innovations, despite inherent limitations at many levels in the Policy, the Law and the Programs.

BACKGROUND

The initial development of mental health services in the first few decades of immediate postindependence India had been on sequential developments of expansion of the General Hospital Psychiatry Units (GHPUs) mainly with academic departments, increasing the number of postgraduate courses' seats in Psychiatry, reform of a few "mental hospitals", slow but steady growth of the private sector, and the launch of the National Mental Health Programme (NMHP) in 1982. The NMHP, despite its broad and ambitious conceptual framework for "reaching the unreached", did not have any recognition of the need for mental health services for the destitute or homeless persons with mental illness (HPMIs) on the streets. Indeed, the Indian Lunacy Act of

1912 which continued to govern and regulate the mental health services till 1980s not only used the term "wandering lunatics" for these persons but also carried the approach of seeing these persons as criminals or at least social "nuisance". The much awaited reformative Mental Health Act of 1987 did improve the nomenclature to "mentally ill persons" alongside improvement in many such other terms, but continued to see the need for intervention only in situations of such a person if "found wandering" or believed "to be dangerous". Although the 1987 Act provided for the mentally ill persons being taken into protection, the tacit assumption, it can be surmised, had been that such persons be taken up for treatment more for the society's need, as compared to any societal obligation toward such PMIs. In actual practice, the implementation of the provisions of the act, in the absence of a "care" model or a *rights*-based approach, and due to lack of any operationalization became more for protecting the society than the concerned PMI. As part of a public interest litigation (PIL), for *homeless populations with mental illnesses*, the Hon'ble High Court of Delhi had ensured that the police headquarters issues a standard operating procedure (SOP) for the police personnel, with specific guidelines for a more proactive orientation to the role of the police for HPMIs and homebound PMIs. The availability of this SOP did help a little, but largely the "blind spot" in policy, legislation, and program remained quite reflective of the social attitudes toward all mental illnesses and persons afflicted by these, more so for those with disabling and visibly unpleasant *severe mental disorders* (SMDs) (seen as psychoses in that time), even more so for those persons with such problems who happened to be on the streets. The Mental Health Policy document of 2014 makes some pertinent observations about the social reality of mentally ill homeless populations, although there are no specific recommendations.[1]

SOCIAL REALITY

The negative attitudes in the society toward PMIs get reflected in many ways, not only with disregard for their *rights* but also by active discrimination and marginalization. The frequent prevalent pattern of depicting PMIs in popular media such as films and television in highly distorted negative light is also the other almost ubiquitous experience of anyone or of any such PMI at the street corner or on the roads, being chased by a group of children often throwing stones and indulging in other means of ridicule. The sight of a haggard and weather-beaten person wearing rags and with extremely poor hygiene, clearly not aware of the miserable living conditions around, evoking sympathy or pity from onlookers is not an uncommon sight or memory of any sensitive citizen, specially in urban and semiurban areas. Some decades ago, one may have come across such HPMIs occasionally in small cities or townships, and possibly in hundreds or thousands in major cities or megalopolises; by now in the 21st century, this phenomenon has not only increased exponentially but also assumed alarming proportions.

MAGNITUDE OF THE NEED FOR SERVICES

Although reliable scientific or epidemiological estimation is difficult and unavailable, the next best manner of assessing the extent of the problem is collective population estimates by consensus amongst the teams and agencies working on the issue. One recent nationwide consultation and review of almost all such programs placed the magnitude of the problem of HPMIs at minimally 1–2 lakhs (hundred thousand) persons in the country and could be much larger even up to 3 lakhs. The specific provision of mental health care as a right in the Mental Healthcare Act (MHA) of 2017, implemented from May 2018, requires that more specific and assertive attention be paid to the service needs of all unreached PMIs, specially those on the streets and in homeless situations.[2]

SERVICE INITIATIVES FOR HOMELESS PERSONS WITH MENTAL ILLNESS IN MAJOR CITIES

No sensitive person in any part of the world could have been left untouched or can remain unaffected at the sight of HPMI on the streets. There have been notable and praiseworthy initiatives for HPMIs, from nongovernmental organization (NGO) teams and sensitive mental health professionals as well as recovering PMIs, notwithstanding the policy gap. The turn of the century and the two decades after that have seen different programs in some of the major cities across the country, following the pioneering initiatives by a few sensitive individuals in major cities such as Mumbai (then Bombay) and Chennai (then Madras) in the 1980s and 1990s for rescue and treatment of HPMIs, followed by similar programs in other megalopolises of Delhi, Kolkata, and Bengaluru in the early part of the 21st century. The earliest initiative came from Ramon Magsaysay Award winner of 2017, Dr Bharat Vatwani, a psychiatrist in Mumbai, in the form of Shraddha Rehabilitation Foundation way back in 1985, followed by The Banyan in Chennai by Vandana Gopikumar, a professional social worker, and Vaishnavi Jayakumar, a mental health activist. Similar initiative in Kolkata came from concerned citizens with support from local psychiatrists in the form of "Ishwar Sankalpa" in 2007, along with the support of NGO activists and a few socially committed psychiatrists such as Dr Prabir Paul and Dr RR Ghosh Roy.

Service Initiatives in Delhi, the National Capital

The national capital of Delhi had witnessed the first major initiative in 1992 by one NGO, Sudinalaya, sincerely working for prevention of human trafficking with the social commitment of a voluntary social worker Smt. Sreerupa Mitra Chaudhary. Her team used to rescue homeless, mentally ill women and provide shelter and treatment with the ultimate goal of rehabilitation. At the turn of the century, in 2000 a newly formed NGO "Aashray Adhikar Abhiyan (AAA)", working for the broad spectrum of rights of the homeless populations, approached Institute of Human Behaviour and Allied Sciences (IHBAS) for the PMIs in Delhi. An extensive field-based needs assessment study carried out by IHBAS and AAA in September, 2000 led to an *outreach service* being launched in the heart of the old city of Delhi, in Jama Masjid area the same year, which integrated mental health and substance abuse services with general health services at the street level in a low-cost model.[3,4] The experience of this initiative has continued for two decades leading to health services being delivered for homeless populations at one location, in Jama Masjid area which has the largest congregation of homeless populations. With the active support from the state agency for legal aid and the Delhi State Legal Services Authority (DSLSA), the treatment of homeless persons with SMDs became operational with legally sound procedure adopted by joint action of the NGO team, IHBAS hospital team, and the DSLSA legal team at the street level leading to treatment of such persons without hospitalization. The legally sound procedure was in accordance with the provisions of the Mental Health Act, 1987[5] (Sections 24, 25, and specifically 29), with follow-up care with active monitoring by the NGO teams. In the first year, it had been possible to treat 49 such persons,[6] and in the decade from 2009 to 2020 just before the pandemic, nearly 500 such persons. The initiative for community based treatment, quite similar to the community-based treatment order (CTO) substance use-related services, and indeed, general health services.

With the outreach mental health services for the homeless populations at Jama Masjid location, the basic idea had been incorporated as part of the NMHP/District Mental Health Programme (DMHP) components for the state of Delhi, with initiatives from IHBAS and concurrence of the state government and the central government. This had actually also been included in the final report of the evaluation of the DMHP submitted by the Indian Council of Market Research (ICMR) to the Ministry of Health and Family Welfare, Government of India in 2009.[7]

The other initiative by IHBAS was meant to reach out to PMIs in homeless situations beyond the one location of Jama Masjid and was started as a pilot in 2012, with two mobile mental health units (MMHUs), each comprising a mental health team with an ambulance for rescue and engagement of such persons with due clinical diligence and legally correct procedure. During the recent pandemic, this initiative has been extended to a network of eleven such units across the city-state of Delhi, with one team proposed to serve each district. This network, made operational in 2021, is mandated to provide rescue services for HPMIs and those in family settings as well as provide home based aftercare in suitable cases and crisis support/intervention. The experience generated from this innovative program can be suitably modified and adopted for other states.

RECENT DEVELOPMENTS
National Mental Health Policy 2014

The increasing realization and consistent advocacy from various groups has contributed to recognition of the need for services for homeless populations in the National Mental Health Policy of India published in 2014, citing the homeless populations as one of the *vulnerable populations*.

"There are several linkages between homelessness and mental ill-health. Homelessness can occur as an adverse consequence of mental health problem. Persons could either be abandoned by resource-poor, helpless or uncaring family or wander away in the absence of accessible and appropriate mental health care. Conversely, the stress of living on the streets and sleeping rough can contribute to the risk of developing mental health problem.

Person(s) with mental health problem, high support needs, and no caregivers (either due to death or abandonment by family or caregiver) are specially vulnerable. In the absence of existing caregivers, there is almost no provision for care and support of these persons."

(Ministry of Health and Family Welfare, Government of India, 2014— Paragraph 4.3.2, page 7 of the Policy Document)

These observations pertain more directly to the impact of homelessness on mental health, most commonly in terms of common mental disorders (CMDs) such as depression and anxiety disorders. The service needs of this kind can be seen as the issues of HPMIs, which may also include some persons with SMDs and substance use disorders, but largely would involve persons who can be expected to avail of the outreach services once these are made available. The other service need, even more difficult and less recognized, would include mentally ill homeless persons (MIHPs) rendered so mainly on account of SMDs as mentioned in the policy document. This service need would entail more proactive and intersectoral approach, fortunately with some very good demonstrable models across the country.

Mental Healthcare Act, 2017[8]

The new law for regulation of mental health services enacted in 2017, and implemented from May 2018, seems to continue the tradition of laying the large part of responsibility for engaging PMIs, specially those with SMDs on the local police—with similar and yet different provisions for those living with families at home, or in "private residence" in their jurisdiction (Section 101), and those "wandering at large" within the limits of the police station (Section 100). It is noteworthy that the law continues to use the term "wandering lunatic" reminiscent of the Indian Lunacy Act of 1912 and shies away from using the more empathic term "homeless" in the major provisions of this section specifically meant for such persons, except for the last two of the seven subsections, wherein the "wandering" person suddenly gets referred to as "homeless", although the terms "homeless" and "wandering" are referred to as almost synonymous, ignoring the fact that any person with SMD is most unlikely to be "wandering" of free will or choice and is ever so often in homeless situation because of the effects of the mental illness and/or the inconsiderate attitude of the society at large.

One positive aspect is that for HPMIs in the new law of 2017 the term "detention" has been dropped and the action by the local police for such persons is to be seen as being "taken under protection" as per the provisions under Section 100. The 1987 Act provided for "medical detention".

The most common interpretation for provisions for admission of a judicial order under Section 102, subsequent to action by the police under Section 100, is that these are similar to the provisions for persons taken for action under Section 101. There has been some difference of opinion across magisterial courts about this aspect and the provisions of Section 100(5) require to be interpreted and applied uniformly.

Section 100(5) provides that *"the medical officer in charge of the public mental health establishment shall be responsible for arranging the assessment of the person and the needs of the person with mental illness will be addressed as per other provisions of this Act as applicable in the particular circumstances".*

One interpretation of this provision is that in cases wherein the medical officer in charge of the public mental health establishment feels the necessity and/or appropriateness for an order by metropolitan/judicial magistrate, for admission of which the same can be requested. The other interpretation, on record by a few such courts in Delhi and possibly other states too, has been that there is no role for a court of law and the decision for admission can be made and should be made by the concerned medical officer in charge of public mental health establishment. This view negates the need for judicial oversight for admissions proposed to be made in such situations and has potentially dangerous implications for misuse of the provisions for admission to any public mental health establishment on gender-based or property-related considerations.

This and some other aspects about the ground level implementation of the provisions of the new law, i.e., MHA 2017, in general, and specifically about mental health services for HPMIs remain to be settled in due course. These can be expected to happen through case laws with time and/or through amendments.

It can be safely said that the new law, MHA 2017, for all the controversies it has generated and the aspirational and ambitious character, seems to be not so different from the previous law, MHA 1987. One glaring aspect is the lack of any provision other than the Section 100, which in itself is not too innovative or forward-looking, and a very few other provisions like the provision for use of ambulance services for PMIs. One of the most striking provisions in the legal obligation of the government for Universal Health Coverage (UHC), viz., *"right to access mental healthcare"* in Section 18 even ahead of any such legal provision for *"right to access healthcare"*. Keeping the larger dimensions of this provision aside, the applicability of this provision and the operationalization of this "right", by common sense as well as adequate data and experience generated till now, require specific attention to promotion of mental health services for homeless populations.

National Mental Health Programme-District Mental Health Programme (NMHP-DMHP): Latest Available Guidelines

The operationalization of the legal provisions as noted above can be reasonably expected to occur through the mental health program of the government. As it so happens, except for a few indirect references to the need for focusing on the homeless, very little seems to have translated to action points for mental health services for the homeless populations, in the NMHP or its major vehicle the DMHP. The NMHP in India having been among the first few such outreach programs in 1982, and the DMHP initiated in the 1990s, and by now claimed to cover all the districts across the nation, has been updated and revised from time to time incorporating the emerging mental health service needs. The last set of guidelines issued by the Ministry of Health and Family Welfare in 2015 has no mention of the need for outreach services for the HPMIs, while providing specific funding, howsoever minimal, for related needs like day care centers and residential care centers—the need assessment for such centers to be made based on long-stay patients (LSPs) in hospitals. The National Health Mission (NHM), the source for flexipool of funding for the NMHP, does refer to the need to cover vulnerable populations including the "homeless".

The promising possibility is for some level of mitigation of this gap, as part of the recent Tele-MANAS (Tele Mental Health Assistance and Networking Across States)[9] program of the Government of India, by National Institute of Mental Health and Neurosciences (NIMHANS), Bengaluru, with participation of the states and the union territories. The initial information, at least from a few states, is that the tele-counseling program recently initiated is open to being availed by homeless populations and service utilization trends seem encouraging. Some aspects of the mental health service needs of the homeless populations will be possible to be met with, although the

Tele-MANAS program or any other component of government-supported outreach will require to be fine-tuned to meet the service need of PMIs with SMDs, with its legal dimensions.

The utilization of mental health services provided through the routine DMHP activities and even the Tele-MANAS services with emerging innovations can be expected to occur in the HPMIs, but the approach required for the more "difficult to reach" PMIs who are rendered homeless or MIHPs with SMDs would have to be much more of the "assertive outreach".

RECENT REVIEW OF NATIONAL SCENARIO

Different models for intervention in different cities and states in the past few decades have attempted to reach out for providing services to the homeless populations, often being initiated and conducted by NGOs, occasionally in partnership with or cooperation from government organizations. The ongoing work in this area was discussed and reviewed recently in 2019 at a National Seminar organized by IHBAS and the State Mental Health Authority (SMHA) of Delhi, in partnership with the National Legal Services Authority (NALSA) with DSLSA and the Indian Psychiatric Society (IPS), supported the Delhi Psychiatric Society (DPS) and the Indian Association of Private Psychiatry (Delhi Chapter). The conclusions and the recommendations of this seminar with participation by psychiatrists and other mental health professionals as well as the NGO teams working in this area along with legal activists, judicial officers, and Hon'ble judges of the state high courts and Hon'ble Supreme Court, as officials of NALSA, DSLSA, and other state legal services authorities summarize the current situation and the recommendations as action points. Review of 12 such programs at this "National Seminar for Homeless and Other Unreached Persons with Mental Illnesses" has identified the essential components of "good practice" models.[2]

Conclusions and Recommendations of National Seminar

- The magnitude of the problem of HPMIs is estimated to be at least 10 lakh persons across the country, possibly much larger.
- The extent and magnitude of the problem of "homebound" PMIs could not even be estimated in numbers, but was agreed to be quite significant and perhaps even larger than the number of HPMIs.
- Routine practice of mental health as well as the legal provisions do not adequately address the needs of the HPMIs or the homebound PMIs and their families.
- The activities of the NMHP or its major vehicle for service delivery, viz., the DMHP tend to leave these PMIs largely unattended.

- Specific activities for homeless populations be encouraged to be incorporated in the implementation of NMHP/DMHP and be included in the national program.
- The problem of homelessness and PMIs needs to be recognized as being reciprocal and bidirectional. Quite a large part of PMIs being rendered homeless is due to deinstitutionalization, decreasing ability and/or willingness of families for long-term care of PMIs, and absence of alternative models for community-based living.
- At the same time, there are many PMIs who continue to live with their families in India often with adequate care, but equally crucial is the problem of homebound PMIs, contributed to by total lack of engagement in treatment or absence of long-term continuous care, leading to violation of *rights* of PMIs in family settings too.
- Long-stay homes and halfway home are still lacking in most parts of the country. There is an urgent need to encourage all forms of activities for aftercare homes and different models of community-based independent living and supported and assisted living.
- There is a widespread apprehension that the provisions of MHA, 2017 may further contribute to difficulties in engagement of PMIs in treatment as well as their long-term care, thus contributing to the problems of HPMIs and homebound PMIs.
- The provision of mental health care and protection of the rights of PMIs living in nonmental health residential care settings also need to be ensured, e.g., old age homes, homes for women, child care institutions (CCIs), prisons, etc.
- In accordance with the *priority areas* identified for NALSA in 2015, there is a huge potential role for legal services going beyond legal aid. A specific scheme needs to be developed for implementation. At the state level, the State Legal Services Authority (SLAs) and the SMHAs should collaborate with each other.
- Manual for police to be prepared for dealing with HPMI or homebound PMI.
- Manual to be prepared for judicial officers for appropriate implementation of MHA, 2017.
- All-round efforts need to be made for ensuring *civil, political,* and *economic rights* of PMIs, specially for homeless populations. Intersectoral coordination is necessary to be ensured, through administrative or judicial mechanisms.
- In the long-term, efforts need to be made not only to ensure mental health services for homeless populations with mental illnesses, and other unreached populations, but also for *prevention* of homelessness on account of mental illnesses.

- The *components of good practice models*, identified based on the *review* of experience till now, would be desirable to be followed for future endeavors.

Components of Good Practice Models

All programs reviewed and the models followed are found to carry the following components which are identified as *components of good practice models*.

- Community-based teams or organization, generally as NGO, either as the nodal agency or one of the active partners
- Intersectoral coordination across agencies being central to any proactive or assertive outreach program for HPMIs and homebound PMIs
- Active collaboration between community teams and mental health teams, with definitive role of the legal agencies
- Involvement of local police and civic administration
- Such coordination and collaboration being difficult but possible to be achieved with sustained effort
- Campaigns for increasing awareness and reducing the stigma associated with mental illnesses and PMIs as well as about the real situation about homelessness
- There is a need for residential services or inpatient services, in the program or as a backup service, with effective pharmacological and psychosocial components.
- Ongoing continuous efforts at rehabilitation and reintegration for family-based or community-based living are central to any such program, so as to avoid long-term stay or institutionalization.
- Regular sensitization for all categories of staff members and volunteers, for the nature of work required as well as for their own well-being

FUTURE DIRECTIONS

- *Gaps and possible actions at policy level:* The significant gaps at various levels for this mental health service need are important to be recognized and acted upon and to start with at the policy level. It is helpful that the National Mental Health Policy has recognized the issue of *homelessness*, and yet as discussed earlier, the policy document, but the need for more clear recognition of the need for more assertive outreach often with involuntary hospitalization or closely monitored community-based program is much higher, since it requires collaboration across teams in health, social, police, and judiciary.
- *Gaps and possible actions in the legal framework:* The new law, MHA 2017, is progressive inasmuch as it moves beyond the erstwhile provisions of those PMIs being taken into "medical custody", and yet is limited to the

extent that it now postulates PMIs who may be "incapable of taking care of themselves" to be taken into protective care; the entire responsibility is left to the local police. This provision while it may seem necessary for human rights concerns, the ground reality is that the police force with all their myriad responsibilities is neither able nor inclined to attend to the mental health needs as much as is appropriate.

- *Legal provision for CTO:* The situation of "difficult to reach" PMIs and the need for long-term treatment for effective stabilization would merit consideration of legal provisions and the idea of CTO, as is available in some countries.
- *Gaps and possible actions in the programs:* Based on the experience generated in Delhi as well as in other states, the NMHP and DMHP modules need to include the provision of assertive outreach for HPMIs. The obligation of the government for this group of the most disadvantaged and marginalized persons cannot be over emphasized.
- *Assertive mobile mental health services:* Cumulative experience across the country, in the past few decades has adequate basis for more assertive and mobile mental health services for the rescue and engagement of HPMIs as well as the other equally difficult group of "homebound" PMIs. The MMHU model followed in Delhi or a suitable variant of that would seem necessary in an intersectoral mode, with more direct responsibility being taken by the public sector in mental health.

The dehumanizing condition of homeless populations is starting to get its due attention and within that larger concern, there needs to be specific effort to ensure that the now legally provided *right to access mental healthcare* accrues to the group of persons who are arguably the most marginalized population group in the larger policies and programs for the disadvantaged populations. On the other hand, all parts of the mental health service sector and specifically the government sector also need to recognize and respond to this heretofore neglected group.

In summary, this collective *blind spot* of a fundamental service need deserves to get much more emphasis than it has as a basic humanitarian consideration.

CONCLUSION

The public health approach to mental health, has its own set of priorities; and recent advances which require to be understood and applied. The mental health services for homeless populations is one such final frontier to be addressed. The logical sequential step to the strategy of deinstitutionalization, has to be "prevention of hospitalization", and indeed prevention of homelessness on account of mental illness. The larger phenomenon of homelessness and the movement for the Rights of these populations surely needs intersectionality, but even the smaller but more compelling issue of ensuring comprehensive mental health services for homeless populations, deserves to be seen in the larger perspective. The much acclaimed provision of Right to Access Mental Healthcare, already in place in the Indian Law, and likely to become a reality in most parts of the World, might face its toughest challenge in the context of the homeless populations. The manner in which mental health professionals, including psychiatrists, respond to this challenge, with willingness to step out of the confines of their sphere of work, may well contribute to the further advancement and acceptance of the discipline of mental health. The relatively small in size, and yet robust experience in India in the last few decades in this area, has the potential to be upscaled to reach all those in need, and also provide a framework for such programs in other countries across the World.

TAKE-HOME POINTS

- Routine clinical work of mental health professionals, including psychiatrists, does not make them aware of the reality of homeless persons with mental illness (PMIs), although it is becoming a major challenge for public mental health.
- Initiatives for services for homeless mentally ill persons, have emanated from individual psychiatrists, mental health teams from institutions, NGOs and social sector organizations, with or without involvement of legal entities/ judicial bodies.
- Some demonstrable models of care have been established in different locations, with identifiable components of good practice.
- There is scope and potential for many more initiatives as per local situation and in context of the needs.
- There is some increasing recognition of the issue in mental health policy, law and the programs, and yet the blind spot remains in actual meaningful action points.
- Services for homeless mentally ill persons, need to be integrated with the Government's mental health programs.
- Assertive outreach services, including mobile services for rescue and engagement, need to be in place for effectively ensuring the Right to Access Mental Healthcare.
- Prevention of homelessness on account of mental illness can be next level of goal setting.
- On all counts, mental health services for homeless populations should be a priority.

REFERENCES

1. Ministry of Health and Family Welfare. (2014). New Pathways New Hope: National Mental Health Policy of India. [online] Available from https://nhm.gov.in/images/pdf/National_Health_Mental_Policy.pdf [Last accessed May, 2023].
2. Desai NG, Singh V, Jahanara MG, Yannavar P (2019). Report of National Seminar for Homeless and Other Unreached Persons with Mental Illnesses (PMIs) by IHBAS and Delhi SMHA, with NALSA & DSLSA with DPS and IAPP (Delhi Chapter), IHBAS, Delhi.
3. Desai NG, Kaur P, Bhardwaj J, Singh N, Singh IP, Selhore N, et al. Health Care Beyond Zero—Ensuring a Basic Right for the Homeless, Delhi. Aashray Adhikar Abhiyaan (AAA) Delhi. 2003.

4. Desai NG, Shivalkar R, Kuar P, Jahanara MG, Kumar S, Tripathi CB, et al. (2008). Situation Analysis of Homeless Women in Delhi with special reference to Mental Health and Psychosocial Aspects. Study Carried out by IHBAS for National Commission for Women (NCW), IHBAS, Delhi.
5. Ministry of Health and Family Welfare. (1987). Mental Health Act of India. [online] Available from https://lddashboard.legislative.gov.in/sites/default/files/A1987-14.pdf [Last accessed May, 2023].
6. Desai NG, Kaur P, Menon A, Shivalkar R, Kumar P, Kumar S, Yadav A. (2010). Intersectoral Joint Initiative by IHBAS, AAA & DLSA for Treatment of Homeless Persons with Severe Mental Illness: Making a Difference. IHBAS, Delhi.
7. Indian Council of Market Research (ICMR) (2009). Evaluation of the District Mental Health Porgramme: Final Report Submitted to the Ministry of Health and Family Welfare, Govt of India, Delhi.
8. Ministry of Health and Family Welfare. (2017). Mental Healthcare Act, 2017. [online] Available from https://egazette.nic.in/WriteReadData/2017/175248.pdf [Last accessed May, 2023].
9. Ministry of Health and Family Welfare. (2022). Tele MANAS Programme. [online] Available from https://telemanas.mohfw.gov.in/#/home [Last accessed May, 2023].

CHAPTER 15

Cyberpsychiatry

Rajarshi Chakravarty, Subir Bhattacharjee, Arabinda Brahma

INTRODUCTION

Cyber space is presently our new society. Constantly changing technology, internet, and newer application platforms are giving us new ways of living and interacting with the virtual world. How we behave and interact in web space and how it changes or shapes our future behavior, is a bidirectional phenomenon that needs to be understood and studied, presently emerging as a newer area of psychiatry, called cyberpsychiatry.

CYBER SPACE AND PSYCHIATRY: A BIDIRECTIONAL RELATIONSHIP

First Direction: How Internet affects our Mental Health?

The importance of Internet in our lives today cannot be undermined. But excessive use of Internet can almost present with various psychological disorders ranging from anxiety, depression, sleep disorder, and even substance dependence-like issues.

The Internet Use Disorder can be studied in the following headings: (1) Social Media, (2) Cybersex and Internet Pornography, (3) Information overload, and (4) Internet Gaming Disorder.

Impact of Social Media on Mental Health

It is very difficult nowadays to imagine a day, leave alone a life without interacting in social media. Platforms like Orkut have become defunct while others like Facebook, Instagram, and others are expanding and are widely popular.

Facebook is by far one the most popular social media platform with 1.7 billion monthly users and 1.1 billion logins/day in 2016. The area of concern is 71% of adolescents aged 13-17 years age use Facebook.[1]

- An estimated 28% of all time online is spent on social networking. Indians on an average spend 2.4 h/day on social networking sites.

- 22% of teens log on to a social media site more than 10 times a day, and more than half of adolescents log on to a social media site more than once a day.
- In 2014, Facebook estimated that the average user spends 8.3 hours a month on the site.
- A study found out that "Facebook chatting", "wall posting", and "picture uploading" were the modes preferred by young Facebook users.

Advantages: Advantages include creativity, content sharing, learning, social support, and increasing communication.[1]

Disadvantages: Disadvantages include Facebook addiction (FAD)[1] and Facebook intrusion disorder.[1] Symptoms include thinking about Facebook while not using it, being unable to reduce screen time and feeling of distress when offline. Other psychosocial problems include increased feeling of isolation, increased jealousy, and dissatisfaction with intimate relationships, low self-esteem, fear of missing out (FOMO), depression and anxiety, and poor quality of sleep. A report by American Academy of Pediatrics stated that Facebook use can lead to depression.[1] Instagram use has often been associated with worsening of bulimia and negative body images.[2]

Causes: Sriwilai et al. showed that lower mindfulness and use of emotion-focused coping are correlated with FAD.[3] Brailovskaia et al. found that FAD was positively correlated with trait narcissism and negative mental health variable (depression and anxiety).[4] Casale et al. found out Narcissism needing admiration correlated positively with FAD.[5] Another study found high prevalence of social anxiety in Facebook users and positive correlation of scores with FAD rating scales.[6]

Cybersex Addiction

A working definition of cybersex addiction should include symptoms like loss of control, preoccupation, withdrawal, and continuous engagement in online sexual activities despite negative consequences.[7] Cybersex has a bigger implication: internet pornography, searching sexual information, sex-toys, as well as sexual partners on the web.[7] It is not related to hypersexuality/sexual addiction as it deals with online sexual activities only.[7]

The impact can be threefold: socio-interpersonal, psychological, and legal.

Socio-interpersonal: For married people cybersex addiction can adversely impact their spouse and children. A study from Indonesia showed that 22.3% of partners considered divorce or separation because of cybersex as they felt ignored, rejected, and lost faith on their partners after knowing they were using cybersex. 68% complained decreased interest in sexual activity as they felt weak in comparison to the people shown on cybersex. Another important consideration is the impact of children who may accidentally see the sites or see parents masturbating. As a consequence of this addiction, children are often neglected and abused. Children exposed to such content may become traumatized, abusive, and addiction prone. It impairs their social and sexual development as they have unrealistic expectation from their future partners. The addicted person may also lose close friends or relatives who disapprove these activities.

Psychological: Squirrell[8] researched 1,325 people of the United States and Australia, who spent 12 hours a week related to online sexual activity. The study showed that 27% of subjects experienced severe depression, 30% experienced high anxiety, and 35% felt depressed with their activities. The severity to depression and anxiety correlated directly with amount of time spent on cybersex activities. Boies et al.[9] surveyed students in 2004 and found that students not involved in cybersex had higher social and environmental support than students who used the internet to satisfy their sexual needs.

Legal consequences: Online pornography can increase sexual aggression by as much as four times that leads to violent sexual practices and subsequent incarceration. Preoccupation with cybersex may cause loss of job. People may lose lots of money on online sexual intimacy platforms and thus resort to criminal activities to continue cybersex. Cyber stalking is another criminal activity which is a direct result of cybersex.

Information Overload

Overload describes an individual's subjective perception and evaluation of the number of information, people, or objects that are beyond one's capability to process.[10]

Here the information accessed by individual is beyond his scope of processing or accommodating it.[11] Students may be subjected to information overload as a result of teaching curriculum. It can occur across various other domains besides social media such as online shopping, online healthcare information searches, and mobile technologies. Online healthcare information searches are particularly relevant in this COVID-19 era. People who have lower health literacy or confidence in health information seeking express greater information overload as regards to COVID-19 pandemic. Those who suffer from information overload go through Heuristic processing (superficial, not critically examined) and can be subjected to severe anxiety and may also spread rumours. Jacoby et al. found that performance at first increases amongst them, but decreases drastically soon after as the information overload occurs.[12] All this may lead to Internet discontinuation or website anxiety and cause severe stain in users reduce cognitive thresholds and lower ability to process new information.

Internet Gaming Disorder

Often occurs in conjunction with social media use (use of same virtual interaction in multiple player formats) and augments its effects on mental health. Though it may contribute to cognitive functioning, various reports are coming up on resultant dysfunctional behavior. Users develop tolerance and withdrawal and even deceive others about time spent on games thus suggesting it is a behavioral addiction.

Study showed that social media use correlated positively with gaming disorder with social media use. Male gender and younger age were identifiable risk factors. Gaming disorders seemed to exacerbate symptoms of depression, anxiety, and stress thereby forming a vicious cycle. The effects were more significant when compared with the effect of social media use.[13] An Iranian study[14] revealed that Internet gaming was causing increased prevalence of insomnia and obesity in adolescents.

Reverse-direction: How Psychiatric Disorders affect Internet Use?

Schizophrenia and Psychosis

Interpersonal relationship difficulty is a key feature of schizotypal personality disorder and they have been found to use the Internet with a particular interest in social interaction on the web. Schizophrenia patients also show marked social anxiety and they found internet social platforms as an easier way for communication.[15] Another study found that they value and use Internet like general population, with the same advantages of easy and quick access, broad spectrum of available information, and the anonymity of Internet use without feeling devalued or unsafe.[16] But due to attention deficit and delusional interpretations sometimes it become difficult to use Internet freely.[17] They often access to a certain amount of information as reasonable and guard themselves against excess information. They showed some ambivalence regarding the need for information and also struggled to achieve a subjectively adequate distance from illness-related topics.[16]

Depression

Researchers found that people with depression tend to express their needs on internet implicitly, frequently disclosing personal problems, and indirectly asking for help on social media.

In online support groups, they seek more emotional-support content compared to nonterminal physical conditions.[18] Depression often co-occurs with internet addiction and vice-versa. Low self-esteem, low motivation, social avoidance, and fear of negative evaluation in depressed patients lead to excessive and addictive usage of internet in them.[19]

Bipolar Disorder

Researchers found that one in five patients with bipolar disorder (BD) screened positive for problematic use of internet (PUI). They found a significant association between PUI and lifetime traumatic events and highlighted the relevance of the comorbidity between post-traumatic stress disorders and PUI in subjects with BD.[20]

CONCLUSION

- The importance and contribution of cyber-world in our day-to-day lives cannot be overlooked.
- A lot of time and emotions have been invested on social media platforms. While there are some good effects of social media, some mental health issues are coming up like Facebook Addiction and Facebook Intrusion Disorder. These are accompanied by anxiety, depression, loss of sleep and self-esteem and jealousy. Instagram can lead to body image disturbances.
- Other problems include online pornography which cause breakdown of marriage/relationships, parental neglect as well as major depressive and anxiety disorder as psychological fallout. The legal consequences include stalking, stealing of money and other information by blackmailing victim.
- Covid-19 added a unique problem of information overload especially in those with poor health literacy. This can lead to severe anxiety, Internet stoppage and spreading of rumors.
- Internet gaming is also common among young males. It increases anxiety and depression and shows tolerance, thereby proving to be a variant of behavioral addiction.
- Last but not least, interaction between mental health and cyberworld is bidirectional. Depressed and anxious people are particularly prone to social media and pornographic addiction. Some trait narcissism were also observed among social media users.
- Psychotic people tend to collect information according to their delusional beliefs and that may aggravate illness. As they perform poorly on direct social interaction they tend to use social media more.

TAKE-HOME POINTS

- Cyber space is presently our new society, and there is significant increase in daily-use time.
- A bidirectional relationship exists between cyber space and psychiatry.
- Excessive use of Internet has various psychological consequences ranging from anxiety, depression, sleep disorder, and even substance dependence-like issues.
- The impact of cybersex addiction can be threefold: Socio-interpersonal, psychological, and legal.
- Information overload can cause severe anxiety in students.
- Social media overuse has positive correlation with internet gaming disorder.
- Schizophrenic patients though use Internet like others but often guard themselves from excessive information and disease-related information.
- Depressive patients seek more emotional-support content on social platforms.

REFERENCES

1. Adriana K. Facebook Use and Negative Behavioral and Mental Health Outcomes: A Literature Review. J Addict Res. 2018;10(1):375.
2. Padalino F, Camerini A. Instagram use and Body Dissatisfaction—The Mediating Role of Upward Social Comparison with Peers and Influencers among Young Females. Int J Environ Res Public Health. 2022;19:1543.
3. Sriwilai K, Charoensukmongol P. Face it, don't Facebook it: Impacts of social media addiction on mindfulness, coping strategies and the consequence on emotion exhaustion. Stress Health. 2015;32:427-34.
4. Brailovskaia J, Magraf J. Facebook addiction disorder among German students—a longitudinal approach. Plos One. 2017;12:1-15.
5. Casale S, Fioravanti G. Why narcissists are at risk for developing Facebook Addiction: The need to be admired and the need to belong. Addict Behav. 2018;76:312-18.
6. Shaw A, Timpano K, Tran T, Joorman J. Correlates of facebook usage patterns: The relationships between passive facebook use, social anxiety symptoms and brooding. Comput Ham Behav. 2015;48:575-80.
7. Snagowski J, Brand M. Symptoms of cybersex addiction can be linked to both approaching and avoiding pornographic stimuli: results from an analog sample of regular cybersex users. Front Psychol. 2015;6:653.
8. Squirrell M. Psychological characteristics of individuals who engage in online sexual activity (OSA). 2011.
9. Boies SC, Cooper A, Osborne CS. Variation in internet-related problems and psychosocial functioning in online sexual activities: implications for social and sexual development of young adults. Cyberpsychol Behav. 2004;7(2):207-30.
10. Saegart S. Cognitive overload and behavioral constraint. Environ Design Res. 1973;2:254-60.
11. Farhoomand A, Drury DH. Managerial information overload. Commun ACM. 2002;45(10):127-31.
12. Jacoby J, Speller DE, Kohn CA. Brand choice behaviour as a function of information load. J Market Res. 1971;11(1):63-9.

13. Pontes HM. Investigating the differential effects of social networking site addiction and Internet Gaming Disorder on Psychological Health. J Behav Addict. 2017;6(4):601-10.
14. Zamani E, Hedayati N. Effect of Addiction to Computer Games on Physical and Mental Health of Female and Male Students of Guidance School in city of Isfahan. Addict Health. 2009 Fall;1(2):98-104.
15. Mittal VA, Tessner KD, Walker EF. Elevated social Internet use and schizotypal personality disorder in adolescents. Schizophr Res. 2007;94(1-3):50-7.
16. Schrank B, Sibitz I, Unger A, Amering M. How Patients With Schizophrenia Use the Internet: Qualitative Study. J Med Internet Res. 2010;12(5): e70.
17. Kalk NJ, Pothier DD. Patient information on schizophrenia on the Internet. Psychiatric Bulletin. 2008;32:409-11.
18. Deetjen U, Powell, JA. Informational and Emotional Elements in Online Support Groups: A Bayesian Approach to Large-Scale Content Analysis. J Am Med Inform Assoc. 2016;23:508-13.
19. Yang CK, Choe BM, Baity M, Lee JH, Cho JS. SCL-90-R and 16PF profiles of senior high school students with excessive internet use. Can J Psychiatry. 2005;50:407-14.
20. Carmassi C, Bertelloni CA, Cordone A, Dell'Oste V, Pedrinelli V, Barberi FM, et al. Problematic Use of the Internet in Subjects with Bipolar Disorder: Relationship with Posttraumatic Stress Symptoms. Front Psychiatry. 2021;12:646385.

CHAPTER 16

Recent Indian Laws in Psychiatry

Raveesh BN, Guru S Gowda, Ravindra Neelakanthappa Munoli

INTRODUCTION

India's judicial procedure and administration date back to 400 BC with Arthashastra and 100 AD with Manusmriti. In Ancient India, Law was considered to be a religious prescription. This custom was disrupted when the British imposed uniform English laws in India. Currently, many of the laws enacted by the British are still in effect in India. As a result, the foundations of most legislation in general, as well as respect for people with mental illnesses (PMIs), may be traced back to British times.[1] Following India's independence, the Mental Health Act of 1987 and the Persons with Disability Act of 1995 were enacted to take care of PMIs. Furthermore, after India signed the United Nations Convention on the Rights of Persons with Disabilities (UNCRPD) in 2008, it became mandatory to amend all disability legislation to bring it in line with the UNCRPD.[2] As a result, this millennium has seen the enactment of the Rights of Persons with Disabilities Act, 2016 (RPWD Act, 2016) and the Mental Healthcare Act, 2017 (MHCA, 2017). The RPWD Act, 2016 and MHCA, 2017 emphases have moved to the protection of PMIs and their rights in society. Additionally, the chapter will focus on the Juvenile Justice (Care and Protection of Children) Act of 2015; the Protection of Children from Sexual Offences (POCSO) Act of 2012; the Digital Information Security in Healthcare Act of 2018; and Telemedicine Practice Guidelines 2020 and their relevance to psychiatric practice

THE RIGHTS OF PERSONS WITH DISABILITIES ACT, 2016

The Persons with Disability Act of 1995 was limited to seven disabilities like blindness, low vision, hearing impairment, cured leprosy, mental retardation, and mental illness. It was based on medical model and did not emphasize the right of a person with a disability. The RPWD Act, 2016 was based on biopsychosocial model and increased disability conditions from 7 to 21. The RPWD Act, 2016 covers people with cerebral palsy, dwarfism, muscular dystrophy, chronic neurological disorders (like Parkinson's disease and multiple sclerosis), blood disorders (like hemophilia, thalassemia, and sickle cell disease), acid attack victims, speech and language disability, and intellectual disability (ID), which includes specific learning disability (SLD) and an autism spectrum disorder.[3] This has made it possible for more people with disability conditions to receive welfare benefits under the Act. Furthermore, the RPWD Act, 2016 is more focused on the rights of people with disabilities, appointing a limited guardian and a push for an inclusive approach in higher education, vocational training, agricultural land, housing, self-employment, and Job by increasing reservations to 5% and supportive accommodation.[4,5]

THE MENTAL HEALTHCARE ACT, 2017

The Mental Healthcare Act, which the government passed in 2017, was seen as a good step toward helping the millions of people with mental illness in India. It aims to protect, advance, and uphold the rights of people with mental illness and make it the state's responsibility to provide its citizens with affordable mental health care at the community level.[6] The most important changes in MHCA, 2017 are the right of a person with mental illness, advance directive, nominated representative, and setting up mental health authority at central and state levels and review board at the district level. The heart and soul of the MHCA, 2017 is the right of a person with mental illness. These include:

- Everyone has the right to access mental health care and treatment.
- Government-run or -funded mental health services should be available and accessible at the community level.
- Everyone with a mental illness has the right to live with dignity.
- People who are mentally ill should not be treated differently because of their gender, race, religion, culture, sexual orientation, caste, social class, disability, or political views.
- Its emphasis is on the right to privacy when it comes to a person's mental health, treatment, mental health care, and physical health care.
- Make it illegal to use a picture or other information about a person with mental illness in the media without that person's permission.
- The right to choose the person who would be responsible for making decisions about his care and hospital admission.
- People with mental illness will also be protected from cruel and degrading treatment.
- A person with a mental illness who is homeless and below the poverty line gets free care and treatment.

Advance directive: A person with a mental illness who is major (18 years) can decide how their condition will be treated in the future by placing their wishes in writing, as well as whom they want to nominate as representative. The advance directive should be signed by a doctor or registered with the Mental Health Review Board.

A nominated representative is a major (18 years), related by blood or adoption, friend, or appointed by mental health review board (MHRB) to make treatment decisions for a person with mental illness when the patient cannot make decisions on their own.

Mental health authority: This Act gives the government the power to set up the Central Mental Health Authority at the national level and the State Mental Health Authority in each State.

Decriminalizing suicide: The MHCA presumes suicide attempters are assumed to be under much stress. MHCA directs the government to offer care, treatment, and rehabilitation to lessen the risk of recurrence rather than a fine and simple prison sentence that could last up to a year as per Section 309 of the Indian Penal Code. This medicalization and decriminalization of suicide aids the individual in seeking help and improve epidemiological data, planning, and resource allocation. This is one of the landmark steps in the MHCA.[7]

Prohibitions: The MHCA, 2017 restricts procedures such as sterilization (of men or women used to treat mental illness), unmodified electroconvulsive therapy (ECT), seclusion, and chaining. This Act also sets rules for researching PMI and using restraints and neurosurgical therapy.

THE JUVENILE JUSTICE (CARE AND PROTECTION OF CHILDREN) ACT, 2015

This law was enacted in 2015 for children (less than 18 years of age) who have alleged and found to conflict with the law and as well as Juvenile Justice (JJ) Act looks into children in need of care and protection by catering to their basic needs through proper care, protection, development, treatment, social reintegration, by adopting a child-friendly approach in the adjudication.[8] There is a link between the mental health of children who break the law and the bad things they do. This could be because they are both more likely to get sick or because one illness makes the other worse. If you do not deal with these interconnected factors, you end up with repeat offences and bad functional outcomes. So, it is essential to help these young people with their mental health needs.

Similarly, children who are in trouble with the law or need care and protection are more likely to have mental health and substance use problems. In the same way, children with mental health problems are more likely to get into trouble with the juvenile justice system. Unfortunately, people who care for these kids in observation homes or child care centers are often not trained or skilled, and they do not get enough help from mental health professionals (MHPs) to understand and meet the psychological needs of these kids. In some ways, this is also true for the people on the justice system board and the officers of the district's child police protection unit. This is a big problem on the way to giving holistic and complete care to all kids who come into contact with the juvenile justice system. The JJ of 2015 gives this issue the attention it deserves. It says that no social worker can be appointed to the JJ Board or the Child Welfare Committee (CWC) unless they have experience in education or a degree in child psychology, psychiatry, sociology, or law and are working as a professional. There are bidirectional connections between the juvenile justice system and the mental health of the children involved. Following are the places where there is a role of MHP for children.

- The JJ Act of 2015 mandates a preliminary assessment of the mental and physical capacity of a 16–18-year-old juvenile who is accused of committing a serious offence.
- JJ board can also ask for the help of mental health specialists to receive the proper care, treatment, and psychosocial reintegration.
- MHPs play a crucial role in addressing the mental health issues of orphan children both before and after adoption.
- Similarly to the MHCA, the JJ Act of 2015 necessitates juveniles in contact with or likely to come into contact with juvenile justice system to maintain their confidentiality.

Aside from their role as above roles in the juvenile justice system, MHPs can make a big difference in the areas of prevention, therapy, and rehabilitation.[9]

THE PROTECTION OF CHILDREN FROM SEXUAL OFFENCES ACT, 2012

The POCSO Act was passed in 2012 and is a landmark law against child sexual abuse in India.[10] The POCSO Act says that anyone younger than 18 years is a child and protects all children from sexual assault, sexual harassment, and pornography.[11] It makes heinous crimes against children under the age of 18 years a crime and gives offenders harsh punishments. The salient points of the POCSO Act and its relevance to psychiatric practice are:

- An MHP has a legal obligation to disclose to the state, particularly minors who have been sexually assaulted and come to the therapeutic alliance by violating the privacy, confidentiality, and autonomy.
- The state must establish Special Courts, and the cases registered under POCSO case should be tried in a Special Court.
- To protect the privacy of a child and his/her family, the law prohibits the disclosure of a child's identity, including his name, address, photograph, family details, school, neighbourhood, or any other particulars that may lead to the disclosure of a child's identity in any media report, without the permission of the Court.
- If the offence was committed, attempted, or is likely to be committed by a person living in the same or shared household with the child, CWC

would decide within 3 days whether the child needs to be removed from the custody of his family or shared household and placed in a children's home or a shelter home.
- The judge of the Special Court can ask MHP to help with the case as an expert witness.

Parents or the child's primary caretaker (if the parents are not around) must be told about the abuse and how it affects the child,[12] and a third party (like the police, CWC, or the Court) must get involved, it breaks up the therapeutic relationship and the trust and confidence that have been built up in the care.[13] In India, the social, religious, and (traditionally) stereotypical ways of doing things make it hard to accept, report, or get help for sexual abuse.

DIGITAL INFORMATION SECURITY IN HEALTHCARE ACT, 2018

The main goal of this Act is to protect, secure, and standardize digital health information. This Act controls how digital health data connected to personally perceptible information is made, collected, stored, sent, and accessed. It keeps track of all the health information about a person's physical and mental health, as well as the health services they have received, any body parts or bodily substances they have donated, any testing or examination of a body part or bodily substance, information gathered while giving health services, and information about any clinical facility they have visited.[14]

TELEMEDICINE PRACTICE GUIDELINES 2020

In India, telemedicine practice guidelines give a framework for the telemedicine practice of medicine. On May 12, 2020, the government published its rules in the gazette.[15] The Indian Medical Council (Professional Conduct, Etiquette, and Ethics) Regulations, 2002 include the "Telemedicine Practice Guidelines" as "Appendix 5". However, it is also clear that these rules do not apply when digital technology is used to do surgery or other invasive procedures remotely. Even though the current telemedicine rules in India are incomplete, they could be used as a place to start. They have tried to ensure that teleconsultation services are already available in India.[16]

Popular platforms like WhatsApp, Facebook, and Skype can be used for telepsychiatry consultations because the Telemedicine Practice Guidelines 2020 allow it. However, the patient and the psychiatrist must feel safe and respect their privacy. Therefore, for any information, like a summary, pictures, audio recordings, or video recordings, to be posted or shared, the patients must give their written, informed consent. However, psychiatrists should not do this, and patients should be told not to record or transfer any part of the consultation process or content in the media or social networks.[17]

CONCLUSION

Indian laws and mental health interphase are common. In this millennium, the RPWD Act, 2016; the MHCA, 2017; the Juvenile Justice (Care and Protection of Children) Act of 2015; the POCSO Act of 2012; the Digital Information Security in Healthcare Act of 2018; and Telemedicine Practice Guidelines 2020 have all had a strong influence on psychiatric practice. This ranges from child care and protection to ensuring the safety and confidentiality of a child, a person with mental illness, and advocating right person with mental illness. Additionally, Telemedicine Practice Guidelines 2020 and the Digital Information Security in Healthcare Act of 2018 gave a legal framework practice of psychiatry in an online platform.

TAKE-HOME POINTS

- The RPWD Act, 2016 and MHCA, 2017 emphases on protection of PMIs and their rights in society.
- The RPWD Act, 2016 was based on biopsychosocial model and include 21 disability conditions.
- The RPWD Act, 2016 provides the framework for guardianship for person with mental disability.
- The MHCA, 2017 restricts procedures such as sterilization, unmodified electroconvulsive therapy (ECT), seclusion, and chaining.
- The JJ Act of 2015 mandates a preliminary assessment of the mental and physical capacity of a 16–18-year-old juvenile who is accused of committing a serious offence.
- Popular platforms like WhatsApp, Facebook, and Skype can be used for telepsychiatry consultations under the Telemedicine Practice Guidelines 2020.

REFERENCES

1. Narayan CL, Shikha D. Indian legal system and mental health. Indian J Psychiatry. 2013;55(Suppl 2):S177-81.
2. WHO. (2006). Convention on the Rights of Persons with Disabilities. [online] Available from https://www.ohchr.org/en/instruments-mechanisms/instruments/convention-rights-persons-disabilities [Last accessed March, 2023].
3. The Rights of Persons with Disabilities Act, 2016. [online] Available from https://legislative.gov.in/actsofparliamentfromtheyear/rights-persons-disabilities-act-2016 [Last accessed March, 2023].
4. Balakrishnan A, Kulkarni K, Moirangthem S, Kumar CN, Math SB, Murthy P. The Rights of Persons with Disabilities Act 2016: Mental Health Implications. Indian J Psychol Med. 2019;41(2):119-25.
5. Narayan CL, John T. The Rights of Persons with Disabilities Act, 2016: Does it address the needs of the persons with mental illness and their families. Indian J Psychiatry. 2017;59(1):17-20.
6. The Mental Healthcare Act, 2017. [online] Available from https://www.indiacode.nic.in/bitstream/123456789/2249/1/A2017-10.pdf. [Last accessed March, 2023].

7. Sneha V, Madhusudhan S, Prashanth NR, Chandrashekar H. Decriminalization of suicide as per Section 115 of Mental Health Care Act 2017. Indian J Psychiatry. 2018;60(1):147-8.
8. The Juvenile Justice (Care and Protection of Children) ACT, 2015. [online] Available from https://cara.nic.in/PDF/JJ%20act%202015.pdf [Last accessed March, 2023].
9. Snehil G, Sagar R. Juvenile Justice System, Juvenile Mental Health, and the Role of MHPs: Challenges and Opportunities. Indian J Psychol Med. 2020;42(3):304-10.
10. The Protection of Child Sexual Offenses (POCSO) Act was passed in 2012. [online] Available from https://wcd.nic.in/sites/default/files/POCSO%20Act%2C%202012.pdf [Last accessed March, 2023].
11. Jus Corpus. POCSO Act and Its Interpretation. [online] Available from https://www.juscorpus.com/pocso-act-and-its-interpretation/ [Last accessed March, 2023].
12. Sagar R. Child Sexual Abuse: Need for a preventive framework in the Indian context. J Ment Health Hum Behav. 2014;19(2):53-5.
13. Sowmya BT, Seshadri SP, Srinath S, Girimaji S, Sagar JV. Clinical characteristics of children presenting with a history of sexual abuse to a tertiary care center in India. Asian J Psychiatry. 2016;29;19:44-9.
14. Pahwa N. (2018). Summary: Digital Information Security in Healthcare Act (DISHA) to enable electronic health records. [online] Available from https://www.medianama.com/2018/03/223-disha-electronic-health-records/ [Last accessed March, 2023].
15. Board of Governors in supersession of the Medical Council of India. (2020). Telemedicine Practice Guidelines. [online] Available from https://www.mohfw.gov.in/pdf/Telemedicine.pdf [Last accessed March, 2023].
16. Venkatesh U, Aravind GP, Velmurugan AA. Telemedicine practice guidelines in India: Global implications in the wake of the COVID-19 pandemic. World Med Health Policy. 2022;14(3):589-99.
17. Raveesh BN, Munoli RN. Ethical and legal aspects of telepsychiatry. Indian J Psychol Med. 2020;42(5 Suppl):63S-69S.

CHAPTER 17

Newer Drugs in Psychiatry

Imon Paul, Anamika Das

INTRODUCTION

Mental illness is one of the leading causes of disability worldwide, having far reaching physical, social, and economic consequences. This is particularly relevant during the current coronavirus disease 2019 (COVID-19) pandemic where the aftermath of social isolation, economic uncertainties, and anxiety about the illness have all contributed to the worsening of mental health.

Acknowledging the devastating impact of psychiatric and neurological disorders, the global impetus in research focusing on neurosciences has led to significant advances in the understanding about complex neuronal circuits and their association with psychopathology. Despite this improved insight, there remains dearth of truly novel neuropsychiatric drugs.

In this chapter the newer drugs that have come up for various psychiatric disorders in the last decade have been discussed.

ORGANIC DISORDERS INCLUDING DEMENTIA

Pimavanserin

It is an atypical antipsychotic currently indicated for management of delusions and hallucinations in Parkinson's disease psychosis. It is a 5HT2A receptor inverse agonist and antagonist and also acts at the 5HT2C receptor. Pimavanserin is metabolized to an active N-desmethylated metabolite by the cytochrome P450 system (mainly CYP3A4 and CYP3A5). As with other atypical antipsychotics, it increases the risk of mortality in elderly patients with dementia. The common adverse effects reported are peripheral edema, nausea, and confusion. Unlike other antipsychotics it does not worsen motor symptoms in patients with Parkinsonism probably because it lacks affinity for dopamine, histamine, muscarinic, or adrenergic receptors. The recommended dosage is 34 mg/day.[1] In a randomized double-blind placebo-controlled trial, pimavanserin showed benefit in patients with Parkinson disease psychosis[2] and it is being investigated in dementia-related psychosis.

PSYCHOSIS AND MOOD DISORDERS

Cariprazine

It is a new antipsychotic drug, which received Food and Drug Administration (FDA) approval in September 2015 for the treatment of schizophrenia and bipolar disorder (manic and mixed episodes) in adults[3] and subsequently for expanded use in the treatment of bipolar depression. It is a D3 and D2 receptor partial agonist and also binds to 5HT2B, 5HT1A, and 5HT2A serotonin receptors. What makes this molecule unique is its high affinity for D3 receptor which is even higher than that of dopamine. This differs significantly from other antipsychotics whose D3 blockade can be reversed by dopamine. The dopamine D3 autoreceptor blockade by cariprazine is speculated to be the reason for its procognitive activity and role in negative symptoms of psychosis. The pharmacokinetics of cariprazine shows that it has a half-life (t1/2) of 2-4 days but its active metabolite didesmethyl cariprazine has a t1/2 of 1-3 weeks, which is the longest among all atypical antipsychotics, thus making it a long-acting oral agent. This is advantageous for patients who are noncompliant to treatment by preventing immediate relapse.[4] Cariprazine is metabolized mainly by the CYP3A4 enzyme and significant drug interactions can occur with strong CYP3A4 inhibitors or inducers. It should be used with caution in patients with known cardiovascular disorders, hepatic impairment, and severe renal impairment. The common adverse effects include extrapyramidal symptoms, insomnia, headache, and akathisia.[5] Cariprazine is available in dosages of 1.5 mg, 3 mg, 4.5 mg, and 6 mg.

Cariprazine has shown efficacy in the treatment of negative symptoms of schizophrenia in comparison to risperidone on the basis of PANSS (positive and negative syndrome scale) negative subscale items and all PANSS-derived factors.[6] In a post hoc analysis of three pooled phase II/III studies, it was seen that cariprazine was more effective than placebo in terms of improvement in all five factor domains of PANSS.[7]

A systematic review and meta-analysis of cariprazine in the treatment of bipolar disorder showed that it is well tolerated and efficacious in treating acute manic and mixed episodes. Cariprazine also showed efficacy in management of acute depressive episode in bipolar disorder but with a smaller effect size. The use of cariprazine as prophylactic treatment in bipolar disorder needs more research.[8]

Brexpiprazole

This is a new serotonin dopamine activity modulator with structural similarity to aripiprazole. However, it has lower agonist activity at D2 receptors compared to aripiprazole leading to lower incidence of activating side effects like akathisia. It shows antagonism of 5HT2A and α1B receptors and agonism of 5HT1A receptors, thus reducing akathisia and extrapyramidal side effects

(EPS) mediated by D2 receptor blockade. When compared to aripiprazole, reduced binding at H1 receptor decreases antihistaminic side effects correlating with less sedation and weight gain.[9] It was approved by the US FDA in 2015 for the treatment of schizophrenia and adjunctive treatment of depressive disorder.[10] Brexpiprazole is highly protein bound and has 95% oral bioavailability. It is mainly metabolized by CYP3A4 and CYP2D6 enzymes. The dose ranges from 1 to 4 mg.[9]

Efficacy data for schizophrenia shows that 2 mg and 4 mg brexpiprazole were efficacious in the treatment of patients with acute schizophrenia.[11] Another multicenter randomized trial established the safety and efficacy of 4 mg brexpiprazole in treating acute schizophrenia.[12] However, both of the abovementioned short-term trials were limited by absence of an active comparator.

In a randomized, double blind, phase 3 trial, 3 mg brexpiprazole showed efficacy versus placebo as an adjunct to antidepressants in major depression.[13] Similarly, in another study, 2 mg brexpiprazole was efficacious as adjunctive treatment in patients with depression.[14]

A systematic review concluded that 2–4 mg brexpiprazole was efficacious in treating schizophrenia and at dosage of 2 mg it was useful as adjunctive treatment in depressive disorder.[15]

Lumateperone

Lumateperone is a unique molecule, which acts on dopamine, serotonin, and glutamate neurotransmission. It combines 5HT2A receptor antagonism with modulation of glutamate [N-methyl-D-aspartate (NMDA)] receptor subtype 2B. It is a presynaptic D2 partial agonist and postsynaptic D2 antagonist. Lack of affinity for muscarinic or histaminic rectors leads to reduced propensity for sedation, weight gain, and metabolic side effects. It is indicated for treatment of schizophrenia in adult patients and is being investigated for bipolar depression.[10,16]

In a short-term randomized trial on 450 patients, lumateperone showed significant improvement in symptoms of schizophrenia (as measured by the PANSS and Clinical Global Impression-Severity of Illness score) in comparison to placebo.[17] In another randomized, placebo controlled and active controlled (risperidone) trial on 335 patients with acute schizophrenia, lumateperone showed improvement in the PANSS score while secondary analysis was indicative of improvement in depressive and negative symptom domains.[18] In an open label antipsychotic switch study on adults with stable schizophrenia, lumateperone was tolerated well with significant reduction of cardiometabolic side effects and EPS compared to previous antipsychotics.[19]

Lumateperone (42 mg/day) was significantly superior to placebo in improving depressive symptoms in a randomized controlled trial of patients with bipolar (Bipolar I and II) depression. Treatment emergent side effects were comparable to placebo except somnolence and nausea, which was higher in the drug group.[20]

Long-acting Injectables of Second-generation Antipsychotics

- *Aripiprazole lauroxil:* A prodrug of aripiprazole; it is converted to aripiprazole via enzyme-mediated hydrolysis. It works mainly on the D2 receptors like the parent drug and is metabolized through cytochrome P450 isoenzymes 3A4 and 2D6. The dosage is 882 mg at an interval of every 6 weeks. The side effect profile is similar to oral aripiprazole.[10]
- *3-month formulation of paliperidone:* The new 3-month formulation has a significantly longer dosing interval and can be beneficial for patients with frequent noncompliance by preventing relapse. The efficacy, tolerability, and pharmacokinetic profile are similar to 1 month preparation.[10]

Deutetrabenazine and Valbenazine

Both these molecules are indicated for treatment of tardive dyskinesia (TD)—an abnormal involuntary movement disorder associated with the use of neuroleptics. They belong to vesicular monoamine transporter type 2 (VMAT2) inhibitors. KINECT studies on valbenazine (25-100 mg) and ARM-TD and AIM-TD studies on deutetrabenazine (12-48 mg) showed them to be efficacious and well tolerated in the treatment of TD. Insomnia, headache, somnolence, and diarrhea are the common side effects. Valbenazine has to be administered with caution if the patient is on strong inducers of CYP3A4 or has severe renal impairment. Deutetrabenazine is contraindicated in patients with suicidality, depression, and hepatic impairment and it can worsen depression and suicidality in patients suffering from Huntington's disease.[21]

Ketamine

The racemic mixture of (R, S) ketamine acts as a glutamatergic modulator and thus exerts its rapid antidepressant effect. Ketamine inhibits NMDA receptors present in gamma aminobutyric acid (GABA)ergic interneurons and increases synaptic glutamate release by lowering inhibitory tone of pyramidal neurons via the GABAergic interneurons. This glutamate burst is responsible for the rapid antidepressant effect. It also causes intracellular changes in protein expression, leading to increased level of brain-derived neurotrophic factor (BDNF) by deactivation of calcium/calmodulin-dependent kinase and dephosphorylation of eukaryotic elongation factor 2. This antagonism at NMDA receptor accompanied by AMPA receptor modulation causes changes in synaptic plasticity resulting in synaptic spine remodeling and antidepressant effect. Ketamine can be given via intravenous

(IV), intramuscular (IM), intranasal (IN), and oral routes. The bioavailability is maximum when ketamine is administered IV or IM and most studies of ketamine in depression used IV administration.[22,23]

Multiple placebo-controlled trials have demonstrated the efficacy of ketamine as an antidepressant in both unipolar and bipolar depression. Meta-analysis of studies has shown the rapid effect to start after about 40 minutes of infusion of a single subanesthetic dose of ketamine, with peak reaching at 24 hours and weaning of effects by 10–12 days. The long-term antidepressant action and the effect of repeated administration of ketamine are still uncertain and warrant further research.[23,24]

Ketamine has a rapid antisuicidal response and suicidal ideation in various psychiatric disorders can be treated with ketamine.[23] A recent randomized control trial to investigate the antisuicidal effect of ketamine in the short term and at 6 weeks showed that ketamine caused rapid remission of suicidal ideation with limited adverse effects and the antisuicidal benefit was maintained to some extent at 6 weeks.[25] A systematic review and meta-analysis of 25 reports involving 15 independent trials on patients with predominantly affective disorders showed short-term beneficial effects of IV ketamine on suicidality. The effect was maximal on patients with unipolar depression. This effect seemed to be mediated by its antidepressant action although the effect of treatment for depression lasted longer than its antisuicidal effect. Improvement in areas of memory or reduction in symptoms such as pessimism, sadness, and anhedonia are likely to be associated with its antisuicidal effect.[26] Another recent systematic review also concluded that IV ketamine caused rapid and significant reduction in suicidal ideation in patients with baseline suicidality but the long-term efficacy was undetermined.[27]

Esketamine Nasal Spray

Intranasal esketamine (S-enantiomer of ketamine) is indicated for treatment of depression in adults with major depression and acute suicidality. In the ASPIRE studies IN esketamine (84 mg twice weekly) was compared with placebo for 4 weeks along with comprehensive standard of care and esketamine plus standard of care treatment rapidly improved symptoms of depression in patients with major depression and acute suicidality.[28]

Brexanolone

Postpartum depression is an underreported condition with serious adverse impact on the mother and newborn as well as the family and society at large. There is a rapid fluctuation of endocrine hormones and neuroactive steroids in the peripartum period which is implicated in the causation of postpartum depression. Brexanolone was developed as an IV proprietary formulation of allopregnanolone, a neuroactive steroid and endogenous metabolite of progesterone. It is speculated to regulate neuronal excitability via its action on GABA-A receptors. There occurs an increase in allopregnanolone levels in pregnancy followed by sudden decline during childbirth. Brexanolone be administered as a continuous infusion over a period of 60 hours to restore stable serum levels comparable with third trimester concentrations in postpartum mothers.[29]

A recent review of randomized clinical trials of brexanolone in postpartum depression concluded that brexanolone was more efficacious than placebo in rapid reduction of depressive symptoms at the end of 60 hours infusion of the drug and that this antidepressant benefit was maintained up to 1 month. However, longer term efficacy and safety data with brexanolone is lacking. As the IV formulation of brexanolone can limit its usage, an oral analog, zuranolone (SAGE-217), is being developed and clinical trials are underway.[30]

Vortioxetine

It is a relatively new drug for treatment of depressive disorders in adults. In can effectively manage both acute depression as well as prevent relapse of episodes. The drug has multimodal activity on various receptors— agonism at 5HT1A, antagonism at 5HT1D, 5HT3, 5HT7, partial agonism at 5HT1B, and serotonin transporter inhibition. The molecule has a long half-life of about 57 hours which can prevent discontinuation syndrome in case of abrupt cessation and it reaches steady state in 14 days. It is mainly metabolized by CYP2D6 enzyme and dose adjustment is needed with concomitant administration of CYP2D6 inhibitors or inducers. The available dosages are 5, 10, 15, and 20 mg, with the initial starting dose in adults being 10 mg/day, which can be increased to 20 mg/day as per response and tolerability. Vortioxetine has a unique procognitive role, which may even occur independent of its antidepressant action. Another major advantage is the lesser incidence of sexual side effects, which improves compliance to treatment.[31] Efficacy data shows the molecule to be effective and safe in the treatment of adults with major depression.[32,33] Another meta-analysis of 10 placebo-controlled trials concluded that vortioxetine improved depressive and anxiety symptoms in patients of major depression with comorbid high levels of anxiety.[34]

Vilazodone

It is an antidepressant, which targets multiple monoamine transporters or receptors. The main mechanism of action is selective serotonin reuptake inhibition combined with partial agonism at 5HT1A; thus, it is regarded as serotonin partial agonist reuptake inhibitor (SPARI). It can be initiated at a dosage of 10 mg/day with gradual increase to 40 mg/day. It is metabolized by the CYP3A4 system and drug interactions can occur with CYP3A4 inhibitors or inducers. Vilazodone should be taken with food to improve bioavailability and prevent gastrointestinal side effects. Presynaptic 5HT1A autoreceptor activation decreases serotonin secretion but can be desensitized with chronic stimulation. Compared to conventional selective serotonin reuptake inhibitors, vilazodone causes faster and greater desensitization of 5HT1A autoreceptors, which helps in faster onset of action and reduces the therapeutic time lag. Activation at postsynaptic 5HT1A receptors leads to increased dopamine thus reducing sexual side effects.[35]

The efficacy profile shows that vilazodone is efficacious in the treatment of depressive disorder with a favorable weight gain profile in the short term.[36] A systematic review and network meta-analysis demonstrated that the efficacy of vilazodone is comparable to other second-generation antidepressants.[37]

Sublingual Dexmedetomidine

Agitation is commonly present in various psychiatric disorders and is a challenge for the treating team. The sublingual formulation of dexmedetomidine, an alpha-2 adrenergic receptor agonist, is a promising treatment option for managing agitation.[38,39] A multicentric, randomized clinical trial on agitated patients with bipolar disorder demonstrated that administering a single dose of sublingual dexmedetomidine (120 μg or 180 μg) resulted in significant decline in agitation at 2 hours compared to placebo.[40]

SLEEP DISORDERS

Dual Orexin Receptor Antagonist

Lemborexant, suvorexant, and daridorexant are the new molecules indicated for the treatment of insomnia. They improve sleep onset (subjective and objective), sleep maintenance, and sleep quality. Lemborexant is also under study for irregular sleep wake rhythm disorder in patients with Alzheimer's disease. The orexin/hypocretin system promotes wakefulness through various mechanisms. Antagonism in the OX1R and OX2R receptors by these molecules thus helps in sleep by antagonizing the wake drive. Details of the three molecules are discussed in **Table 1**.[41-44]

NOVEL THERAPIES STILL IN PIPELINE

It is essential to focus on new drug discovery either through translation of neurocircuitry knowledge to treatment opportunities or by garnering more knowledge from existing drug mechanisms. The pathophysiology of psychiatric disorders needs to be understood in greater detail. NEWMEDS (Novel Methods Leading to New Medications in Depression and Schizophrenia), a European project, has been created for overcoming this problem.[45]

TABLE 1: Dual orexin receptor antagonists and their characteristics.

Molecule	Lemborexant	Suvorexant	Daridorexant
Recommended starting dose (adults and older adults)	5 mg	10 mg	25/50 mg
Dose range	5–10 mg	10–20 mg	25–50 mg
When to be taken	Immediately before sleeping and at least 7 hours before planned wake time	Within 30 minutes of going to bed and at least 7 hours before planned wake time	Within 30 minutes of going to bed and at least 7 hours before planned wake time
Half-life (t½)	17–19 hours	12 hours	8 hours
Potential drug reactions	• Moderate CYP3A inhibitors not to be prescribed concomitantly • Dose reduction is needed with mild inhibitors	Moderate inhibitors can be used with lower dosage	• Moderate inhibitors can be used with lower dosage • Should be avoided with inducers of CYP3A
Contraindications	Narcolepsy, severe hepatic impairment	Narcolepsy, severe hepatic impairment	Narcolepsy, severe hepatic impairment
Side effects	Day time somnolence	Day time somnolence, fatigue, abnormal dreams	Day time somnolence, complex sleep behaviors—sleep walking, sleep driving, hypnopompic and hypnogogic hallucinations, possible worsening of depressive and suicidal symptoms

A few other promising therapeutic agents in various phases of clinical trials have been enumerated below.

- The endocannabinoid system has evolved as a potential target for treatment of schizophrenia. Cannabidiol is a plant-derived cannabinoid, which has proved beneficial for psychosis in small scale clinical studies.[46]
- *Glutamatergic system in schizophrenia:* Dysfunction of NMDA receptor is currently implicated in pathophysiology of schizophrenia. The NMDA

receptor hypofunction theory has given rise to the treatment opportunity by activating metabotropic glutamate receptors (mGluRs). The group II mGluRs and subtype 5 GluR have come out to be novel targets for cognitive deficits in schizophrenia.[47]

- *Glutamatergic agents in mood disorders:*[22] Ketamine is the prototype agent for depression, which has been discussed. There are novel molecules, which act as glutamatergic modulators and are currently under study. Some of them are:
  - *Dextromethorphan:* Currently used as cough suppressant; it acts as NMDA receptor antagonist (nonselective and noncompetitive) and is being studied for depression.
  - *Nuedexta (dextromethorphan 20 mg + quinidine 10 mg):* Currently FDA approved for pseudobulbar effect. This drug is also undergoing trials for use in depression. Quinidine being a potent inhibitor of CYP2D6—the main pathway for dextromethorphan metabolism, the combination allows for higher bioavailability of dextromethorphan.
  - *Axsome (AXS-05—dextromethorphan + bupropion):* Currently designated as fast-track by FDA for treatment-resistant depression; this combination has shown efficacy as antidepressant in phase III trials.
  - *Dextromethadone:* Isomer of methadone and NMDA receptor antagonist with lower affinity to mu and delta opioid receptors. Currently undergoing phase III trials as an antidepressant. The major concern is abuse potential.
  - *D-cycloserine:* A broad-spectrum antibiotic and acts as glycine site modulator of NMDA receptor.
  - *Rapastinel and apimostinel:* IV glycine site modulator with rapid antidepressant effects at 1–2 hours.

CONCLUSION

Mental and behavioral disorders are a major cause for disability worldwide, necessitating research on newer psychotherapeutic agents. Though research on these areas is ongoing but major breakthroughs are still anticipated. Drugs with fewer adverse effects and better efficacy needs to be designed for better compliance and effectivity. Finding newer molecular targets, repurposing medicines to decrease side effects are other strategies that can be employed. The last decade has seen development of some novel psychiatric agents and many are in pipeline. The impetus in research should be focused on translational neurosciences as psychopharmacology will be gaining huge importance in future.

TAKE-HOME POINTS

- Psychiatric disorders are amongst the leading causes of disability worldwide.
- There is immediate need for improving impetus in research on translational neurosciences aimed at discovery of novel psychiatric drugs with improved efficacy and minimal side effects.
- New therapeutic options include truly novel agents, existing drugs repurposed on the basis of improved understanding of psychiatric illnesses, and medications aimed at new molecular targets rather than the conventional ones.
- In the last decade some promising new agents for various psychiatric disorders include cariprazine, brexipiprazole, lumateperone, es-ketamine nasal spray, IV brexanolone, vortioxetine, vilazodone, sublingual dexmedetomidine, and dual orexin receptor antagonists. Multiple drugs targeting the cannabinoid system and glutamatergic system are under trial.

REFERENCES

1. Hunter NS, Anderson KC, Cox A. Pimavanserin. Drugs Today (Barc). 2015;51(11):645-52.
2. Cummings J, Isaacson S, Mills R, Williams H, Chi-Burris K, Corbett A, et al. Pimavanserin for patients with Parkinson's disease psychosis: a randomised, placebo-controlled phase 3 trial. The Lancet. 2014;383.
3. Cariprazine [package insert]. US Food and Drug Administration website. [online] Available from http://www.accessdata.fda.gov/drugsatfda_docs/nda/2015/204370Orig2s000TOC.cfm [Last accessed March, 2023].
4. Stahl SM. Mechanism of action of cariprazine. CNS Spectr. 2016;21(2):123-7.
5. Earley W, Durgam S, Lu K, Laszlovszky I, Debelle M, Kane JM. Safety and tolerability of cariprazine in patients with acute exacerbation of schizophrenia: a pooled analysis of four phase II/III randomized, double-blind, placebo-controlled studies. Int Clin Psychopharmacol. 2017;32(6):319.
6. Fleischhacker W, Galderisi S, Laszlovszky I, Szatmári B, Barabássy Á, Acsai K, et al. The efficacy of cariprazine in negative symptoms of schizophrenia: Post hoc analyses of PANSS individual items and PANSS-derived factors. Eur Psychiatry. 2019;58:1-9.
7. Marder S, Fleischhacker WW, Earley W, Lu K, Zhong Y, Németh G, et al. Efficacy of cariprazine across symptom domains in patients with acute exacerbation of schizophrenia: pooled analyses from 3 phase II/III studies. Eur Neuropsychopharmacol. 2019;29(1):127-36.
8. Pinto JV, Saraf G, Vigo D, Keramatian K, Chakrabarty T, Yatham LN. Cariprazine in the treatment of Bipolar Disorder: A systematic review and meta-analysis. Bipolar Disord. 2020;22(4):360-71.
9. Stahl SM. Mechanism of action of brexpiprazole: comparison with aripiprazole. CNS Spectr. 2016;21(1):1-6.
10. Ceskova E, Silhan P. Novel treatment options in depression and psychosis. Neuropsychiatr Dis Treat. 2018;14:741-7.
11. Correll CU, Skuban A, Hobart M, Ouyang J, Weiller E, Weiss C, et al. Efficacy of brexpiprazole in patients with acute schizophrenia: review of three randomized, double-blind, placebo-controlled studies. Schizophr Res. 2016;174(1-3):82-92.

12. Kane JM, Skuban A, Ouyang J, Hobart M, Pfister S, McQuade RD, et al. A multicenter, randomized, double-blind, controlled phase 3 trial of fixed-dose brexpiprazole for the treatment of adults with acute schizophrenia. Schizophr Res. 2015;164(1-3):127-35.
13. Thase ME, Youakim JM, Skuban A, Hobart M, Zhang P, McQuade RD, et al. Adjunctive brexpiprazole 1 and 3 mg for patients with major depressive disorder following inadequate response to antidepressants: a phase 3, randomized, double-blind study. J Clin Psychiatry. 2015;76(9):465.
14. Thase ME, Youakim JM, Skuban A, Hobart M, Augustine C, Zhang P, et al. Efficacy and safety of adjunctive brexpiprazole 2 mg in major depressive disorder: a phase 3, randomized, placebo-controlled study in patients with inadequate response to antidepressants. J Clin Psychiatry. 2015;76(9):6108.
15. Citrome L. Brexpiprazole for schizophrenia and as adjunct for major depressive disorder: a systematic review of the efficacy and safety profile for this newly approved antipsychotic–what is the number needed to treat, number needed to harm and likelihood to be helped or harmed? Int J Clin Pract. 2015;69(9):978-97.
16. Barman R, Majumder P, Doifode T, Kablinger A. Newer antipsychotics: Brexpiprazole, cariprazine, and lumateperone: A pledge or another unkept promise? World J Psychiatry. 2021;11(12):1228.
17. Correll CU, Davis RE, Weingart M, Saillard J, O'Gorman C, Kane JM, et al. Efficacy and safety of lumateperone for treatment of schizophrenia: a randomized clinical trial. JAMA Psychiatry. 2020;77(4):349-58.
18. Lieberman JA, Davis RE, Correll CU, Goff DC, Kane JM, Tamminga CA, et al. ITI-007 for the treatment of schizophrenia: a 4-week randomized, double-blind, controlled trial. Biol Psychiatry. 2016;79(12):952-61.
19. Correll CU, Vanover KE, Davis RE, Chen R, Satlin A, Mates S. Safety and tolerability of lumateperone 42 mg: An open-label antipsychotic switch study in outpatients with stable schizophrenia. Schizophr Res. 2021;228:198-205.
20. Calabrese JR, Durgam S, Satlin A, Vanover KE, Davis RE, Chen R, et al. Efficacy and safety of lumateperone for major depressive episodes associated with bipolar I or bipolar II disorder: a phase 3 randomized placebo-controlled trial. Am J Psychiatry. 2021;178(12):1098-106.
21. Touma KT, Scarff JR. Valbenazine and deutetrabenazine for tardive dyskinesia. Innov Clin Neurosci. 2018;15(5-6):13.
22. Henter ID, Park LT, Zarate CA. Novel glutamatergic modulators for the treatment of mood disorders: current status. CNS Drugs. 2021;35(5):527-43.
23. Caddy C, Giaroli G, White TP, Shergill SS, Tracy DK. Ketamine as the prototype glutamatergic antidepressant: pharmacodynamic actions, and a systematic review and meta-analysis of efficacy. Ther Adv Psychopharmacol. 2014;4(2):75-99.
24. Kishimoto T, Chawla JM, Hagi K, Zarate CA, Kane JM, Bauer M, et al. Single-dose infusion ketamine and non-ketamine N-methyl-d-aspartate receptor antagonists for unipolar and bipolar depression: a meta-analysis of efficacy, safety and time trajectories. Psychol Med. 2016;46(7):1459-72.
25. Abbar M, Demattei C, El-Hage W, Llorca PM, Samalin L, Demaricourt P, et al. Ketamine for the acute treatment of severe suicidal ideation: double blind, randomised placebo controlled trial. BMJ. 2022;376:e067194.

26. Witt K, Potts J, Hubers A, Grunebaum MF, Murrough JW, Loo C, et al. Ketamine for suicidal ideation in adults with psychiatric disorders: a systematic review and meta-analysis of treatment trials. Aust N Z J Psychiatry. 2020;54(1):29-45.
27. Siegel AN, Di Vincenzo JD, Brietzke E, Gill H, Rodrigues NB, Lui LM, et al. Antisuicidal and antidepressant effects of ketamine and esketamine in patients with baseline suicidality: A systematic review. J Psychiatr Res. 2021;137:426-36.
28. Canuso CM, Ionescu DF, Li X, Qiu X, Lane R, Turkoz I, et al. Esketamine nasal spray for the rapid reduction of depressive symptoms in major depressive disorder with acute suicidal ideation or behavior. J Clin Psychopharmacol. 2021;41(5):516.
29. Frieder A, Fersh M, Hainline R, Deligiannidis KM. Pharmacotherapy of postpartum depression: current approaches and novel drug development. CNS Drugs. 2019;33(3):265-82.
30. Faden J, Citrome L. Intravenous brexanolone for postpartum depression: what it is, how well does it work, and will it be used? Ther Adv Psychopharmacol. 2020;10:2045125320968658.
31. Paul I. Newer Updates in Psychiatry: Focus on Vortioxetine. Indian J Private Psychiatry. 2018;12(2):62-5.
32. Thase ME, Mahableshwarkar AR, Dragheim M, Loft H, Vieta E. A meta-analysis of randomized, placebo-controlled trials of vortioxetine for the treatment of major depressive disorder in adults. Eur Neuropsychopharmacol. 2016;26(6):979-93.
33. Cipriani A, Furukawa TA, Salanti G, Chaimani A, Atkinson LZ, Ogawa Y, et al. Comparative Efficacy and Acceptability of 21 Antidepressant Drugs for the Acute Treatment of Adults With Major Depressive Disorder: A Systematic Review and Network Meta-Analysis. Focus (Am Psychiatr Publ). 2018;16(4):420-9.
34. Baldwin DS, Florea I, Jacobsen PL, Zhong W, Nomikos GG. A meta-analysis of the efficacy of vortioxetine in patients with major depressive disorder (MDD) and high levels of anxiety symptoms. J Affect Disord. 2016;206:140-50.
35. Wang SM, Han C, Lee SJ, Patkar AA, Masand PS, Pae CU. Vilazodone for the treatment of depression: an update. Chonnam Med J. 2016;52(2):91-100.
36. Citrome L. Vilazodone for major depressive disorder: a systematic review of the efficacy and safety profile for this newly approved antidepressant–what is the number needed to treat, number needed to harm and likelihood to be helped or harmed? Int J Clin Pract. 2012;66(4):356-68.
37. Wagner G, Schultes MT, Titscher V, Teufer B, Klerings I, Gartlehner G. Efficacy and safety of levomilnacipran, vilazodone and vortioxetine compared with other second-generation antidepressants for major depressive disorder in adults: a systematic review and network meta-analysis. J Affect Disord. 2018;228:1-2.
38. Citrome L. Dexmedetomidine sublingual film for agitation. Curr Psychiatry. 2022;21(6):34-8.
39. Almeida M, Cicolello K, Hanson A, DeCavalcante G, DeOliveira GS. Treatment of acute agitation associated with excited catatonia using dexmedetomidine: case series and literature review. Prim Care Companion CNS Disord. 2021;23(5):20cr02899.
40. Preskorn SH, Zeller S, Citrome L, Finman J, Goldberg JF, Fava M, et al. Effect of sublingual dexmedetomidine vs placebo on acute agitation associated with bipolar disorder: a randomized clinical trial. JAMA. 2022;327(8):727-36.

41. Kuriyama A, Tabata H. Suvorexant for the treatment of primary insomnia: a systematic review and meta-analysis. Sleep Med Rev. 2017;35:1-7.
42. Scott LJ. Lemborexant: first approval. Drugs. 2020;80(4):425-32.
43. Rhyne DN, Anderson SL. Suvorexant in insomnia: efficacy, safety and place in therapy. Ther Adv Drug Saf. 2015;6(5):189-95.
44. Markham A. Daridorexant: First Approval. Drugs. 2022:1-7.
45. Filippo C, Leggio GM, Salvatore S, Filippo D. New drugs in psychiatry: focus on new pharmacological targets. F1000Res. 2017;6:397.
46. Leweke FM, Mueller JK, Lange B, Rohleder C. Therapeutic potential of cannabinoids in psychosis. Biol Psychiatry. 2016;79(7):604-12.
47. Hashimoto K, Malchow B, Falkai P, Schmitt A. Glutamate modulators as potential therapeutic drugs in schizophrenia and affective disorders. Eur Arch Psychiatry Clin Neurosci. 2013;263(5):367-77.

CHAPTER 18

Changing Perspectives in Psychiatry Training in India

Henal Shah, Kishor M

INTRODUCTION

Globally, there is a tsunami of changes in higher education ranging from demands to have efficient, faster, and robust training, increased workforce accountability, the ability to lead teams, and, while working locally, be globally relevant and abreast of the exponential growth of information. This has been coupled with coronavirus disease 2019 (COVID-19), which paralyzed many systems, necessitating drastic changes in education systems and service provision. Educational disruptions and changes in undergraduate, postgraduate, and continuing medical education (CME) have occurred. In India, parallel to the effect of global changes, there has been the introduction of an outcome-based education system, namely competency-based medical education (CBME).

UNDERGRADUATE PSYCHIATRY EDUCATION

With the introduction of UG CBME, the psychiatry training was more organized. There are 117 competencies outlined for psychiatry.[1] Didactic teaching is 25 hours; 10 hours are for integrated teaching and seminars. The level and type of integration are described as the competency where integration is possible vertically and horizontally. The concept of self-directed learning is spelled out for the first time, and 5 hours are demarcated for the same. Clinical posting is for 2 weeks each during the second and third minor years. While these are the curriculum's strengths, the downside is the absence of the requirement of any psychiatry skill as essential for certification.[2]

With the advent of this new step, the Indian Psychiatric Society (IPS) UG committee compiled a book describing the sequence of lectures and practical guidelines for implementing the new curriculum in all the country's medical colleges. This book was to support the faculty to charter unknown waters and was to be scaffolded by faculty training. The latter was affected by COVID and the diversion of psychiatry teachers to be part of the team facing the pandemic. To add to this burden was the sudden need to train students online and be digitally savvy, a competency that many faculty and students did not possess.

The challenges in psychiatry training were taken up by teachers across India, who explored many ways to enhance undergraduate training even during the pandemic, such as innovative online clinical sessions and engaging theory sessions. IPS Faculty Training Taskforce propagated and published guidelines.[3] Many psychiatry teachers and students shared their experiences with online teaching-learning on the popular platform such as Sunday Special 60 minutes with Psychiatry Teachers, which was a novel joint initiative of the IPS Faculty Training Task Force, IPS UG and PG Education Subcommittee, and Indian Teachers of Psychiatry (IToP) Forum supported by Minds United for Health Sciences and Humanity Trust, Mysuru, Karnataka.[4] Systematic surveys on online teaching-learning were also carried out, and findings were reflected in the same platform for enhanced psychiatry training.

However, with COVID, UG training took a backseat. A few batches of undergraduate students have had minimal or no exposure to psychiatry. Either lecture classes did not occur or were conducted virtually. The learning from these classes could have been more effective. Clinical postings were cancelled and shortened, and often students were posted to emergency and COVID duties. These were lost opportunities that could have far-reaching repercussions for the field. It was a missed chance to learn psychiatry, sensitize students to mental health, and dispel many myths students have about our field. It was also a loss of a critical window to encourage bright young students to pursue psychiatry. Undergraduate psychiatry has also introduced foundation courses, simulation laboratories, and AETCOM (Attitude, Ethics, and Communication).[5] These were other possibilities for psychiatry faculty to interact with students and discuss and inspire students to consider psychiatry as a career option. The internship, another occasion to interact with patients, see them improve, and appreciate the role of psychiatry, was skipped with students being routed for COVID duties.

While formal training in UG psychiatry was affected, the experience of the pandemic resulted in the community valuing the importance of mental health. A booklet was prepared on equipping doctors to face the pandemic where there was no mention of mental health. This resulted in an uproar in the newspaper and finally an inclusion of this chapter by National Medical Commission (NMC).[6]

Another significant move is the introduction of NeXT as an examination to decide entry in PG, which will also be required for all medical graduates who have completed MBBS abroad.[7] This is an essential step in improving standards across the country. It is also a window to increase the representation of psychiatry in this examination. The UG, PG education, and faculty training had a closed group discussion with many psychiatry department chairs to decide on a plan to lobby for the same. The request letter is forwarded to IPS officials to take the following steps to discuss with NMC.

POSTGRADUATE PSYCHIATRY EDUCATION

Similar to UG education, the most significant changes recently are the disruption of conventional psychiatry training due to the COVID-19 pandemic and the implementation of CBME. This has put the entire focus on psychiatry teachers, who had to suddenly adapt to online teaching–learning during the COVID-19 pandemic while simultaneously focusing on training. It is important to note that implementing the National Education Policy in the coming years will also alter the landscape of psychiatry training in this subcontinent. Thus, there is an urgent need to review and document changing perspectives in psychiatry training in India. PG curriculum described the competencies and provided a logbook outline to monitor and document the learning. NMC advised the need and length of various types of rotations.[8]

Many batches, though, learned the resilience required to face the pandemic; they missed the chance to interact and learn psychiatry during a period of the residency. Formal didactic teaching was suspended for a short time and later initiated in a digital format. In a significant development, a first of its kind in the world of psychiatry training, a scholarship for psychiatry teachers (IToP STEPS—Scholarship for Teachers towards Enrichment of Psychiatry Teaching Skills) was initiated in India.[9] A fully sponsored program conducted online for enthusiastic faculty who had to apply and be selected through interviews by a group of psychiatry education experts from India and abroad began in 2020. Interestingly, this was an initiative of a nongovernment organization (NGO), Minds United for Health Sciences and Humanity Trust, funded by Infosys Foundation.[10] This online faculty training enhanced the psychiatry training and demonstrated innovative ways of the faculty development program.[11]

The pandemic also posed challenges in the postgraduate examination process. Novel ways of documenting the suggestions from the psychiatry teachers were undertaken by IPS Faculty Training Task Force and IPS PG Education Subcommittee through online meets, and possible ways of conducting examinations in the middle of the pandemic were discussed.[12.] Case scenario-based examination through online mode was highlighted. It is interesting to note that the NMC had guidelines similar to that of psychiatry teachers. This process demonstrates that all components of psychiatry training can be addressed even in uncertain times when psychiatry teachers across the country are involved and innovative ways emerge. Mock examinations on a digital platform were conducted by the

IPS PG, UG, and faculty training committee along with the Department of Psychiatry, Nair Hospital. The summary of learning was:
- The need for training and practice is high, with 1,061 students registering. Over the three days of the training, at the end of the day there were 450–500 participants logged in and interacting. Many departments organized collective viewing to discuss and encourage peer and collaborative learning.
- The virtual mode makes it much simpler to have representations of students and examiners across the country. Both examiners and examinees were enthusiastic about participating.
- The immediate comments revealed there was immense learning.
- There is variability in learning, especially during the pandemic and learners need more support to master the interpretation of radiological findings, EEG, and psychological tests.
- Besides students, many young psychiatrists in practice and junior faculty found this revision very useful.
- Such programs help improve standards, and faculty must reflect on the best ways to assess competencies.
- National bodies such as IPS should continue improving academic standards and supporting teachers and students.

The country, including NMC, also woke up to the need for psychiatrists, and therefore increased the number of students allocated to teachers and the number of departments that could initiate the training for postgraduate students. While this is an excellent move, the number of teachers required to run a department decreased. While the load of patients has multiplied, and the effort required to implement CBME is time intensive, there is a dip in faculty requirements as prescribed by NMC. This will have an impact on the quality of education. This is another area where the national body IPS is lobbying with NMC.

The implementation of Mental Healthcare Act (MHCA) and its ramifications are other important landmarks in the service and training of psychiatrists. This act has many strengths and challenges, and for effective implementation, it is necessary to train our future psychiatrists in the nuances of the law.[13]

SUPERSPECIALTY/SUBSPECIALTY EDUCATION

Addiction, geriatric psychiatry, and child and adolescent mental health have specialized training. In the recent past, there have been fellowships of 1 year that have started, especially for child and adolescent psychiatry. Psychiatry departments/universities and a national child and adolescent mental health association initiated these. This has increased the skills of many psychiatry students in dealing with common disorders in Child and Adolescent Mental Health (CAMH).

CONTINUING PSYCHIATRY EDUCATION

The NMC has mandated the need for CME and a requirement to regularly submit proof to acquire reaccreditation. With the onset of COVID, there has been a deluge of accredited online CME conferences and training. These are on varied topics, satisfying the needs of various groups, and have been attended well.

GLOBAL OPPORTUNITIES FOR LEARNING

With the exponential rise in the use of digital platforms, many avenues for training have appeared. These vary from short- to long-term courses ranging from cognitive behavioral therapy (CBT) to many other therapies. The exodus of psychiatrists to foreign lands had decreased during COVID and is again gathering steam. The wide acceptance of Indians reflects the appreciation and trust in their competencies.

CONCLUSION

We are at a cusp for many long-reaching changes in education in psychiatry. The new curriculum, the perceived need for mental health specialists in the aftermath of COVID, the effective use of technology, and the increase in the training of faculty herald a time for improvement in psychiatry education. The mandate rests on the shoulders of each psychiatrist and the national bodies to fuel the momentum and seize the opportunity to raise the benchmark of standards in psychiatry education and care.

TAKE-HOME POINTS

- Psychiatry education in UG and PG is on the cusp of transformation.
- Competency-based psychiatry education is here to stay, and the national body has a role in supporting faculty and helping in their training.
- Technology will have a role in education.
- IPS must continuously liaison with NMC to strengthen the call for robust training and representation in summative examinations.

REFERENCES

1. National Medical Council. (2018). Competency Based Undergraduate Curriculum for the Indian Medical Graduate, Volume 1-3. [online] Available from https://www.nmc.org.in/wp-content/uploads/2020/01/UG-Curriculum-Vol-II.pdf. [Last accessed March, 2023].
2. Jacob KS. Medical Council of India's New competency-based curriculum for medical graduates: a critical appraisal. Indian J Psychol Med. 2019;41:203-9.
3. Kishor M. What to Teach and how to teach medical students in the middle of COVID-19? Guidance for Teachers in Psychiatry. Indian J Psychol Med. 2021;43(4):357-9.

4. Launch of Sunday Special 60 Minutes with psychiatry teachers. [online] Available from https://youtu.be/_HBh7njcrFA [Last accessed March, 2023].
5. National Medical Council. AETCOM. [online] Available from https://www.nmc.org.in/wp-content/uploads/2020/01/AETCOM_book.pdf. [Last accessed March, 2023].
6. National Medical Council. (2018). Module on Pandemic Management from: National Medical Council. Competency Based Undergraduate Curriculum for the Indian Medical Graduate, Volume 2. [online] Available from https://www.nmc.org.in/wp-content/uploads/2020/09/Pandemic-MGT-Module-UG.pdf [Last accessed March, 2023].
7. National Exit Test (NEXT Exam). [online] Available from https://www.mbbsadmissionabroad.in/national-exit-test-next-exam [Last accessed March, 2023].
8. Guidelines for Competency-based Postgraduate Training Programme for MD in Psychiatry. [online] Available from https://www.nmc.org.in/wp-content/uploads/2019/09/MD-Psychiatry.pdf. [Last accessed March, 2023].
9. IToP STEPS. Indian Teachers of Psychiatry. [online] Available from http://indianteachersofpsychiatry.com [Last accessed March, 2023].
10. Minds United for Health Sciences and Humanity Trust. Indian Teachers of Psychiatry. [online] Available from http://indianteachersofpsychiatry.com [Last accessed March, 2023].
11. Kar SK, Dere SS, Mishra DK, Das G. Training of psychiatry teachers on teaching skills: Needs, innovations and initiatives. Asian J Psychiatr. 2022;72:103108.
12. Kishor M, Shah H, Chandran S, Mysore AV, Kumar A, Menon V, et al. Psychiatry postgraduate examinations for 2020 in the middle of COVID19 crisis: Suggestions from Indian teachers of psychiatry. Indian J Psychiatry. 2020;62:431-4.
13. The Mental health Care Act, 2017. [online] Available from https://legislative.gov.in/sites/default/files/A2017-10.pdf. [Last accessed March, 2023].

CHAPTER 19

Treating Addiction: Multidimensional Approach and Prevention to Relapse

Senjam Gojendra Singh, Rajkumar Lenin Singh

INTRODUCTION

Drug addiction is a serious mental disorder having lapsing and relapsing course and often require multidimensional approach, which include both pharmacological and psychological approach.[1]

Prolong drug exposure on brain lead to uncontrollable drug craving, seeking for drug compulsively, development of tolerance, presence of withdrawal symptoms on stopping drug, and drug use in presence of socio-occupational dysfunction or any physical or mental illness.

NEUROBIOLOGY OF ADDICTION

Before going to management, basic understanding of addiction at neurobiological level is must. Usually, person start drinking alcohol impulsively in initial phase, later on repeated impulsive behavioral pattern of drug abuse, the securing of its supply, leads to compulsive pattern of behavior. The neurocircuit involved in impulsivity is an extrapolation from the ventral striatum to the thalamus, then from thalamus to ventromedial prefrontal cortex (VMPFC), and from VMPFC back to the ventral striatum, in other words impulsivity is a ventrally dependent learning system, and over time, however, these behaviors migrate dorsally as a result of a process of neuroadaptations and neuroplasticity. Neurocircuit involved in compulsive behavior is an extrapolation from the dorsal striatum to the thalamus, then from thalamus to orbitofrontal cortex (OFC), and from OFC back to the dorsal striatum.[2]

Prevention

Prevention of addiction aims at avoidance of intake of drug causing serious health and social consequences. It can be achieved in two ways, first reduce sources of drug (on the basis of principle that decreased obtainability of illicit drugs reduces the chances for abuse and dependence) and reduce demand (disease prevention and raise health awareness). Supply reduction aimed at dropping and production of source of illicit drugs by destroying poppy plants (opium crops), introducing replacement crops, interrupting drug trafficking route, and illicit drug dealers. The term demand reduction is trying to prevent people taking illicit drugs by implementing policies and programs in the community level, providing education to drug users about their harmful effects and giving in time treatment to drug users.[3]

Brief Intervention

Brief intervention is an organized, client-centered nonjudgmental therapy using multiple counselling sessions by a trained interventionist of shorter duration.[4] Brief Intervention (BI) aims complete abstinence or to lessen a person's illicit drug use to harmless level. This is different from brief therapies, which aim client engagement, assessment, and rapid implementation of change strategies. Usually, brief interventions are of shorter duration than brief therapies.[5] The model used in BI goes by the abbreviation FRAMES, which was first developed by Miller and Rollnick.

Detoxification

Depending upon severity of drug addiction, and the type of withdrawal presentation usually management can be of two types, outdoor and indoor care. Usually patients having severe withdrawal, refusal for food, any physical comorbidity, history of multiple relapses, and any life-threatening condition are planned for inpatient care. Treatment medications such as lorazepam chlordiazepoxide or diazepam with high dose of thiamine are used for detoxification in alcohol use disorder patients. Opioid used disorder patients are usually detoxified with either buprenorphine, methadone, or tramadol. Usually, the duration of indoor management is 10–14 days.

Antipsychotics, antianxiety medications, antidepressants, and mood stabilizers may be used when patients have co-occurring mental disorders, such as bipolar disorder, schizophrenia, depression, and anxiety disorders.

LAPSE VS RELAPSE

Lapse also called as sometimes "slip" is the preliminary contravention of problematic behavior after attempting to quit substance use. This ultimately led to sustained transgressions to a level that is close to earlier quitting behavior and is defined as a "relapse". Another probable consequence of a lapse is that the client may succeed to refrain and thus continue to go onward in a positive change, "prolapse".[6]

RELAPSE PREVENTION

Relapse prevention (RP) is a plan of action for lessening the probability and severity of relapse following the stopping or reduction of problematic behaviours.[6] RP is a cognitive-based behavioral tactic with an aim of recognizing and addressing high-risk conditions for relapse and helping individuals in maintaining appropriate behavioral changes.

It has two specific purposes: (1) Preventing a preliminary lapse and maintaining abstinence or harm reduction treatment goals; (2) Providing lapse management if a lapse happens such that additional relapses can be prohibited.[1]

Usually RP is managed pharmacologically by anticraving and nonpharmacologically by different psychotherapies.

Anticraving Medications

Anticraving medications started irrespective of what kind of care a patient is receiving, i.e., outdoor or indoor care. Naltrexone is a Food and Drug Administration (FDA)-approved medication used to stop alcohol drinking.[7] It is an opioid receptor antagonist, mainly blocking μ opioid receptors, thus reducing the rewarding effect of alcohol and opioid on brain. The starting dose is 50 mg/day after a test dose of 25 mg. Patient should be observed for any side effects or any sign of opioid withdrawal symptoms. Naltrexone is contraindicated in acute hepatitis or liver failure. Another agent which can be used as anticraving is acamprosate, which is also FDA approved. Baclofen can also be used as anticraving, though it is not approved by FDA. The duration of anticraving can be from 6 months to 1 year.

In case of opioid-dependence syndrome after a definite wash out period of drug which is usually 5 days in case of short-acting opioids and 10 days after long-acting opioids such as methadone, anticraving started. However, in case of alcohol use disorder anticraving medication can be started in detoxification phase.

Aversive Therapies

Disulfiram is a second-line option in patients one of three drugs approved by the FDA for the treatment of alcohol dependence. Started with a dose of 250 mg/day, with caution as it causes disulfiram-ethanol reaction (DER) result from inhibition of metabolism of acetaldehyde to acetate by inhibition of aldehyde dehydrogenase when patient take alcohol, which can be fatal and cause serious consequences. DER can happen with drugs such as metronidazole and ornidazole also, so physicians should be careful regarding prescribing these medications to an alcohol use disorder patient.[8]

Motivational Enhancement Therapy

Motivational enhancement therapy (MET) is a systematic approach to evoke change in individuals. It is a short-term drug or alcohol addiction treatment that is designed to support clients to recognize and build on personal strengths to help change damaging drug abusing or drinking behaviors. It focuses in encouraging a patient to develop a negative view of their abuse, along with a desire to change their behavior. MET is typically conducted as individual counselling, though family members may also be present and engaged.

Motivational enhancement therapy is typically brief, limited to two to four sessions that each last one hour. MET extensively supports the stages of change: transtheoretical model. It consists of a linear pattern of the stages of change, which includes four stages namely precontemplation, contemplation, action, and maintenance. But in most individuals, this do not progress linearly and it led to relapse.[9]

Chronic use of drug can lead partial or complete social and occupational disruption of individual, and it requires utmost importance to manage these areas to achieve comprehensive management of patient. Evidence-based psychosocial interventions are available, which can promote behavior change.[10]

Cognitive Behavioral Therapy

Cognitive behavioral therapy (CBT) is commonly evaluated as the most successful method of treatment of drug and alcohol population.[11] CBT can help in those individuals who have sort of cognitive distortions, persistent stressor, which enable the person to remain in the state illness phase. Usually, cognitive strategies employed are allowing and challenging malfunctional thoughts about illicit drugs and identifying outwardly inappropriate decisions that lead to a relapse.[12]

Managing Enabling

Managing enabling can be challenging in case of family dysfunction and is typically associated with a family member's alcohol or drug abuse.[13] In patient having multiple relapses enabling should be suspected. Instead of helping, family members can enable person to continue using substance. Identifying enabling could be a difficult task and proper management is necessary to avoid multiple relapses.

CONCLUSION

Drug addiction is a complex but treatable brain disease which affects multiple brain circuits including reward and motivation, learning and memory and behavior. It has lapsing and relapsing course and often require both pharmacological and psychological approach. Drug addiction treatment varies depending on the type of drug and the characteristics of the patients. The success of the treatment also depends on addressing individual's drug abuse and other associated medical, psychological, social issues.

TAKE-HOME POINTS

- Drug addiction is a chronic, complex disease but a treatable medical condition.
- Drug addiction results from a complex interaction among genes, various brain circuits and the environment.
- The first step in overcoming an addiction is taking a decision to change.
- No single treatment is appropriate for everyone in addiction management.
- Effective treatment means to address the multiple needs of the individual, not just his or her drug abuse problem.
- Drug addiction treatment often requires medications combined with counseling and other behavioral therapies.
- Seeking help from social support groups such as self help groups is sometimes helpful.

REFERENCES

1. Menon J, Kandasamy A. Relapse prevention. Indian J Psychiatry. 2018;60:473-8.
2. Stahl SM, Stahl SM (Eds). Stahl's Essential Psychopharmacology, 4th edition. Cambridge University Press; 2013.
3. Medina-Mora ME. Prevention of substance abuse: a brief overview. World Psychiatry. 2005;4(1):25.
4. Roche A, Freeman T. Brief interventions: Good in theory but weak in practice. Drug Alcohol Rev. 2004;23:11-8.
5. Fleming MF, Mundt MP, French MT. Brief physician advice for problem drinkers: long-term efficacy and benefit-cost analysis. Alcohol Clin Exp Res. 2002;26:36-43.
6. Marlatt GA, Donovan DM. Relapse prevention: Maintenance strategies in treatment of addictive behaviours, 2nd edition. Guilford Press; 2005.
7. Shen WW. Clinical psychopharmacology for the 21st century, third edition. Taipei: Ho-Chi Publishing Company; 2011.
8. Medication for the Treatment of Alcohol Use Disorder: A Brief Guide. [online] Available from https://store.samhsa.gov/sites/default/files/d7/priv/sma15-4907.pdf [Last accessed March, 2023].
9. Prochaska JO, DiClemente CC. Toward a comprehensive model of change. In: WR Miller, N Heather (Eds). Treating Addictive Behaviors: Processes of Change. Plenum Press. 1986. pp. 3-27.
10. Hubbard RL, Craddock SG, Flynn PM, Anderson J, Etheridge RM. Overview of 1-year follow-up outcomes in the drug abuse treatment outcome study (DATOS). Psychol Addict Behav. 1997;11:261-78.
11. McRae AL, Budney AJ, Brady KT. Treatment of marijuana dependence: a review of the literature. J Subst Abuse Treat. 2003;24:369-76.
12. Jhanjee S. Evidence based psychosocial interventions in substance use. Indian J Psychol Med. 2014;36(2):112-8.
13. Rotunda RJ, Doman K. Partner enabling of substance use disorders: critical review and future directions. Am J Fam Ther. 2001;29(4):257-70.

CHAPTER 20

Early Prevention in Psychiatry

Ravichandra Karkal, Ganesh Kini K, Mohan Raju S

"The prevention of any disease is the prevention of psychiatric disorders. Anyone who teaches preventive medicine teaches preventive psychiatry; he can do no other".

–Paul V Lemkau, 1965

■ INTRODUCTION

Preventive psychiatry is the branch of psychiatry that aims at developing individual, familial, social, economic, legal, political, and medical measures for health promotion, protection from specific mental illnesses, early diagnosis and effective treatment of mental illness, disability limitation, and rehabilitation.[1] Mental disorders are a major reason for global disease burden and 1 in 7 Indians were affected by psychiatric disorders in 2017. The contribution of mental disorders to disability-adjusted life years (DALYs) almost doubled in 2017 (2.5%) as compared to 1990 (4.7%).[2] Existing treatments reduce the disease burden only by about 40% even under optimal conditions.[3] In addition, most mental disorders have an onset before the age of 18 years.[4] A meta-analysis of 18,282 children found that a fifth of these children had a diagnosable mental health disorder before the age of 7 years.[5] Childhood and adolescence are critical stages of life for mental health because of greater sensitivity and vulnerability of early brain development. They are a crucial period for developing social and emotional skills that contribute to adult mental well-being. Traditionally mental health services are inefficient in providing services to young individuals.[6] Emergence of psychiatric disorders will invariably have impact on the developmental trajectory of an individual and have long-term consequences on social, family, educational, and vocational areas. Prevention of these disorders is perhaps one of the most effective ways to reduce the burden to the individual and to the healthcare system. Preventive approaches are traditionally seen to be cheaper than treatment interventions, can be delivered by nonspecialists, and can be delivered to larger numbers making them best suited for a lower middle-income country like ours. Thus, prevention is the only sustainable option for the field of mental health care. Some of the puzzling questions facing the field of preventive psychiatry are: Which approaches will be beneficial? When to intervene? Who are the key groups that will benefit? How to deliver at scale and across the life span? and are there any potential harmful effects of these early prevention approaches?[7]

COMMON FRAMEWORKS FOR PREVENTIVE EFFORTS

Current preventive approaches for mental health are based on a biopsychosocial understanding of mental illnesses. The public health framework in preventive medicine classifies preventions into: (1) primary prevention, which aims at stopping mental health problems before they start; (2) secondary prevention, which aims at supporting those at higher risk of experiencing mental health problems; and (3) tertiary prevention, which aims at helping people living with mental health problems stay well. The current World Health Organization (WHO) framework includes universal, selective, and indicated preventive interventions under the primary prevention paradigm, which focus on who receives the intervention.[8] Universal prevention is targeted at the larger population regardless of its risk status. Selective prevention, on the other hand, is targeted at individuals who are at a higher risk of developing a mental disorder because of one or more risk factors. Indicated prevention, on the contrary, is targeted at those individuals who do not currently meet diagnostic criteria for a disorder but show some detectable signs or symptoms, or biological markers indicating a predisposition for a certain disorder. Experts also identify that the conceptual boundaries between preventive interventions and treatments are blurred in the early stages of management.[9]

TRANSDIAGNOSTIC MODEL TO IDENTIFY AT-RISK GROUPS

Early prevention in psychiatry began with a narrow focus on individuals at high risk of developing psychotic disorders. The "prodrome" was initially understood as a state where symptoms existed in lower intensity than a categorical diagnosis and it would inevitably lead to a full-blown disorder. Over the last few decades, we have moved to "at-risk mental state" concept for the prevention of mental disorders. Research has shown that in addition to transition to psychosis, or persistent subthreshold psychotic symptoms, "at-risk mental states" can progress to persistent mood, anxiety, personality, and substance use disorders (SUDs). Risk factors are pluripotent and during development may lead to a range of psychopathologies. For example, Adverse Childhood Experiences (ACEs) may contribute to several mental disorders. A transdiagnostic Clinical High-Risk Mental States (CHARMS) paradigm may be able to capture not only psychotic disorders but subthreshold bipolar and borderline personality symptoms as well as depression.[6]

THE INTERPLAY OF RISK AND PROTECTIVE FACTORS

Environmental risk factors increase susceptibility to mental disorders and are characterized by small effect sizes. They may include antenatal factors (poor maternal nutrition, exposure to drugs, maternal infections, and stress), birth complications, social risks (poverty, immigration, social isolation, and disadvantage), angiotensin-converting enzymes (ACEs) (parental neglect, physical, emotional, and sexual abuse), stressful life events, and substance use. Risk factors tend to occur together and have synergistic effect leading to a vicious cycle. Epigenetic changes support this "facilitation effect"; for example, victims of childhood trauma show epigenetic changes in serotonin transporter and glucocorticoid receptor genes.[10]

Literacy, healthy lifestyle, adaptability, positive attachment, parent–child interaction, healthy school and work environments, good coping skills, healthy interpersonal relationships, and community support are protective factors. These environmental risk and protective factors interact with the genetics of the individual inducing neurobiological changes, and then modulating the individual's ability to adapt to stress. This interplay of environmental factors across the lifespan opens opportunities for preventive interventions—biological, psychological, family-related, or social.[11]

UNIVERSAL PREVENTIVE INTERVENTIONS

Universal prevention aims at promoting normal neurodevelopment by addressing genetic risk and protective factors. WHO Health Promoting School framework has shown public health benefits at population level.[12] Brief intervention with video feedback to new parents may promote positive parenting and improve parental sensitivity.[13] A meta-analysis assessing 213 school-based programs for ages 5–18 years has shown to be effective in improving socioemotional skills, attitudes, behaviors, and academic performance.[14] Universal psychoeducation and psychological interventions have shown some evidence in improving affective and anxiety symptoms.[15] School-based interventions minimize risk of bullying and peer rejection. Lifetime omega-3 fatty acid, vitamin, sulforaphane, and prebiotic supplementation help reduce putative risk factors such as neuroinflammation, oxidative stress, and gut dysbiosis.[6]

Self-administered questionnaires such as the Prodromal Questionnaire and Kessler Psychological Distress Scale have been used to identify surrogate markers for psychosis, bipolar, depressive, and anxiety disorders. Childhood behavioral problems are associated with later development of psychoses. One study looked at supplementation of phosphatidylcholine in healthy pregnant women and found that their children showed fewer attention problems and less social withdrawal at 40 months of age thus potentially altering the risk of later development of psychosis.[16] A randomized controlled trial (RCT) looked at the effect of folate and long-chain polyunsaturated fatty acid (PUFA) supplementation in pregnant women. Children born to such mothers showed improved neurocognitive biomarkers.[17]

In one study the cohort of children who had Good Behavior Game (GBG) intervention during their first grade had significantly lower incidence of SUDs when followed up at age 19–21 when compared with children who received the standard intervention.[18]

A meta-analysis of prospective cohort studies confirmed that physical activity could confer protection against the emergence of anxiety regardless of demographic factors.[19] Physical activity was found to be specially protective in agoraphobia and post-traumatic stress disorder (PTSD). Several universal preventive interventions, which include psychoeducation, psychotherapy, and art therapy among others, have been tested for their effectiveness to promote good mental health in young people. One meta-analysis confirmed the efficacy of these interventions in young people.[20]

The Lancet Commission on Dementia Prevention, Intervention, and Care[21] estimated that 35% of the dementia could be prevented by modifying nine risk factors: Early life education, midlife hypertension, obesity, hearing loss, old-age smoking, depression, physical inactivity, diabetes, and social isolation. In a Cochrane Database Systematic Review of three high quality RCTs looking at the effect of omega-3 long-chain PUFA for the prevention of cognitive decline and dementia, the authors concluded that there is no benefit of omega-3 PUFA supplementation on cognitive function in cognitively healthy older people.[22] The Prevención con Dieta Mediterránea (PREDIMED) trial investigated for the effect of Mediterranean diet on cognitive function in cognitively healthy participants. It was noted that a Mediterranean diet supplemented with olive oil or nuts was associated with improvement in cognitive function.[23] RCTs have not found *Ginkgo biloba* to be an effective cognitive enhancer.[24]

SELECTIVE PREVENTIVE INTERVENTIONS

Selective prevention strategies target subsets of the total population that are considered at risk for mental health problems by virtue of their membership in a particular segment of the population. It targets the entire subgroup regardless of the degree of risk of any individual within the group. These interventions require significant understanding of the association between specific genetic and nongenetic factors and incidence of mental disorders. Preventive efforts focus on addressing social risk factors, emotional problems, promoting resilience, facilitating early detection, and ensuring access to services.[11]

Familial vulnerability, especially parental mental illness and SUDs, is the most implementable target for selective screening interventions. Genetic vulnerability, for example, 22q11.2 deletion syndrome, offers a promising human model for studying psychosis risk factors. One European study found that the transition rate to psychosis was higher for the ultrahigh risk (UHR) group compared to the non-UHR group with 22q11.2 deletion syndrome.[25] However, the study highlighted additional predictors such as baseline verbal IQ and presence of anxiety disorder for transition to psychosis. One meta-analysis found that selective psychoeducational interventions may have a small effect on reducing the severity and incidence of depression in patients' children.[26] However, the efficacy of psychosocial interventions in young individuals with a family vulnerability for psychotic, bipolar, or anxiety disorders is currently not known.

One umbrella review found two peripheral biomarkers, viz. decreased pyridoxal levels and elevated awakening cortisol levels to be reliably associated with psychosis, bipolar disorder, and depression.[27] A meta-analysis found that selective psychological interventions could reduce anxiety in women who experienced intimate partner violence.[28] Another meta-analysis which reviewed the efficacy of selective psychological interventions for young people found psychoeducation to be the most effective intervention in improving affective symptoms.[20] A systematic review and a network meta-analysis of school-based interventions found weak evidence for cognitive behavioral interventions in reducing anxiety; however, no intervention was seen to be effective in preventing depression.[29] One systematic review of meta-analyses found evidence for effectiveness of exercise intervention in depressive symptoms in at-risk youths.[30] Hydrocortisone has been shown to be effective in preventing PTSD in adults after a traumatic event.[31]

The screening, brief intervention, and referral to treatment (SBIRT) model has been tried with some success for adolescents who have started using substances but have not developed SUDs. In a systematic review of the effectiveness of SBIRT in emergency department, the reviewers found that Brief Interventions were effective in reducing the negative consequences of alcohol such as driving under influence of alcohol and subsequent injuries, at least in the short term.[32] These Brief Interventions can perhaps be implemented at the school level and can be supplemented with frequent follow up at substance use clinics.

Vitamin E (2,000 IU/day) has been proven to slow the functional decline in patients with mild to moderate Alzheimer's disease by reducing oxidative stress.[33] However, another study has shown no benefit in patients with mild cognitive impairment.[34] B vitamins (via lowering of homocysteine) have not shown significant lowering of cognitive decline.[35] Vitamin D acts as a neuroprotective factor by influencing the output of several neurotrophic factors. Low levels of vitamin D seem to pose a higher risk for Alzheimer's disease.[36] However, this meta-analysis not only included RCTs but also cross-sectional studies, cohort studies, and case–control studies.

INDICATED PREVENTIVE INTERVENTIONS

There is a growing body of evidence for indicated preventive interventions in reducing the incidence of psychotic, bipolar, and common mental disorders in young people.

An international online survey of 47 centers offering services to 22,248 individuals at clinical high risk for psychosis (CHR-P) concluded that primary indicated prevention of psychosis in CHR-P individuals was possible but the implementation of CHR-P services was heterogenous and constrained by pragmatic challenges.[37] Indicated prevention for psychosis has the potential to improve the presenting symptoms, delay or prevent the onset of symptoms, reduce healthcare access, and duration of untreated psychosis.[38] Researchers have so far focused on antipsychotic medications such as olanzapine and risperidone, dietary interventions such as omega-3 fatty acids, psychological interventions such as cognitive behavioral therapy (CBT), supportive counselling, and integrated psychological therapy. A 2018 network meta-analysis found no robust evidence to favor any intervention in preventing transition to psychosis.[39]

N-methyl-D-aspartate (NMDA) receptor modulating compounds such as glycine and D-serine are potential treatments in individuals with high risk for schizophrenia. Glycine was noted to produce reduction in positive symptoms with large effect size.[40] D-serine was noted to produce statistically significant reduction in negative symptoms in patients with prodromal symptoms of schizophrenia.[41] The biggest limitations of both the trials were the small sample size. In one small double-blind randomized clinical trial, 16 patients at CHR-P received a single oral dose of 600 mg of cannabidiol (CBD). It was noted that the blood oxygen level-dependent (BOLD) functional magnetic resonance imaging (fMRI) signal activation noted in medial temporal, mid brain, and striatal regions was intermediate when compared to control and patients who received a placebo.[42] Cognitive training in patients at high risk for psychosis with cognitive deficits shows improvement in functional and social outcomes. In one study auditory cognitive training was noted to produce statistically significant improvements in social functioning.[43] Another study, where patients received intensive cognitive training, noted significant improvement in verbal memory.[44]

Indicated prevention in bipolar disorder is relatively new with its support base lagging behind that for CHR-P. Bipolar at-risk individuals are represented by young help-seeking clinical samples (mean age 16–23 years) including a subset of CHR-P individuals. One study which used MRI data from a multicenter study to assess structural gray alterations in 263 help-seeking young adults (age 15–35 years) from seven study sites found that the cortex was significantly thinner in high-risk individuals compared to those in the no-risk group. This is in line with previous findings in patients with the established disorder.[45] Two RCTs conducted among adolescents and young adults presenting with genetic risk for affective disorder and attenuated affective symptoms suggested probable benefits from family-focused and cognitive behavioral interventions to recover from attenuated symptoms. However, these interventions did not help in reducing the severity of affective symptoms or preventing the onset of bipolar disorder.[46,47]

Research on indicated prevention of depression and anxiety disorders in young people is limited. There are no established clinical high-risk criteria to assess young people with an increased risk of depression (without bipolar risk features) or anxiety disorders. One study that used systematic review, meta-analysis, and meta regression found that psychological and or educational interventions had a small but significant benefit for anxiety prevention in all populations evaluated.[48] A review of the joint efficacy of universal, selective, and indicated preventive strategies used with children and adolescents showed reduction of risk of disorder onset and reduction of symptom levels for internalizing disorders for up to 12 months.[15]

Cognitive behavioral therapy-based interventions are shown to be effective for preventing PTSD in individuals showing acute stress after a traumatic event.[49] CBT-based strategies are also shown to be effective in preventing eating disorders in young individuals with subthreshold symptoms.[31] Parent management training have shown efficacy in preventing externalizing disorders in children with high antisocial behavior.[50]

Anonymity provided by digital platforms helps in engaging teenagers and young adults who have SUDs. In one such digital program for quitting e-cigarettes, researchers followed up a cohort of 27,000 teenagers and young adults.[51] At the end of 14 days, 60.8% of the participants had either reduced or stopped e-cigarettes. There was high engagement with the program despite the knowledge that they were engaging in a conversation with a bot. A scoping review of indicated online preventive interventions revealed effectiveness in reducing subclinical symptoms of various mental illnesses and improve several outcome measures such as quality of life and mindfulness.[52]

A recent systematic review from 2018 which included Advanced Cognitive Training for Independent and Vital Elderly (ACTIVE) trial concluded that the evidence to show that cognitive training done to prevent/delay the onset of dementia is insufficient.[53] In preclinical models, statins have been known to reduce inflammatory cytokine release from astrocytes and endothelial cells, induced by fibrillary beta-amyloid, which is known to cause cell death.[54] However, a Cochrane Database Systematic Review from 2016 found that there was no difference between statins and placebo on five different cognitive tests.[55] Acetylcholinesterase inhibitors such as donepezil,[56] rivastigmine,[57] and galantamine[58] have all proven to be unsuccessful in preventing dementia in patients with mild cognitive impairment. Nonsteroidal anti-inflammatory drugs have not shown benefits in cognitively healthy adults and in case of naproxen and celecoxib showed higher hazard ratios.[59,60] In June, 2021 the United States Food and Drug Administration (US FDA) approved aducanumab for treatment of patients with mild cognitive impairment or mild dementia stage of Alzheimer's disease.[61] The approval was provided based on evidence from two randomized, double blind, placebo-controlled trials by Biogen (n = 3,285). 80% of the participants, in both the trials, were patients with mild cognitive impairment. However, experts who have reviewed the data from the two trials have questioned the approval, stating that only one of the trials could obtain the primary end point relative to the placebo.[62] Meanwhile other monoclonal antibodies such as lecanemab, solanezumab, crenezumab, donanemab, and gantenerumab are in various stages of clinical trials/review process for approval.[63]

CHALLENGES IN THE EFFICIENT IMPLEMENTATION OF EARLY PREVENTION

There are hindrances to effective implementation of prevention strategies in mental health. The risk and protective factors contributing to mental health are small and too many to quantify. They are nonspecific and may lead to a host of disorders. Even with the advances in neurosciences, neuroimaging, molecular techniques, and genomics we are yet to discern clear pathways that lead to a specific International Classification of Diseases/Diagnostic and Statistical Manual of Mental Disorders (ICD/DSM) diagnosis. There is absence of reliable biomarkers and validated screening tools to deploy at scale. As these prevention efforts do not have short-term returns, they are relatively unattractive to researchers. Poor understanding of long-term economic savings makes it less feasible for policy makers. Interventions are difficult to implement in low-resource settings and in populations with lack of access to care. One must be mindful of potential harms of treatment, especially pharmacological in false positive cases or individuals with temporary symptoms.[11]

CONCLUSION

Efforts to develop curative remedies for psychiatric disorders have been met with limited success. Mental health professionals have become cognizant of the need for a paradigmatic shift in the management of psychiatric disorders through early preventive strategies. There is a dearth of reliable biomarkers and assessment tools to identify these "at-risk states". In addition, there is sparse evidence of the benefits of available treatment options for these high-risk individuals. Yet it is too early to overlook the role of early prevention in psychiatry.

TAKE-HOME POINTS

- Early prevention strategies in psychiatry exist and are effective.
- Implementation of these strategies is limited by nascent understanding of developmental psychopathology across the lifespan and lack of reliable biomarkers for early detection.
- A transdiagnostic CHARMS model will help identify at-risk individuals.
- Universal, selective, and indicated preventive interventions have shown effectiveness in promoting mental health and preventing mental disorders.
- Policy makers need to realize the potential of early prevention in psychiatry and make investments in structurally integrated, multicomponent interventions.

REFERENCES

1. Campbell RJ. Campbell's Psychiatric Dictionary, 9th edition. Oxford, New York: Oxford University Press; 2009.
2. Sagar R, Dandona R, Gururaj G, Dhaliwal RS, Singh A, Ferrari A, et al. The burden of mental disorders across the states of India: the Global Burden of Disease Study 1990-2017. Lancet Psychiatry. 2020;7:148-61.
3. Andrews G, Issakidis C, Sanderson K, Corry J, Lapsley H. Utilising survey data to inform public policy: comparison of the cost-effectiveness of treatment of ten mental disorders. Br J Psychiatry. 2004;184: 526-33.
4. Kim-Cohen J, Caspi A, Moffitt TE, Harrington H, Milne BJ, Poulton R. Prior juvenile diagnoses in adults with mental disorder: developmental follow-back of a prospective-longitudinal cohort. Arch Gen Psychiatry. 2003;60:709-17.
5. Vasileva M, Graf RK, Reinelt T, Petermann U, Petermann F. Research review: a meta-analysis of the international prevalence and comorbidity of mental disorders in children between 1 and 7 years. J Child Psychol Psychiatry. 2021;62:372-81.
6. Colizzi M, Lasalvia A, Ruggeri M. Prevention and early intervention in youth mental health: is it time for a multidisciplinary and trans-diagnostic model for care? Int J Ment Health Syst. 2020;14: 23.
7. Holmes EA, Ghaderi A, Harmer CJ, Ramchandani PG, Cuijpers P, Morrison AP, et al. The Lancet Psychiatry Commission on psychological treatments research in tomorrow's science. Lancet Psychiatry. 2018;5(3):237-86.
8. WHO. Prevention of Mental Disorders. Geneva: World Health Organization. [online] Available from https://public.ebookcentral.proquest.com/choice/publicfullrecord.aspx?p=4978589 [Last accessed March, 2023].
9. Fusar-Poli P, Correll CU, Arango C, Berk M, Patel V, Ioannidis JPA. Preventive psychiatry: a blueprint for improving the mental health of young people. World Psychiatry. 2021;20:200-21.
10. Teicher MH, Samson JA, Anderson CM, Ohashi K. The effects of childhood maltreatment on brain structure, function and connectivity. Nat Rev Neurosci. 2016;17:652-66.
11. Arango C, Díaz-Caneja CM, McGorry PD, Rapoport J, Sommer IE, Vorstman JA, et al. Preventive strategies for mental health. Lancet Psychiatry. 2018;5:591-604.
12. Langford R, Bonell CP, Jones HE, Pouliou T, Murphy SM, Waters E, et al. The WHO Health Promoting School framework for improving the health and

13. well-being of students and their academic achievement. Cochrane Database Syst Rev. 2014;(4):CD008958.
13. Juffer F, Bakermans Kranenburg MJ, Van Ijzendoorn MH. Promoting Positive Parenting: An Attachment-Based Intervention. Routledge & CRC Press. [online] Available from https://www.routledge.com/Promoting-Positive-Parenting-An-Attachment-Based-Intervention/Juffer-Bakermans-Kranenburg-Ijzendoorn/p/book/9780805863529 [Last accessed March, 2023].
14. Durlak JA, Weissberg RP, Dymnicki AB, Taylor RD, Schellinger KB. The impact of enhancing students' social and emotional learning: a meta-analysis of school-based universal interventions. Child Dev. 2011;82:405-32.
15. Stockings EA, Degenhardt L, Dobbins T, Lee YY, Erskine HE, Whiteford HA, et al. Preventing depression and anxiety in young people: a review of the joint efficacy of universal, selective and indicated prevention. Psychol Med. 2016;46:11-26.
16. Ross RG, Hunter SK, Hoffman MC, McCarthy L, Chambers BM, Law AJ, et al. Perinatal phosphatidylcholine supplementation and early childhood behavior problems: evidence for CHRNA7 Moderation. Am J Psychiatry. 2016;173:509-16.
17. Catena A, Muñoz-Machicao JA, Torres-Espínola FJ, Martínez-Zaldívar C, Diaz-Piedra C, Gil A, et al. Folate and long-chain polyunsaturated fatty acid supplementation during pregnancy has long-term effects on the attention system of 8.5-y-old offspring: a randomized controlled trial. Am J Clin Nutr. 2016;103:115-27.
18. Kellam SG, Mackenzie AC, Brown CH, Poduska JM, Wang W, Petras H, et al. The good behavior game and the future of prevention and treatment. Addict Sci Clin Pract. 2011;6:73-84.
19. Schuch FB, Stubbs B, Meyer J, Heissel A, Zech P, Vancampfort D, et al. Physical activity protects from incident anxiety: a meta-analysis of prospective cohort studies. Depress Anxiety. 2019;36:846-58.
20. Salazar de Pablo G, De Micheli A, Solmi M, Oliver D, Catalan A, Verdino V, et al. Universal and selective interventions to prevent poor mental health outcomes in young people: systematic review and meta-analysis. Harv Rev Psychiatry. 2021;29:196-15.
21. Livingston G, Sommerlad A, Orgeta V, Costafreda SG, Huntley J, Ames D, et al. Dementia prevention, intervention, and care. Lancet. 2017;390:2673-734.
22. Sydenham E, Dangour AD, Lim WS. Omega 3 fatty acid for the prevention of cognitive decline and dementia. Cochrane Database Syst Rev. 2012;CD005379.
23. Valls-Pedret C, Sala-Vila A, Serra-Mir M, Corella D, de la Torre R, Martínez-González MÁ, et al. Mediterranean diet and age-related cognitive decline: a Randomized Clinical Trial. JAMA Intern Med. 2015;175:1094-103.
24. DeKosky ST, Williamson JD, Fitzpatrick AL, Kronmal RA, Ives DG, Saxton JA, et al. Ginkgo biloba for prevention of dementia: a randomized controlled trial. JAMA. 2008;300:2253-62.
25. Schneider M, Armando M, Pontillo M, Vicari S, Debbané M, Schultze-Lutter F, et al. Ultra high risk status and transition to psychosis in 22q11.2 deletion syndrome. World Psychiatry. 2016;15:259-65.
26. Loechner J, Starman K, Galuschka K, Tamm J, Schulte-Körne G, Rubel J, et al. Preventing depression in the offspring of parents with depression: a systematic review and meta-analysis of randomized controlled trials. Clin Psychol Rev. 2018;60:1-14.

27. Carvalho AF, Solmi M, Sanches M, Machado MO, Stubbs B, Ajnakina O, et al. Evidence-based umbrella review of 162 peripheral biomarkers for major mental disorders. Transl Psychiatry. 2020;10:152.
28. Keynejad RC, Hanlon C, Howard LM. Psychological interventions for common mental disorders in women experiencing intimate partner violence in low-income and middle-income countries: a systematic review and meta-analysis. Lancet Psychiatry. 2020;7:173-90.
29. Caldwell DM, Davies SR, Hetrick SE, Palmer JC, Caro P, López-López JA, et al. School-based interventions to prevent anxiety and depression in children and young people: a systematic review and network meta-analysis. Lancet Psychiatry. 2019;6:1011-20.
30. Hu MX, Turner D, Generaal E, Bos D, Ikram MK, Ikram MA, et al. Exercise interventions for the prevention of depression: a systematic review of meta-analyses. BMC Public Health. 2020;20:1255.
31. Astill Wright L, Sijbrandij M, Sinnerton R, Lewis C, Roberts NP, Bisson JI. Pharmacological prevention and early treatment of post-traumatic stress disorder and acute stress disorder: a systematic review and meta-analysis. Transl Psychiatry. 2019;9:1-10.
32. Barata IA, Shandro J, Montgomery M, Polansky R, Sachs CJ, Duber HC, et al. Effectiveness of SBIRT for alcohol use disorders in the emergency department: a systematic review. West J Emerg Med. 2017;18(6):1143-52.
33. Dysken MW, Sano M, Asthana S, Vertrees JE, Pallaki M, Llorente M, et al. Effect of vitamin E and memantine on functional decline in Alzheimer disease: the TEAM-AD VA cooperative randomized trial. JAMA. 2014;311:33-44.
34. Petersen RC, Thomas RG, Grundman M, Bennett D, Doody R, Ferris S, et al. Vitamin E and donepezil for the treatment of mild cognitive impairment. N Engl J Med. 2005;352:2379-88.
35. Clarke R, Bennett D, Parish S, Lewington S, Skeaff M, Eussen SJ, et al. Effects of homocysteine lowering with B vitamins on cognitive aging: meta-analysis of 11 trials with cognitive data on 22,000 individuals. Am J Clin Nutr. 2014;100:657-66.
36. Balion C, Griffith LE, Strifler L, Henderson M, Patterson C, Heckman G, et al. Vitamin D, cognition, and dementia: a systematic review and meta-analysis. Neurology. 2012;79:1397-405.
37. Kotlicka-Antczak M, Podgórski M, Oliver D, Maric NP, Valmaggia L, Fusar-Poli P. Worldwide implementation of clinical services for the prevention of psychosis: The IEPA early intervention in mental health survey. Early Interv Psychiatry. 2020;14:741-50.
38. Fusar-Poli P, McGorry PD, Kane JM. Improving outcomes of first-episode psychosis: an overview. World Psychiatry. 2017;16:251-65.
39. Davies C, Cipriani A, Ioannidis JPA, Radua J, Stahl D, Provenzani U, et al. Lack of evidence to favor specific preventive interventions in psychosis: a network meta-analysis. World Psychiatry. 2018;17:196-209.
40. Woods SW, Walsh BC, Hawkins KA, Miller TJ, Saksa JR, D'Souza DC, et al. Glycine treatment of the risk syndrome for psychosis: report of two pilot studies. Eur Neuropsychopharmacol. 2013;23:931-40.
41. Kantrowitz JT, Woods SW, Petkova E, Cornblatt B, Corcoran CM, Chen H, et al. D-serine for the treatment of negative symptoms in individuals at clinical high risk of schizophrenia: a pilot, double-blind, placebo-controlled, randomised

parallel group mechanistic proof-of-concept trial. Lancet Psychiatry. 2015;2:403-12.
42. Bhattacharyya S, Wilson R, Appiah-Kusi E, O'Neill A, Brammer M, Perez J, et al. Effect of cannabidiol on medial temporal, midbrain, and striatal dysfunction in people at clinical high risk of psychosis: a randomized clinical trial. JAMA Psychiatry. 2018;75:1107-17.
43. Piskulic D, Barbato M, Liu L, Addington J. Pilot study of cognitive remediation therapy on cognition in young people at clinical high risk of psychosis. Psychiatry Res. 2015;225:93-8.
44. Loewy R, Fisher M, Schlosser DA, Biagianti B, Stuart B, Mathalon DH, et al. Intensive auditory cognitive training improves verbal memory in adolescents and young adults at clinical high risk for psychosis. Schizophr Bull. 2016;42 Suppl 1:S118-126.
45. Mikolas P, Bröckel K, Vogelbacher C, Müller DK, Marxen M, Berndt C, et al. Individuals at increased risk for development of bipolar disorder display structural alterations similar to people with manifest disease. Transl Psychiatry. 2021;11:485.
46. Miklowitz DJ, Schneck CD, Walshaw PD, Singh MK, Sullivan AE, Suddath RL, et al. Effects of Family-Focused Therapy vs Enhanced Usual Care for Symptomatic Youths at High Risk for Bipolar Disorder: A Randomized Clinical Trial. JAMA Psychiatry. 2020;77:455-63.
47. Léger M, Wolff V, Kabuth B, Albuisson E, Ligier F. The mood disorder spectrum vs. schizophrenia decision tree: EDIPHAS research into the childhood and adolescence of 205 patients. BMC Psychiatry. 2022;22:194.
48. Moreno-Peral P, Conejo-Cerón S, Rubio-Valera M, Fernández A, Navas-Campaña D, Rodríguez-Morejón A, et al. Effectiveness of Psychological and/or Educational Interventions in the Prevention of Anxiety: a Systematic Review, Meta-analysis, and Meta-regression. JAMA Psychiatry. 2017;74:1021-29.
49. Kliem S, Kröger C. Prevention of chronic PTSD with early cognitive behavioral therapy: a meta-analysis using mixed-effects modeling. Behav Res Ther. 2013;51:753-61.
50. Yap MBH, Morgan AJ, Cairns K, Jorm AF, Hetrick SE, Merry S. Parents in prevention: a meta-analysis of randomized controlled trials of parenting interventions to prevent internalizing problems in children from birth to age 18. Clin Psychol Rev. 2016;50:138-58.
51. Graham AL, Jacobs MA, Amato MS. Engagement and 3-Month Outcomes From a Digital E-Cigarette Cessation Program in a Cohort of 27000 Teens and Young Adults. Nicotin Tob Res. 2020;22:859-60.
52. van Doorn M, Nijhuis LA, Egeler MD, Daams JG, Popma A, van Amelsvoort T, et al. Online indicated preventive mental health interventions for youth: a scoping review. Front Psychiatry. 2021;12:580843.
53. Butler M, McCreedy E, Nelson VA, Desai P, Ratner E, Fink HA, et al. Does cognitive training prevent cognitive decline?: a systematic review. Ann Intern Med. 2018;168:63-8.
54. Griffin JM, Kho D, Graham ES, Nicholson LF, O'Carroll SJ. Statins inhibit fibrillary β-amyloid induced inflammation in a model of the human blood brain barrier. PLoS One. 2016;11:e0157483.

55. McGuinness B, Craig D, Bullock R, Passmore P. Statins for the prevention of dementia. Cochrane Database Syst Rev. 2016;2016(1):CD003160.
56. Birks J, Flicker L. Donepezil for mild cognitive impairment. Cochrane Database Syst Rev. 2006;CD006104.
57. Feldman HH, Ferris S, Winblad B, Sfikas N, Mancione L, He Y, et al. Effect of rivastigmine on delay to diagnosis of Alzheimer's disease from mild cognitive impairment: the InDDEx study. Lancet Neurol. 2007;6:501-12.
58. Winblad B, Gauthier S, Scinto L, Feldman H, Wilcock GK, Truyen L, et al. Safety and efficacy of galantamine in subjects with mild cognitive impairment. Neurology. 2008;70:2024-35.
59. Lyketsos CG, Breitner JCS, Green RC, Martin BK, Meinert C, Piantadosi S, et al.; ADAPT Research Group. Naproxen and celecoxib do not prevent AD in early results from a randomized controlled trial. Neurology. 2007;68:1800-8.
60. Kang JH, Cook N, Manson J, Buring JE, Grodstein F. Low dose aspirin and cognitive function in the women's health study cognitive cohort. BMJ. 2007;334:987.
61. US FDA. Aducanumab (marketed as Aduhelm) Information. [online] Available from https://www.fda.gov/drugs/postmarket-drug-safety-information-patients-and-providers/aducanumab-marketed-aduhelm-information [Last accessed March, 2023].
62. Alexander GC, Emerson S, Kesselheim AS. Evaluation of aducanumab for Alzheimer disease: scientific evidence and regulatory review involving efficacy, safety, and futility. JAMA. 2021;325:1717-8.
63. Decourt B, Boumelhem F, Pope ED 3rd, Shi J, Mari Z, Sabbagh MN. Critical appraisal of amyloid lowering agents in AD. Curr Neurol Neurosci Rep. 2021;21:39.

CHAPTER 21

Ecopsychiatry: An Overview

Astha, Mina Chandra

INTRODUCTION

The environmental determinants of psychiatric disorders are emerging areas of research interest. The conventional etiological explorations for various psychiatric disorders have been largely psychological followed by biological (neurotransmitters, genetics, neuroimaging, etc.). Recent advances are now supporting an environmental contribution to psychiatric disorders beyond the biopsychosocial framework. The emerging field of *ecopsychiatry* is an *"attempt to assess the relationship of environment to mental health"* (Steven Moffik). Coined in late 1970 by American Psychological Association (APA) it came to existence to research population mental health issues that are caused by anthropogenic environmental changes.

Ecopsychology, a term introduced by Theodre Roszak in his book *The Voice of Earth*, advocates for bringing ecological thinking to psychotherapy and changing lifestyle pattern.[1]

It is a well-recognized fact that engaging in physical activity and being in nature both benefit one's physical and emotional well-being. However, biodiversity loss along with deforestation, urbanization, and climate change has raised strong environmental concerns. Air, water, and noise pollution are frequently linked with common mental disorders. Heat waves are related to aggressive behavior. The need for quality urban green space and the effect of changing land use patterns on mental health are being emphasized. The environment therefore can be therapeutic and even pathogenic (Burgess et al; 1988).[2]

METHODOLOGY

A scoping review was conducted to understand the current evidence base on ecopsychiatry. PubMed search was conducted using the following MeSH (medical subject heading) terms singly and in combination: *eco-anxiety, eco-crisis, climate change, PM2.5 depression, urbanization, urban green spaces,* and *land use pattern*. About 1,240 papers were identified by the PubMed search engine. Abstracts of all articles were assessed for relevance to yield 60 articles. Subsequently, the findings reporting in these articles were collated and synthesized.

RESULTS

The etiological contributions of the following environmental factors will be described in this chapter:
- Climate change and natural disaster
- Air pollution
- Noise pollution
- *Urbanization:* Urban green spaces, land use patterns

Climate Change and Natural Disaster

The change in climate is being perceived globally. Rising land surface air temperatures, frequency and intensity of drought, heavy precipitation, wildfire, desertification in some dryland, hurricane, severe storm, and floods[3] are an *"expression of climate variability"*.[4] Such events are forecasted to continue to rise further, with all regions surpassing the previously recorded temperatures.[4] Droughts are expected to become more severe, especially in southern Africa and the Mediterranean region.[4] Wildfires that are known to cause fatal injuries have chronic mental health impact too. Altogether these changes are being considered as a *"mental health crisis"*.[5]

Common mental health disorders have been researched extensively in the light of discrete events of natural disaster.[6] However, environmental degradation has also led to fear of *environmental doom*, i.e., *"eco-anxiety"* and with the changing landscape the term *"solastalgia"* gained popularity.[7]

Mental Health Impacts

American Psychological Association has categorized the impact on mental health into short-term (effects are primarily seen in the aftermath of disasters) and long-term changes (gradual).[8] We will discuss a few briefly **(Table 1)**.
- *Trauma and shock:* Personal injury and loss of loved one and livelihood can affect one deeply. As per Fritze et al. acute stress disorder was most

TABLE 1: Mental health impacts of climate change and natural disasters.

Short-term mental health impacts	Long-term mental health impacts
• Acute stress reaction	• Strains on social relationship
• Aggression	• Loss of autonomy
• Post-traumatic stress disorder (PTSD)	• Loss of identity
• Climate anxiety	• Solastalgia

commonly diagnosed in victims.[9] Depersonalization was reported by 25% of the earthquake survivors (Cardefia and Spiegel, 1993) and 31% of accident survivors (Noyes et al. 1977). 29% of the 1989 Bay Area earthquake survivors (Cardefia and Spiegel, 1993) reported amnesia.[10]

- *Post-traumatic stress disorder:* For majority, the acute symptoms resolve within hours or days but for some it goes on for long. Along with cardinal symptoms of post-traumatic stress disorder (PTSD), high-risk behavior, increased substance use, and suicidal ideations have been also reported.[7]

People living in disaster-prone areas are at a higher risk of having such problems. In a study done by (Kessler et al.),[11] 815 pre-hurricane residents of the areas affected by Hurricane Katrina were interviewed for baseline symptoms of anxiety, PTSD, and suicidality and were followed up to study patterns of recovery. The prevalence significantly increased for PTSD (20.0 vs. 11.8%, $t = 4.0$, $p < 0.001$), serious mental illness (SMI) (14.0 vs. 10.9%), suicidal ideation (6.4 vs. 2.8%, $t = 3.9$, $p < 0.001$), and suicide plans (2.5 vs. 1.0% $t = 3.1$, $p = 0.002$).[11]

Between 2004 and 2017 about 674 disasters occurred in Southeast Asia and two billion were affected between 2000 and 2009 according to the Red Cross Society.[12]

Among victims of Cyclone Fani, Odisha, India, PTSD was found to be 42.9%, severe anxiety (36.7%), depression (16.5%), and suicidal cognitions increased by 14%. However, this study was limited to only 84 participants who were followed up for a month post cyclone (Kar et al).[13]

- *Strains on social relationship:* Damage to livelihood strains the harmonious relationship of family and challenges family dynamics. Factors such as relocations due to disaster, unemployment due to migration, frequent change of schools, or missing academic courses for children can result in parental neglect and increase in child and domestic abuse.[9]

- *Aggression and violence:* The *heat hypothesis* states that hot temperatures increase aggressive motivation.[14] Studies have found link between the two. It can increase *the arousal* in individuals which decrease attention and also reduces *self-regulation* which alters one's cognitive abilities. With global warming "interpersonal violence" and "intergroup aggression" has also increased.[7] One of the oldest psychological explanations for this can be found in *transferred excitation theory of aggression* given by Zillmann. It says that arousal from one source (physiological like heat) can energize some other response.[15]

In an attempt to "Quantifying the Influence of Climate on Human Conflict" Hsiang et al. found that the magnitude of climate's influence on modern conflict is both substantial and statistically significant ($p < 0.001$). Each 1-SD (standard deviation) change in climate toward warmer temperatures or more extreme rainfall increases the frequency of interpersonal violence by 4% and intergroup conflict by 14%.[16]

- *Eco-anxiety/climate anxiety:* Psychologists, environmentalists as well as psychiatrists have put forth their own concepts about climate anxiety. Albrecht coined the term "eco-anxiety" and defined it as *"the generalized sense that the ecological foundations of existence are in the process of collapse".*[17] Anxiety also arises from observing the gradual and seemingly irreversible effects of climate change and from worrying about one's children and future generations. People feel helpless and responsible for not taking efficient steps to stop it.

- *Solastalgia:* Albrecht (2006) coined the term *"solastalgia"* which is an amalgamation of the words *solace* and *nostalgia*.[18] It is defined as an experience of a feeling that one is losing a place that is important to them.[18] This psychological phenomenon is characterized by *a sense of desolation* and loss similar to that experienced by people forced to migrate from their home environment. Loss of relationship to place is a substantial part of climate change. As landscapes change irreversibly, a large number of people tend to harbor this feeling of loss.[7]

- *Other psychiatric disorders:* Apart from mental illness mentioned somatoform disorder and self-harm have also been reported. In a *qualitative* study done by Chowdhury, Brahma et al.,[19] 3,084 households were surveyed for the impact of *increased human–animal conflicts* in Sundarban Reserve Forest. They found that in a span of 15 years 111 persons became victims of animal attacks, of which 73.9% died.

About 51% of widows resulting from these events were in a debilitating condition, 14.6% had major depression followed by *somatoform pain disorder* (14.0%), and 11.2% cases had attempted suicide (55% used pesticides). Sundarbans delta, home to world's largest mangrove area, is experiencing a rise in tidal level. It risks the life of about 8 million people from India and Bangladesh who are directly dependent on its unstable ecosystem.

Air Pollution

Air pollution is a complex mixture of particulate matter (PM), gases, and organic and inorganic compounds present in outdoor and indoor air. PM is defined by the aerodynamic diameter, i.e. >2.5 to <10 µm as coarse particles (PM10); <2.5 µm as fine particles (PM2.5); and <100 nm as ultrafine particulate matter (UFPM)].[20]

Numerous studies have shown a connection between air pollution and respiratory and cardiovascular ailments. Given their toxicity to the central nervous system, air pollution may also contribute to the genesis of mental disorders.

Pathophysiology

Particulate matter exposure has damaging effects on the brain. They set off a chronic inflammatory process beginning with respiratory tracts leading to increased production of pro-inflammatory markers, tumor necrosis factor alpha (TNF-α), reactive oxygen species (ROS), interleukin-1 beta (IL-1β), responsible for neurotoxicity. The ongoing production of ROS and inflammatory markers lead to the worsening of existing medical condition.[21]

In a hypothesized mechanism, these pollutants are also responsible for changes at epigenetic level. For instance, methylation of CLOCK (circadian locomotor output cycles kaput) genes may trigger the onset or exacerbation of psychiatric symptoms. The same genes have been demonstrated to be implicated in the etiology of mood disorders.[22]

Mood Disorder

In a review article of 43 studies by Buoli et al.[21] increased concentration of air pollutants was positively association with onset of depressive symptoms.
- A long-term prospective study from Seoul (study period: 2002–2010, n = 27,270) found *the risk of depression increased with an increase of 10 µg/m³ in PM2.5* [hazard ratio (HR) = 1.59, confidence interval (CI) = 95%)]; (CI: 1.02–2.49, effect size: 0.13/0.26) Kim et al.[23]
- Szyszkowicz (n = 15,556) demonstrated increments in depression-related emergency visits by 6.9% (95% CI: 1.3, 12.9) for carbon monoxide (CO) in warm season; 7.4% (95% CI: 0.5, 14.8) nitrogen dioxide (NO_2) for female patients in warm season; 4.5% (95% CI: 0.1, 9.1) sulfur dioxide (SO_2) for female patients in warm season; 7.2% (95% CI: 2.7, 12.0) PM10 for females in cold season; and 7.2% (95% CI: 2.0, 12.8) for PM2.5 for females in cold season.[24]
- Long-term exposure to *air pollution increases the odds of depression and the use of antidepressants and benzodiazepines*; 2.00 (95% CL:1.37,2.93) for each 10 µg/m³ increase in PM2.5; effect size: 0.13/0.26 (Vert et al., 2017, n = 958)[25]
- However, a review of four large European cohort studies (n = 70,928) i.e., *LifeLines* (the Netherlands), *KORA* (Germany), *HUNT* (Norway), and *FINRISK* (Finland), Zijlema et al., came up with mixed results. Positive associations were found for depression and NO_2 in *LifeLines* odds ratio (OR) = 1.34; 95% CI: 1.17, 1.53 per 10 µg/m³ increase in NO_2), whereas

negative associations were found in HUNT (OR = 0.79; 95% CI: 0.66, 0.94 per 10 µg/m³ increase in NO_2).[26]

The common drawback of the cited studies were that they *failed to account for confounding factors* such as *gender* (women are more susceptible to unipolar depression), *advanced age* (elderly are more susceptible to depression independently from pollution), or *medical comorbidities* (like stroke). Lack of studies from low- and middle-income countries (LMICs) which are known to be highly polluted (annual mean exposure of 48.42 µg/m³)[27] questions the predictive values of available data.

Developmental Disorders

According to a preliminary investigation, increased prenatal exposure to ozone (O_3) and PM2.5 was strongly linked to a higher prevalence of autism diagnoses in offspring (Becerra et al.) (n = 7,063, study period: 1998–2009). The risk of autism increases for each increase in the interquartile range of mean pollutant concentrations during the entire pregnancy, 12–15% relative increase in odds of autism for O_3 [OR = 1.12, 95% CI: 1.06, 1.19; per 11.54 parts per billion (ppb) increase] and PM2.5 (OR = 1.15; 95% CI: 1.06, 1.24; per 4.68 µg/m³ increase).[28]

National Insurance Research Database (NHIRD), a cohort from Taiwan, Jung et al. (n = 49,073; children age <3 years) found early exposure to O_3, CO, and NO_2 *postdelivery to be strongly associated with risk of developing autism spectrum disorder (ASD)* (59% risk increase per 10 ppb increase in O_3 level (95% CI 1.42–1.79), 37% risk increase per 10 ppb in CO (95% CI 1.31–1.4).[29]

Raz et al. (n = 56,289) also found risk of ASD in offspring for each 5.85 ppb increment in the mean pollutant concentrations (NO) during the 9 months after birth (OR: 1.40 CI: 1.09–1.80, ES 0.09/0.19).[30]

The observational period in the above cited studies are highly variable, with some studies focusing on pregnancy and others on early life. The prenatal exposure, occupational risk, and gestational age of study participants were not considered while accumulating data.

There is very limited literature available in context of air pollution and risk of attention-deficit hyperactivity disorder (ADHD). PM10 level was positively correlated with ADHD (OR = 2.07; 95% CI, 1.08–3.99, ES 0.20/0.40) Siddique et al. (n = 900 age: 9–17 years). The study also concluded *that rural children had higher risk of developing ADHD than those coming from urban background*. This study was limited with a small sample size and detection bias in children from rural background.[31]

Min and Min[32] followed up 8,963 infants and found that 314 subjects developed ADHD during the study period. With 1 µg/m³ increase of air pollutants, the HR of childhood ADHD increased to 1.18 (PM10) (95% CI: 1.15-1.21), 1.03 NO_2 (95% CI: 1.02-1.04, ES: 0.05/0.09). Fluegge and Fluegge criticized this study by quoting that exposure to the agricultural and combustion pollutant [nitrous oxide (N_2O)] may be a primary trigger in the onset of neurodevelopmental disorders, such as ADHD and ASD.[33]

Cognitive Decline

The findings on the cognitive impact of air pollution among elderly population concludes that *dose-dependent relationships exist between air pollutants and cognitive performance.*

Neuroimaging has shown that PM2.5 exposure is associated with "smaller brain volumes, white matter hyperintensities, increased rate of infarcts, and necrotic areas in the brain."[34]

A systematic review, Chandra et al. found significant association between exposure to air pollutants and cognitive decline.[35]

Some of the major highlights of the review were:
- A large retrospective cohort study in England (Carey et al.) studied exposure-response relationship between dementia and average annual concentrations of NO_2, $PM_{2.5}$, O_3, and noise levels (n = 1,30,978 aged 50-79 years);[36] positive exposure-response relationship between dementia and all measures of air pollution except O_3, for NO_2; a +7.5 µg/m³ change produced an HR of 1.16 (95% CI 1.05-1.28), for PM2.5 a +0.95 µg/m³, 1.07 (1.02-1.12)
- Oudin et al. found that the risk for incident dementia over a 22-year period (1988-2010) was associated with higher residential exposure to NO_2 (n = 1,469, aged 60-85 years). Participants in the group with the highest exposure to traffic-related air pollution (TRAP) were more likely to be diagnosed with dementia.[27]
- Ailshire and Crimmins, USA, studied 13,996 men and women aged 50 years or older from the 2004 Health and Retirement Study (HRS) survey, residents in areas with higher PM2.5 concentrations were associated with worse cognitive function especially *episodic memory.* (β = −0.26, 95% CI: −0.47, −0.05)[37]
- A cross-sectional study on *Heinz Nixdorf Recall* cohort study conducted in Germany revealed *that long-term residential exposure to PM, NO_2, and traffic noise was negatively correlated with verbal fluency, labyrinth test, immediate and delayed verbal recall, and global cognitive score.*[38] However, misclassification of both noise and air pollution exposure along with residual confounding between these two exposures which share a common source was a major drawback of this study.

Noise Pollution

Environmental noise exposure is as threatening a health hazard as annoying it can be. Its effects are insidious, therefore appear less alarming. The source of noise, its intensity, and proximity to source determine the effects it can have on human physiology. It is known to cause sympathetic and endocrine stress reactions through activation of hypothalamic-pituitary-adrenal (HPA) axis.

In contrast to aircraft noise, which has a detrimental effect on subjective sleep quality, road and railway noise are more likely to awaken people than aircraft noise.[39]

According to a meta-analysis conducted by Hegewald et al., aircraft noise increased depression risks by 12% per 10 dB LDEN (day-evening-night level) (ES = 1.12, 95% CI 1.02-1.23).[40] Surprisingly there are few studies that assess the effect of noise pollution on mental health independently, specially the noise related to road and railways.

Urbanization

Urbanization is a byproduct of globalization, industrialization, and social migration along with economic and political reforms. It is defined as *"the relative increase of the urban population as a proportion of the total population".*[40] From 30% in 1950 to 54% in 2014 and 66% in 2050, the proportion of people living in cities has been rising globally.[41] Uncontrolled urban growth is frequently linked to poverty, environmental damage, and exceeding population needs.

In context of ecopsychiatry, urbanization is an umbrella term that includes urban green space, blue-green space, and land use pattern.

Urban green space serves to enhance the urban environment by offering a variety of locations for recreation and enjoyment. It is defined as *"land that is partly or totally covered with grass, trees, bushes, or other vegetation".* Urban parks and forests are examples of "natural settings" or "natural surfaces" in urban areas. Green space has important advantages such as improving air quality, increasing outdoor activities of residents, and also absorbing the excessive heat and maintaining climate temperature to optimum levels.[42] Researchers generally understand blue-green space as "a composite space made up of blue space represented by rivers and lakes and green space represented by grasslands".[43]

White et al. discovered that residents in metropolitan areas with a relatively high greening level have lower average mental stress and higher life satisfaction. Viewing green landscapes has undeniably proven to have health benefits such as lowering blood pressure and heart rate along with feelings of comfort.[44]

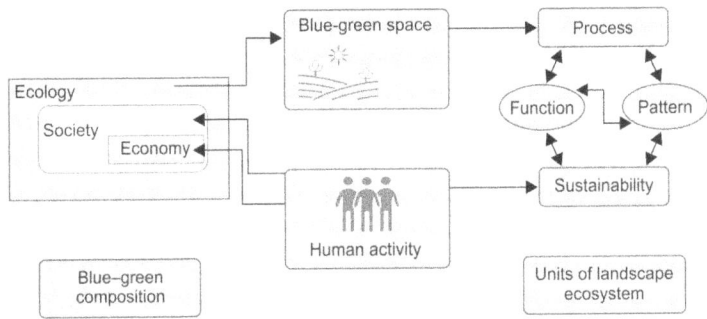

Fig. 1: Interaction between the landscape ecosystem and green spaces.

"Land use change models" are often used to *assess the impact of land cover on biophysical processes*, e.g., climate variability, land degradation, and diversity.

It is a key component of environmental assessment and can be used in multiple ways within the field of land system science. It can be used *to assess the causes of environmental change* on a global scale as well as *"to develop strategies for mitigating or adapting to that change"*. By outlining the land use realities and quantifying the trade-offs involved, land use models have the potential to enhance societal envisioning processes.[45] See **Figure 1** for a pictorial representation of the interaction between the landscape ecosystem and green spaces.

Elderly residents are prevalent in urban locations. By 2050, there will be an estimated 25% of older adults living in cities throughout LMICs, making urban surroundings significant predictors of healthy aging.[46]

A qualitative assessment of urban green spaces was done in India by Adlakha et al. Elderly residents of Delhi and Chennai ($n = 60$, age group >60 years) were interviewed regarding the design of park features, pedestrian infrastructure, and the streetscape. They expressed concerns regarding the lack of *"age-friendly amenities"* and *"safe-walking infrastructure"*. Older people living in high-rise flats valued green space more. Some of them, however, reported active avoidance due to increasing crime and threat to personal safety.

This study clearly indicated that by *reducing loneliness, fostering social cohesion, and strengthening social capital* urban green spaces serve as an important investment for *healthy aging*.[46]

Urban Design and Planning

Policy makers and urban designers together need to adopt policies in order to reduce air, light, and noise pollution, promote walking, cycling, accessible public transportation and health care services in well-organized neighborhoods and common spaces (GAPS framework is depicted in **Figure 2**).[47]

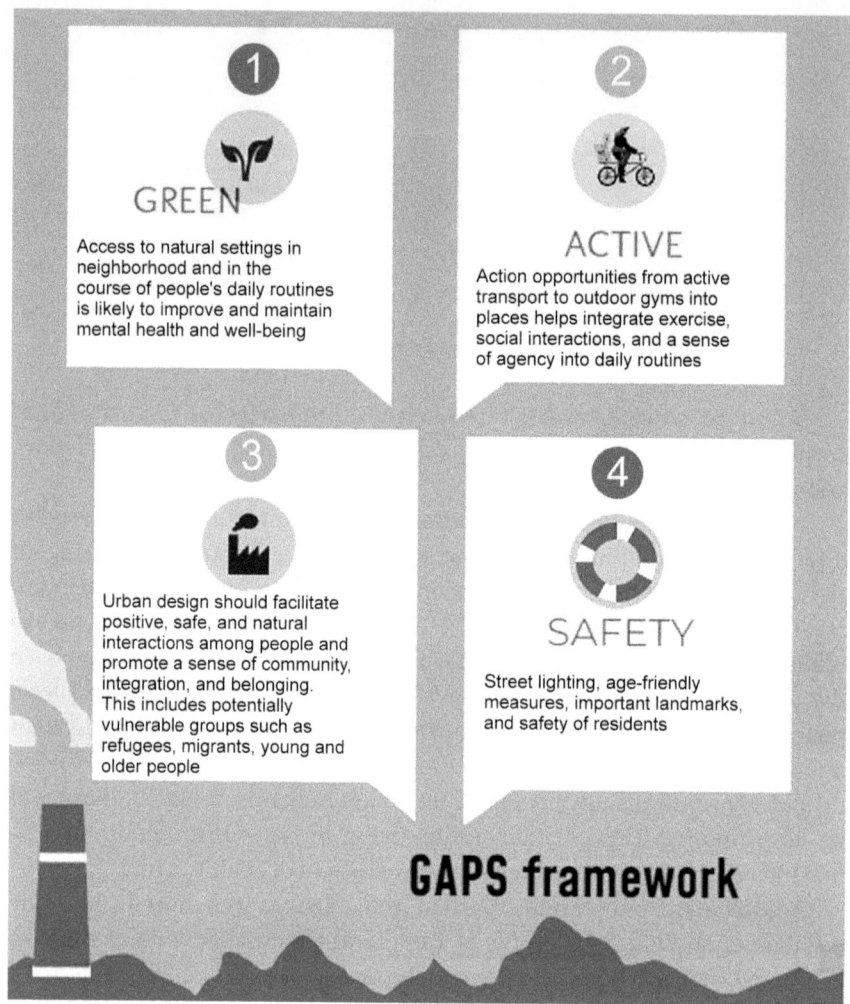

Fig. 2: Model for urban design and planning, i.e., *GAPS* (Green, Active, Pro-social, and Safe place) by the *Centre for Urban Design and Planning*.

Urbanization and Mental Illness

In the 90s, Faris and Dunham, Chicago screened 35,000 hospital admissions for psychosis and reported that risk of psychosis is higher in the city.[48] It has been reinstated thereafter in multiple studies. According to Peen et al.[47] meta-analysis, which included data from 20 population surveys since 1985; 38% higher rates for depression and 21% higher rates for anxiety in urban areas than in rural ones. Pooled OR for total prevalence of any psychiatric disorders = 1.38 (1.17–1.64), $p < 0.001$ and for mood disorders = 1.39 (1.23–1.58), $p < 0.0001$.[47]

TABLE 2: Factors affecting mental health problems in urban population.

Factors that increase mental health problems in urban areas	Preventive measures/urban remediation[47]
• Social stress • Substance abuse • Social isolation • Air and noise pollution • Crime and insecurity • Overcrowding • Cost of living • Low exposure to nature	• Targeted social services • Affordability of housing and transportation • Pro-social places: Parks, public buildings, etc., in order to promote community interactions • Quality green spaces

Sundquist et al. followed up 4 million Swedish residents from densely populated areas to find that they had 68.77% more risk of developing psychosis and 12.20% more risk of developing depression than the residents of less polluted areas. $\beta = 0.81$ (0.058) CI = 95 % HR = 2.25 (2.01–2.52) for psychosis, $\beta = 0.24$ (0.045) CI = 95% HR = 1.27 (1.17–1.39) for depression.[49]

The *AESOP* (Aetiology and Ethnicity in Schizophrenia and Other Psychoses) study, UK, highlighted the incidence of psychosis to be higher in urban areas of London.[48]

As per the National Mental Health Survey of India (2015-16), *prevalence of mood disorders and stress-related disorders in urban areas was two to three times higher than in the populations of rural and semirural areas.*[48]

Possible Etiology of Increased Mental Illness in Urban Setting

Higher prevalence of schizophrenia in urban settings has already been explained by:
- Social drift hypothesis
- Gene-environment interaction
- Exposure to environmental factors
- Detection bias in rural areas

Other contributing factors are summarized in **Table 2**.

CONCLUSION

The environmental determinants of mental health require further research. The available literature suggests deleterious impact of environmental factors on mental health. With the increasing rate of disaster South East Asia and LMIC, and two-third of the elderly people worldwide residing in LMICs, more studies are required to discuss the problem on a global scale. Further evidence base is required before translation at policy level and ground level.

ACKNOWLEDGMENT

We would like to thank Dr Vinay Kumar, President Indian Psychiatry Society, for inspiring us to address this complex topic.

TAKE-HOME POINTS

- The relationship between the built and natural elements of an environment and its relationship with human behavior, interpersonal relationships, and actual mental states is becoming more and more thoroughly documented.
- *Ecopsychiatry* is an "attempt to assess the relationship of environment to mental health".
- *Ecopsychology* is defined as the mind's synergistic relationship between environment and personal well-being; includes ecological thinking to psychotherapy.
- *Eco-anxiety* is a chronic fear of environmental doom.
- *Solastalgia* is anxiety, disorientation and depression from loss of a familiar and loved natural place.
- The effect of climate change on mental health and natural disasters is both acute and insidious. *Heat waves are being linked to aggressive behavior. Acute stress reaction, PTSD and self-harm* are common post disaster sequelae. Relocation, migration and unemployment strain the social relationship leading to a rise in domestic violence in families of victims.
- Air pollutants like PM2.5 has damaging effects on brain. *Dose dependent relationship exists between PM2.5 level and cognitive performance,* onset and worsening of depressive symptoms.
- The increasing rate of urbanization, lack of Urban Green Spaces and changing land use pattern has led to increase in urban mental health problems.
- Urban remediation measures target to increase prosocial places, quality greenspaces, ensure its safety thereby fostering social cohesion and strengthening social capital.

REFERENCES

1. Roszak T, Gomes ME, Kanner AD (Eds). Ecopsychology: Restoring the Earth, Healing the Mind. San Francisco, CA,US: Sierra Club Books; 1995. p. 338, xxiii.
2. Burgess J, Harrison CM, Limb M. People, Parks and the Urban Green: A Study of Popular Meanings and Values for Open Spaces in the City. Urban Studies. 1988;25(6):455-73.
3. Clayton S. Climate Change and Mental Health. Curr Envir Health Rpt. 2021;8: 1-6.
4. Ebi KL, Vanos J, Baldwin JW, Bell JE, Hondula DM, Errett NA, et al. Extreme Weather and Climate Change: Population Health and Health System Implications. Annu Rev Public Health. 2021;42:293-315.
5. Romeu D. Is climate change a mental health crisis? BJPsych Bull. 2021;45(4): 243-5.
6. Lowe SR, Bonumwezi JL, Valdespino-Hayden Z, Galea S. Posttraumatic Stress and Depression in the Aftermath of Environmental Disasters: A Review of Quantitative Studies Published in 2018. Curr Environ Health Rep. 2019;6: 344-60.

7. Clayton S, Manning CM, Krygsman K, Speiser M. Mental Health and Our Changing Climate: Impacts, Implications, and Guidance. Washington, D.C.: American Psychological Association, and ecoAmerica; 2017.
8. Schreiber M. Addressing climate change concerns in practice. Monit Psychol. 2021;52(3):30.
9. Fritze JC, Blashki GA, Burke S, Wiseman J. Hope, despair and transformation: Climate change and the promotion of mental health and wellbeing. Int J Ment Health Syst. 2008;2:13.
10. Koopman C, Classen C, Cardeña E. et al. When disaster strikes, acute stress disorder may follow. J Trauma Stress. 1995;8:29-46.
11. Kessler RC, Galea S, Gruber MJ, Sampson NA, Ursano RJ, Wessely S. Trends in mental illness and suicidality after Hurricane Katrina. Mol Psychiatry. 2008;13(4):374-84.
12. Jang S, Ekyalongo Y, Kim H. Systematic Review of Displacement and Health Impact from Natural Disasters in Southeast Asia. Disaster Med Public Health Prep. 2021;15:105-14.
13. Kar N, Samantaray NN, Kar S, Kar B. Anxiety, Depression, and Post-traumatic Stress a month after 2019 Cyclone Fani in Odisha, India. Disaster Med Public Health Prep. 2022;16(2):670-7.
14. Anderson CA. Heat and violence. Curr Dir Psychol Sci. 2001;10(1):33-8.
15. Zillmann D. Arousal and aggression. In: Geen RG, E. Donnerstein EI (Eds). Aggression: Theoretical and Empirical Reviews, Volume 1: Theoretical and Methodological Issues. New York: Academy Press; 1983. pp. 75-102.
16. Hsiang SM, Burke M, Miguel E. Quantifying the influence of climate on human conflict. Science. 2013;341(6151).
17. Hasbach PH. Therapy in the face of climate change. Ecopsychology. 2015; 7(4):205-10.
18. Silver A, Grek-Martin J. "Now we understand what community really means": Reconceptualizing the role of sense of place in the disaster recovery process. J Environ Psychol [Internet]. 2015;42:32-41.
19. Chowdhury AN, Mondal R, Brahma A, Biswas MK. Eco-psychiatry and environmental conservation: study from Sundarban Delta, India. Environmental Health Insights. 2008 Jan;2:EHI-S935.
20. Calderón-Garcidueñas L, Calderón-Garcidueñas A, Torres-Jardón R, Avila-Ramírez J, Kulesza RJ, Angiulli AD. Air pollution and your brain: what do you need to know right now. Prim Health Care Res Dev. 2015;16(4):329-45.
21. Buoli M, Grassi S, Caldiroli A, Carnevali GS, Mucci F, Iodice S, et al. Is there a link between air pollution and mental disorders? Environ Int. 2018;118: 154-68.
22. Buoli M, Serati M, Grassi S, Pergoli L, Cantone L, Altamura AC, et al. The role of clock genes in the etiology of Major Depressive Disorder: Special Section on "Translational and Neuroscience Studies in Affective Disorders". Section Editor, Maria Nobile MD, PhD. This Section of JAD focuses on the relevance of translational and neuroscience studies in providing a better understanding of the neural basis of affective disorders. The main aim is to briefly summaries relevant research findings in clinical neuroscience with particular regards to specific innovative topics in mood and anxiety disorders. J Affect Disord. 2018;234:351-7.

23. Kim KN, Lim YH, Bae HJ, Kim M, Jung K, Hong YC. Long-term fine particulate matter exposure and majordepressive disorder in a community-based urban cohort. Environmental health perspectives. 2016;124(10):1547-53.
24. Szyszkowicz M. Air pollution and emergency department visits for depression in Edmonton, Canada. Int J Occup Med Environ Health. 2007;20(3):241-5.
25. Vert C, Sánchez-Benavides G, Martínez D, Gotsens X, Gramunt N, Cirach M, et al. Effect of long-term exposure to air pollution on anxiety and depression in adults: a cross-sectional study. International journal of hygiene and environmental health. 2017;220(6):1074-80.
26. Zijlema WL, Wolf K, Emeny R, Ladwig KH, Peters A, Kongsgård H, et al. The association of air pollution and depressed mood in 70,928 individuals from four European cohorts. Int J Hyg Environ Health. 2016;219(2):212-9.
27. Sharma S, Chandra M, Kota SH. Health Effects Associated with PM2.5: a Systematic Review. Curr Pollut Rep. 2020;6(4):345-67.
28. Becerra TA, Wilhelm M, Olsen J, Cockburn M, Ritz B. Ambient air pollution and autism in Los Angeles County, California. Environ Health Perspect. 2013;121(3):380-6.
29. Jung CR, Lin YT, Hwang BF. Air Pollution and Newly Diagnostic Autism Spectrum Disorders: A Population-Based Cohort Study in Taiwan. PLoS One. 2013;8(9):e75510.
30. Raz R, Levine H, Pinto O, Broday DM, Yuval, Weisskopf MG. Traffic-Related Air Pollution and Autism Spectrum Disorder: A Population-Based Nested Case-Control Study in Israel. Am J Epidemiol. 2018;187(4):717-25.
31. Siddique S, Banerjee M, Ray MR, Lahiri T. Attention-deficit hyperactivity disorder in children chronically exposed to high level of vehicular pollution. Eur J Pediatr. 2011;170(7):923-9.
32. Min JY, Min KB. Exposure to ambient PM10 and NO_2 and the incidence of attention-deficit hyperactivity disorder in childhood. Environ Int. 2017;99: 221-7.
33. Fluegge K, Fluegge K. Exposure to ambient PM10 and nitrogen dioxide and ADHD risk: A reply to Min & Min (2017). Environ Int. 2017;103:109-10.
34. Schraufnagel DE, Balmes JR, Cowl CT, de Matteis S, Jung SH, Mortimer K, et al. Air Pollution and Noncommunicable Diseases: A Review by the Forum of International Respiratory Societies' Environmental Committee, Part 2: Air Pollution and Organ Systems. Chest. 2019;155:417-26.
35. Chandra M, Rai CB, Kumari N, Sandhu VK, Chandra K, Krishna M, et al. Air Pollution and Cognitive Impairment across the Life Course in Humans: A Systematic Review with Specific Focus on Income Level of Study Area. Int J Environ Res Public Health. 2022;19(3):1405.
36. Carey IM, Anderson HR, Atkinson RW, Beevers SD, Cook DG, Strachan DP, et al. Are noise and air pollution related to the incidence of dementia? A cohort study in London, England. BMJ Open. 2018;8(9):e022404.
37. Tzivian L, Dlugaj M, Winkler A, Hennig F, Fuks K, Sugiri D, et al. Long-term air pollution and traffic noise exposures and cognitive function:A cross-sectional analysis of the Heinz Nixdorf Recall study. J Toxicol Environ Health A. 2016;79(22-23):1057-69.
38. Tzivian L, Dlugaj M, Winkler A, Weinmayr G, Hennig F, Fuks KB, et al. Long-term air pollution and traffic noise exposures and mild cognitive impairment

in older adults: A cross-sectional analysis of the Heinz Nixdorf recall study. Environ Health Perspect. 2016;124(9):1361-8.
39. Hegewald J, Schubert M, Freiberg A, Starke KR, Augustin F, Riedel-Heller SG, et al. Traffic noise and mental health: A systematic review and meta-analysis. Int J Environ Res Public Health. 2020;17:6175.
40. Bhugra D, Castaldelli-Maia JM, Torales J, Ventriglio A. Megacities, migration, and mental health. Lancet Psychiatry. 2019;6(11):884-5.
41. Bocquier P. World urbanization prospects: An alternative to the UN model of projection compatible with the mobility transition theory. Demographic Research. 2005;12:197-236.
42. Yin C, Yuan M, Lu Y, Huang Y, Liu Y. Effects of urban form on the urban heat island effect based on spatial regression model. Sci Total Environ. 2018;634:696-704.
43. Song S, Wang S, Shi M, Hu S, Xu D. Urban blue-green space landscape ecological health assessment based on the integration of pattern, process, function and sustainability. Sci Rep. 2022;12(1):7707.
44. Chen K, Zhang T, Liu F, Zhang Y, Song Y. How does urban green space impact residents' mental health: A literature review of mediators. Vol. 18, Int J Environ Res Public Health. 2021;18:11746.
45. Veldkamp A, Lambin EF. Predicting land-use change. Agric Ecosyst Environ. 2001;85(1):1-6.
46. Adlakha D, Chandra M, Krishna M, Smith L, Tully MA. Designing age-friendly communities: Exploring qualitative perspectives on urban green spaces and ageing in two Indian megacities. Int J Environ Res Public Health. 2021;18(4):1491.
47. Peen J, Schoevers RA, Beekman AT, Dekker J. The current status of urban-rural differences in psychiatric disorders. Acta Psychiatr Scand. 2010;121(2):84-93.
48. Ventriglio A, Torales J, Castaldelli-Maia JM, De Berardis D, Bhugra D. Urbanization and emerging mental health issues. CNS Spectr. 2021;26(1):43-50.
49. Sundquist K, Frank G, Sundquist J. Urbanisation and incidence of psychosis and depression: Follow-up study of 4.4 million women and men in Sweden. Br J Psychiatry. 2004;184:293-8.

Index

Page numbers followed by *b* refer to box, *f* refer to figure, *fc* refer to flowchart, and *t* refer to table.

A

Aashray Adhikar Abhiyan 146
Abuse in childhood 23
Accelerated transcranial magnetic stimulation 136
Acetaldehyde, metabolism of 191
Acetylcholine 15
Actinobacteria 16
Addiction
　Facebook 157
　neurobiology of 189
　prevention of 189
　treating 189
Adverse Childhood Experiences 195
Age-friendly amenities 215
Aggression
　and violence 209
　transferred excitation theory of 209
Agitation 37, 65, 176
　acute, measures to control 57
Air and noise pollution 217
Air pollutants 210, 213, 208
Aircraft noise 214
Akathisia 63, 65, 171
　medications used in 64*b*
Alcohol 59
Alcoholism, treatment for 52
Allopurinol 104, 105
Alternating current stimulation, transcranial 138
Alzheimer's disease 12*f*, 76, 79, 95, 176, 201
　default mode network in 79
Amantadine 64
Ameliorate 89
Amino acid, degradation of 14
Aminoindanes 31
Aminorex analogs 33
Amitriptyline 108
Amphetamines 28
Amyloid beta 79
Analgesic 116
Anesthesia, dissociative 116
Angel dust 115
Anorexia nervosa 17
Antianxiety medications 190
Anticraving medications 191

Antidepressant 57, 117
　treatment 57
Antiepileptic drugs 107
Antihistamines 60
Anti-inflammatory effects 118
Antipsychotics 190
　atypical 108, 109
　first-generation 61, 62
　long-acting injectables of second-generation 173
　low dose 25, 26
　oral first-generation 58
　oral second-generation 58
　parenteral first-generation 58
　parenteral second-generation 58
　second-generation 61, 62
Anxiety 29, 156
Anxiety disorders 190, 196, 198
　prevention of 200
Anxiety measures to control 57
Aphasia 75
Apimostinel 178
Aripiprazole 25, 61, 104, 105, 106, 108, 110, 113, 171
　lauroxil 173
Armodafinil 108
Aromatic amino acid
　aminotransferase 16
　decarboxylase 16
Asenapine 104, 105, 106, 108
Astrocytes and endothelial cells 200
Asynchronous telemedicine 41
Attention deficit hyperactivity disorder 17, 80
　default mode network in 80
Attenuated psychosis syndrome 22
Auditory verbal hallucinations 77
Auricular neuromodulation 137
Autism 76, 89
　spectrum disorder 12*f*, 17, 79, 90, 94
　default mode network in 79
Autonomic nervous system 13
Autonomy, loss of 208
Aversive therapies 191
Axon guidance 94
Axsome 178
Ayushman Bharat Pradhan Mantri Jan Arogya Yojana 47-49

B

Bacillus 16
Baclofen 60
Bacterial strains 15
Bacteriodetes 12
Bacteroides 12
Bacteroidetes 16
Behavior
    agitated 56, 58
    disruptive 58
Benzodiazepine 35, 58, 60, 61, 64
Benzofuran and indole derivatives 30
Beta-amyloid plaques 79
Beta-blockers 64
Binge eating disorder 70
Biophysical processes 215
Biopsychosocial framework 207
Bipolar depression 96, 112
    acute, molecules and guidelines 108t
    acute, treatment-resistant 110fc
    maintenance with molecules and guidelines 110t
    resistant to maintenance treatment 109
    treatment of 171
Bipolar disorder 6, 17, 90, 92, 101, 106, 160, 171, 190, 198
    maintenance phase 113
    prevention in 199
    systematic treatment enhancement program for 109
    treatment of 171
        refractory 106
        resistant maintenance 101, 111fc
Bipolar mania 112
    treatment-resistant 111fc
    with molecules and guidelines 105t
Blind spot, collective 153
Blood
    disorders 163
    oxygen level 199
Bodily distress disorder 71
Bodily integrity dysphoria 71
Body dysmorphic disorder 68
Body-focused repetitive behavior disorders 69
Bold signal 2
Bonn scale 24
Brain
    activity, understanding of 8
    derived neurotrophic factor 17, 18, 92
        level of 173
    developing 88
    development, early 194
    disorder 75
    natural resonance 137
    organoids 88, 90
    part of 75
    physiological perspective 8
    stimulation techniques 109
    tissue damaged 75
Brexanolone 174
    formulation of 175
Brexpiprazole 171, 172
Bromocriptine 64
Bruxism 29
Bulgarian peasants 11
Buprenorphine 190
Bupropion 92, 108, 178
Burkholderia 16

C

Calcium, deactivation of 173
Calmodulin-dependent kinase 173
Canadian Network for Mood and Anxiety Treatments 96t, 103-105, 108, 110
Cannabidiol 177, 199
Cannabis
    indica 36
    sativa 36
Carbamazepine 104-108
Cardiotoxicity 29
Cardiovascular disorders 171
Cariprazine 108, 171
    meta-analysis of 171
    use of 171
Catatonia 56, 61
Cathinone and pyrovalerone derivatives 29
Celecoxib 108
Cell
    death 94
    differentiation 94
Central executive network 4, 76
Central nervous system 18, 62
Cerebral edema 37
Cerebral palsy 163
Child Welfare Committee 166
Chlorpromazine 104, 105
Cholecystokinin 13
    receptor 13
Cholinesterase inhibitors 61
Cingulate cortex, posterior 76
Climate anxiety 210
Climate change 207
    and natural disaster 208
    mental health impacts of 208t
Climate on human conflict 209
Climate variability 215
    expression of 208
Clonazepam 104, 105
Clostridium 16
Clozapine 57, 65, 104, 105, 106, 108, 113
Cognitive
    behavioral therapy 25, 110, 111, 187, 192, 199, 200

decline 213
deficits in schizophrenia 77
impairment, mild 200, 201
performance 213, 218
therapy 110
training, advanced 200
Complex post-traumatic stress disorder 69
Compulsive sexual behavior disorder 72
Confusion and hypomania 65
Connectome 1
　research of 7
　useful tools and concepts 2
Connectomics and brain in relation to psychiatry 1
Cortical brain changes 89
COVID-19 40, 158, 170, 183
Cranial nerve neuromodulation 138
Crenezumab 201
Crime and insecurity 217
Criminal activity 158
Cyber space 156
　and psychiatry, bidirectional relationship 156
Cyber stalking 158
Cyberpsychiatry 156
Cybersex
　addiction 157
　and internet pornography 156
CYP3A4
　demethylating 122
　enzyme 171
　inhibitors 171
Cyproheptadine 64
Cytochrome P450
　liver enzymes 122
　system 170

D

Daridorexant 177
Decision making 81
Decriminalizing suicide 165
Deep brain stimulation 108, 109
Deep transcranial magnetic stimulation 109, 136
Default mode network 4, 76
　and depression 78
Deficits in social cognition 78
Delhi state legal services authority 146
Delirium 56, 59, 65
Delusional disorder 68
Dementia-related psychosis 170
Depression 6, 76, 78, 156, 159, 190, 200
　long-term 18
　unipolar 96
Depressive disorder
　adjunctive treatment in 172
　major 17, 90, 91
　treatment of 172

Designer drugs 28
Desolation 210
Detoxification 190
Deutetrabenazine 173
Developmental disorders 212
Dexmedetomidine 176
Dextromethadone 178
Dextromethorphan 178
Diaphoresis 65
Diarrhea 65
Diazepam 61, 190
Digital Information Security in Healthcare Act, 2018 167
Digital platforms, use of 187
Diplopia 120
Direct current stimulation, transcranial 138
Disability-adjusted life years 194
Disability limitation 194
Disorders due to addictive behaviors, block 72
Disorders of bodily distress, block 71
Disorders specifically associated with stress, block 69
District Mental Health Programme 146
Disulfiram-ethanol reaction 191
Divalproate 104
Divalproex 105, 106, 107
Donanemab 201
Donepezil 61
Dopamine agonists 15, 92, 64
Dopamine transporter and serotonin transporter 29
Dorsal anterior cingulate cortex 76
Dorsal nexus 78
Dorsal raphe nucleus 79
Dorsolateral prefrontal cortex 76
Dose-dependent relationships 213
Drug
　addiction 189, 193
　exposure 196
　　on brain 189
　orexin receptor antagonist 176
　stopping, withdrawal symptoms 189
　therapy use of ketamine's metabolites 125
Dwarfism 163
Dynamic causal modeling 5
Dystonia, acute 56, 63, 65
　pharmacotherapy of 63b
　treatment for 63

E

Eating disorders
　block 70
　preventing 200
Eco-anxiety 207, 210

Eco-crisis 207
Ecopsychiatry 207
    current evidence base on 207
    emerging field of 207
    methodology 207
Ecopsychology 207, 218
Ecstasy 29
Electrical stimulation, transcranial 134, 137
Electrical, use of 134
Electroconvulsive therapy 64, 104-110
Electromagnetic induction, Faraday's
        principle of 135
Elevated, periods of 101
Emotional skills 194
Enantiomer 122
Endocannabinoid system 177
Enteric nervous system 12
Enteroendocrine cell 13
    in colon 14f
Environmental
    change 215
    doom 208
    noise exposure 214
Epithelium and induce cytokine
        production 18f
Esketamine nasal spray 125, 174
Eukaryotic elongation factor 2,
        dephosphorylation of 173
Euphoria 36
Executive function 81
Extrapyramidal symptoms 171

F

Facebook
    chatting 157
    intrusion disorder 157
Facilitation effect 196
Familial vulnerability 197
Fatty acid
    binding protein levels, abnormal 95
    short-chain 13
Feeding disorders, block 70
Fibrillary beta-amyloid 200
Figure-of-eight coil 135
Fine-tuning connectomes 5
Firmicutes 16
    phyla 12
Flumazenil 60
Fluoxetine 106, 113
Focused ultrasound stimulation,
        transcranial 139
Folic acid 104, 105
Fostering social cohesion 215
Found wandering 144
Fragile X syndrome 90, 94
Free fatty acid 14f
Frequently disclosing personal problems 159

Full-blown disorder 195
Functional connectivity 2, 76
Fusobacteria 16

G

G protein-coupled bile acid receptor 1 14f
Gabapentin 64, 106, 107, 110, 113
Gaming disorder 72
Gamma hydroxybutyrate acid 35
Gamma-aminobutyric acid 15, 18, 23, 35,
        125, 173
Gamma-hydroxyvaleric acid 35
Ganiyari model 42
Gantenerumab 201
Gaps and possible actions in programs 153
Gastrointestinal 13
Gene
    editing, technique of 88
    expression, modulation of 88
    $FOXG1$ lead downstream 94
    function, understand 88
Genetic risk and deterioration syndrome 22
Genome-wide association studies, recent 23
Germ layers 88
Glucagon-like peptide 13, 14f, 14
Glutamate, modulation of 172
Glutamatergic agents in mood
        disorders 178
Glutamatergic modulator 173
Glutamatergic precursors 94
Glutamatergic system in schizophrenia 177
Good practice models, components of 152
Granger causality 5
Graph theory metrics 4
Green spaces 215f
Grey matter reductions 77
Grief disorder, prolonged 70
Gross domestic product 47
Group psychoeducation 111
Gut dysbiosis 16
Gut microbia
    based interventions 18
    products penetrate 18f
    strains 15t
Gut microbiota communicates 13
Gut-brain
    axis 11, 12
    crosstalk 13f
Gut-microbiota to brain 13
Gyral curvature 139

H

Hair pulling 69
Hallucinations 37
Haloperidol 104, 107
Headache 171, 173

Health
　coverage, universal 149
　impact of probiotics on 11
Health insurance
　concept of 47
　policies, types of 47
Healthy controls 90
Heat hypothesis states 209
Helicobacter pylori 17
Hemodynamic response 2
Hemophilia 163
Hepatic impairment 171, 173
Hippo pathway 94
Histamine 15
Histaminic rectors leads 172
Histone deacetylase 14, 14*f*
Hoarding disorder 69
Homelessness, prevention of 151
Human brain comprises 75
Human microbiome 11
Hydroxyindoleacetic acid 16
Hyperalgesia, pathophysiology of 115
Hypericum perform 95
Hyperreflexia 65
Hypochondriacal disorder 68
Hypothalamic-pituitary-adrenal
　axis 18, 214

I

Iatrogenic 56, 62
Iatrogenic emergencies 65
Illness score, severity of 172
Impulse control disorders, block 72
Inconsistencies 80
Independent component analysis 3
Indian health insurance policies 52
Indian Psychiatric Society 45, 150, 183
Indian Teachers of Psychiatry Forum 184
Individual disorders 89
Indole 13
Indole-3
　acetaldehyde 16
　acetamide 16
　acetic acid 16
　acrylic acid 16
　aldehyde 16
　lactic acid 16
　propionic acid 16
　pyruvic acid 16
Indoleamine 2,3-dioxygenase 16
Inflammatory response 118
Information overload 156, 158
Inhibitory control network 81
Insomnia 29, 171, 173
　prevalence of 159
Insula 77

Insurance Regulatory and Development
　Authority of India 50
Intellectual disability 164
Interest, region of 3
Intermittent explosive disorder 72
Intermittent psychosis prodromal
　syndrome 22
International Classification of Diseases 201
Internet
　addiction 81, 160
　gaming disorder 82, 156, 159
　implicitly 159
　pornography 157
　problematic use of 160
Interpersonal and social rhythm therapy 111
Interpersonal relationship 218
　difficulty 159
Interventional psychiatry 139
Intoxication 56
Intra-aural applications 139
Intracellular effector pathways 94
Intranasal esketamine 174
Intrinsic connectivity networks 4
Investigated intrinsic functional
　connectivity 81

J

Juvenile justice act, 2015 165

K

Ketamine 57, 92, 107, 108, 115, 116, 120, 122,
　173, 174
　acts, racemic mixture of (R, S) 173
　antidepressant properties 117
　anti-inflammatory benefits 118
　clinical effects 116
　dissociative anesthetic 124
　half-life values 123
　immediate antidepressant effects 125
　intramuscular administration of 122
　maximum level of 122
　metabolite paradigm 126
　metabolites fast-acting
　　antidepressants 126
　misuse potential of 125
　oral bioavailability 122
　pharmacodynamics 124
　pharmacokinetics 122
　pharmacological targets 124
　plasma levels of 123
　psychotropic side effects 125
　side effects 118
　therapeutic efficacy of 120
　use for recreational purposes 120
Kynurenine aminotransferase 16

L

Lactobacillus rhamnosus JB-1
    supplementation 19
Lamotrigine 106, 107, 113
Land degradation 215
Land use pattern 207
Landscape ecosystem 215*f*
Lapse *vs.* relapse 190
Laryngeal dystonia, acute exacerbation of 63
Leaky guts 17
Learning, global opportunities for 187
Lecanemab 201
Legal consequences 158
Legal highs 28
Lemborexant 177
Levetiracetam 105, 107, 108, 113
Levodopa 64
Levothyroxine 108
Lifestyle pattern, changing 207
Ligands orchestrates multiple signaling
    pathways 93
Light-emitting diodes 138
Light therapy 107
Lip-biting 69
Lipopolysaccharide 13, 14*f*
    induced neuroinflammation 92
Lithium 57, 65, 104, 105, 113
    and lamotrigine 108
    monotherapy 106
Liver function test 64
Living organisms' genes, modify 88
Localization techniques 134
Loneliness, reducing 215
Loperamide 60
Lorazepam 61
    chlordiazepoxide 190
Loxapine 89
Lumateperone 172
Lurasidone 106, 108
Luteolin
    on human, effect of 92
    treatment 92
Lymphoblastoid cell lines 90
Lysergamides 38

M

Magnesium 124
Magnetic neuromodulation 135
Magnetic resonance imaging 75
    diffusion-weighted 2
Magnetic seizure therapy 137
Magnetic stimulation
    repetitive 105
    transcranial 135
Malignant course 6
Mania, acute exacerbation of 58
Maternal immune activation 11, 12*f*
Maternal infections 196
Maternal nutrition, poor 196
Medial dorsal thalamus 78
Medial mystery parietal area 76
Medical custody 152
Medical detention 148
Medical education, competency-based 183
Melatonin 61
Memory 81
    and cognitive impairment 119
    encoding structures 79
Mental and behavioral disorders 178
Mental disorder 189, 194, 209
    incidence of 197
    several 195
    severe 143, 144
Mental health
    authority 165
    care act 45, 145, 164, 147
        implementation of 186
    child and adolescent 186
    crisis 208
    disorder 194
    environmental determinants of 217
    how internet affects 156
    impacts 208
        long-term 208
        of social media on 156
        short-term 208
    insurance in India 47
    prevention strategies in 201
    problem 147
        factors affecting 217*t*
        in urban areas 217
    professionals 165
    services for homeless populations 143
Mental ill-health 147
Mental illness 50, 143, 144, 163, 164, 170, 189
    chronic 101
    coverage of 50
    health insurance for 48, 51
    homeless persons with 143, 144
    in major 145
    treatment of 194
Mental performance 115
Mental states paradigm, clinical high-risk 195
Mental status changes 65
Mentally ill 144
    homeless persons 147
Metabolic acidosis 37
Methadone 60, 190, 191
Microbiota
    activity of 18
    interactions 14*f*
Midazolam 117
Mind, theory of 24
Mind's synergistic relationship 218

Mirtazapine 64
Mitogen-activated protein kinase pathway 94
Mobile mental health services 146, 153
Mobile telepsychiatry model 42
Modafinil 107, 108, 112
Modulating cell proliferation 94
Molecule 177
Monoamine
    depletion 29
    oxidase 16, 29
Mood
    disorder 65, 211
    irritable 101
    stabilizer 106
Motivational enhancement therapy 191, 192
Multiorgan failure 37
Muscular dystrophy 163
Mydriasis 29, 37
Myoclonus 65

N

Naltrexone 191
National Education Policy 185
National Health Mission 149
National Institute for Health and Care Excellence 106
National Institute of Mental Health and Neurosciences 48, 149
    extension for community health 42
National Insurance Research Database 212
National Legal Services Authority 150
National Medical Commission 184
National Mental Health Policy 2014 147
National Mental Health
    Programme 45, 143, 149
    guidelines 149
National Mental Health Survey of India 47, 217
National Trust Act 48
Natural disasters, mental health impacts of 208t
Near infrared spectroscopy 134
Neural plasticity 93
Neural progenitor cells 90
Neural subsystem 5
Neurocircuitry knowledge, translation of 176
Neurocognitive deficits 23
Neurodevelopmental disorder 94
Neuroleptic
    malignant syndrome 56, 63
    use of 173
Neurological disorders 170
    chronic 163
Neurological impairment, severe 37
Neuromodulation and connectomes 7
Neuromodulation techniques 134
Neuron committed cell 90

Neuronal migration 88
Neuronal vacuolation 121
Neuropeptide Y receptor 13
Neurotoxicity 121
Neurotoxin, quinolinic acid 16
Neurotransmitters 15, 15t
Neurotrophin-modulated signaling pathways 94
Nicotinamide adenine dinucleotide 16
Nicotinic acetylcholine receptors 126
Niramaya Health Insurance Scheme 48
Nitric oxide 15
Noise pollution 208, 214
Noninvasive brain stimulation 134
Noninvasive electrical neuromodulation 137
Noninvasive neuromodulatory techniques in psychiatry, newer 134
Nonsteroidal anti-inflammatory drugs 200
    for myalgias 60
Noradrenaline 15
Norepinephrine transporter 29, 33
Novel agents, role of 105
Novel therapies still in pipeline 176
Nuedexta 178
Nuisance 144
Nutraceuticals
    and phytoceuticals 96t
    in psychiatry 94
    role of 87
    use of 105
Nutritional psychiatry 95
Nystagmus 120

O

Obsessive-compulsive disorder
    block 68
    treatment of 135
Olanzapine 25, 61, 105, 106, 108, 113
    and fluoxetine 108
Olfactory reference syndrome 68
Olney's lesions 121
Omega-3
    fatty acid 196
    long-chain 197
Omnipotent 88
Opioid-dependence syndrome 191
Opioids 60
    intoxication, withdrawal in critically ill 59t
Opium crops 190
Orbitofrontal cortex 135, 189
Orexin receptor antagonists, dual 177t
Organic disorders 170
Oxcarbazepine 104
    lithium 104
Oxidative stress regulation 25
Oxygen level dependent 76

Index

P

Paliperidone, 3-month formulation of 173
Parcellation 3, 8
Parietal cortex
  posterior 76
  posterior lateral 78
Parkinson's disease 12f, 163, 170
Paroxetine 108
Pathoconnectomics 5
Peptide YY 14f
Peripheral edema 170
Peripheral effects, direct and indirect 120
Persistent delusional disorder 68
Personalized medicine, concept of 87
Phencyclidine, derived from 115
Phenidate derivatives 32
Phenmetrazine derivatives 33
Phenotypes 91
Phenylcyclohexylamine 115
Phenylethylamines 37
Phenytoin 105, 110, 113
Photic neuromodulation 138
Physical comorbidity 190
Pimavanserin 170
Pioglitazone 108
Piperazines 31
Plasma protein binding ranges 123
Polymerase chain reactions, quantitative 94
Polyunsaturated fatty acids 95
Positive and negative syndrome scale 171
Positron emission tomography 75, 134
Post-traumatic stress disorder 160, 197, 209
  primary symptoms of 69
Potentiation, long-term 18
Pramipexole 107, 108, 112
Pregabalin 64, 104, 105, 108
Preventive efforts, common frameworks for 195
Preventive medicine classifies 195
Prevotella 12
Probiotics and psychiatry 11
Prodromal symptoms, structured interview for 24
Prodromal syndrome, tools for assessing 24
Prodrome 195
  stage, management of 24
Prodrome syndrome
  risk factors of 23
  treat 24
Prohibitions 165
Proinflammatory cytokines 118
Promethazine 64
Proteins serve 94
Proteobacteria 16
Pseudomonas 16
Pseudoresistance 103, 103t
Psychedelics 37

Psychiatric disorders 7, 8, 16, 76, 87, 96t, 210
  deranged microbial profile in 17t
  environmental determinants of 207
  major 22
  pathophysiology of 176
  prevention of 194
  reverse-direction 159
  role in 75
  stem cell models for 90t
  understanding 6
Psychiatric emergency 56
  classification of 56
  pharmacological intervention of 62fc
  pharmacotherapy of 56
  services, demand for 65
Psychiatrist-on-web model, PGI Chandigarh 42
Psychiatry
  branch of 194
  early prevention in 194
  education, undergraduate 183
  newer drugs in 170
  teaching skills 185
Psychiatry training
  challenges in 184
  components of 185
  in India, changing perspectives in 183
Psychoactive effects 118
Psychoeducation, universal 196
Psychological disorders 156
Psychological interventions 25
Psychomimetic effects 115
Psychopathology, triple network model of 80
Psychosis 159
  acute exacerbation of 58
  and mood disorders 171
  clinical high risk for 199
Psychosocial interventions, efficacy of 198
Psychotherapies 109
Psychotic
  disorders 76
  incidence of 199

Q

Quadripulse stimulation 137
Quetiapine 61, 104-106
Quinidine 178

R

Racemic ketamine 117
Random noise stimulation, transcranial 137
Rapamycin, mammalian target of 92
Rapastinel 178
Ras protein signaling pathway 94
Reactive oxygen species 211
Refusal for food 190

Index

Rehabilitation, family-based 143
Relapse prevention 190
Renal failure 37
Renal impairment, severe 171, 173
Research domain criteria 79
    project framework 8
Resistant bipolar depression 106
    level of evidence with modality for 107*t*
    molecule/modality for 104*t*
Resistant bipolar disorder 102
Resistant bipolar mania 103
Resistant depression, acute episode of 106
Respiratory depressive effects, amount of 116
Respiratory failure, prolonged 37
Restrictive food intake disorder 70, 71
Resultant dysfunctional behavior 159
Retrosplenial cortices in rats 121
Rhabdomyolysis 37
Right to access mental healthcare 149
Right ventromedial prefrontal cortex 78
Rights of persons with disabilities
    act, 2016 163
Risk and protective factors, interplay of 196
Risperidone 25, 61, 106, 109
    long-acting injectable 110
Rumination-regurgitation disorder 71
Ruminococcus 12

S

Safe-walking infrastructure 215
Salience network 4
Scale for prodromal symptoms 24
Schemes for persons with disabilities 48
Schizophrenia 6, 17, 22, 65, 76, 77, 78, 89, 90, 96, 159, 190
    acute 172
    default mode network 76
    high risk for 199
    prodromal symptoms of 22
    progression to 24
    social cognition in 78
    symptoms of 172
    treatment of 171, 172
Schizophrenia Research Foundation 41, 42, 46
Schizotypal disorder 68
Schizotypal personality disorder 159
Sclerosis, multiple 163
Sedatives 34, 60
Self-relevant information, processing of 80
Sense of self 77
Separate disorder 81
Sernyl evoked 115
Serotonin 15
Serotonin dopamine activity modulator 171
Serotonin partial agonist reuptake
    inhibitor 175

Serotonin syndrome 37, 64, 65
    management of 65
Sex-toys 157
Sexual
    abuse 196
    activities, online 157
    information, searching 157
    offences act, protection of
        children 2012 166
    partners 157
Shivering 65
Single nucleotide polymorphisms 23
Single-cell sequencing 91
Skin biopsy-derived fibroblasts 88
Skin picking 69
Sleep
    deprivation therapy 108
    disorder 156, 176
Small world network 4
Social cognition plays 24
Social isolation 217
Social media 156
Social reality 144
Social relationship, strains on 208, 209
Social stress 217
Socio-interpersonal 157
Socio-occupational dysfunction, presence of 189
Solace and *nostalgia* 210
Solanezumab 201
Solastalgia 208, 210
Somatoform pain disorder 210
Somnolence 173
Specific learning disability 164
Standard operating procedure 144
State government group health insurance for employees 49
State legal services authority 151
State mental health authority 150
Stem cells 87
    induced pluripotent 88, 90
    role of 87
Stimulants 28
Stimulation
    high-frequency 135
    low-frequency 135
Strengthening social capital 215
Streptomyces 16
Stress
    disorder, acute 208
    reaction, acute 59, 208
Subgenual prefrontal cortex 78
Sublingual dexmedetomidine 176
Subspecialty education 186
Substance
    abuse 217
    induced emergencies 56
    intoxication and withdrawal 59
    use disorders 81, 195

Substrate-type monoamine releasers 29
Suicidal behavior 56, 57
Sulforaphane 26, 196
Superspecialty 186
Supplementary motor area, stimulation of 135
Suvorexant 177
Swavlamban health insurance scheme 48
Synchronized transcranial magnetic stimulation 137
Synchronous telemedicine 41
Synthetic cannabinoids 36
Synthetic opioids 34

T

Tamoxifen 103, 104t, 105t
Tardive dyskinesia, treatment of 173
Task positive networks 77
Tau hyperphosphorylation 79
Tele Mental Health Assistance and Networking Across States 45
Teleconsultation, drug lists type and mode of 44t
Telemedicine delivery systems, types of 41
Telemedicine practice guidelines 43, 167
 for telepsychiatry practice 45
Telemedicine Society of India 45
Telemedicine technology, use of 44
Telepsychiatry
 and health insurance 52
 benefits 40
 operational guidelines 2020 45
Temporoparietal junction 80
 left 135
Thalassemia 163
Theta burst stimulation 136
Thiamine, high dose of 190
Thiophene designer drugs 33
Tissue-specific cells 88
Toll-like receptor 13
Trace-amine-associated-receptor-1 29, 30
Tramadol 190
Transcranial magnetic stimulation, repetitive 104, 110
Trauma and shock 208
Trazodone 64
Treatment order, community-based 146
Treatment-resistant bipolar disorder 101, 112
 approach to management 101
Tremor 65
True resistance 103, 103t
Tryptamine 38
 core structure of 38

Tryptophan 14, 18
 2,3-dioxygenase 16
 hydroxylase 16
 metabolic pathways 16f

U

Ultrasonic neuromodulation 139
Urban design and planning 215
 model for 216f
Urban green spaces 207
Urbanization 214
 and mental illness 216

V

Vagal nerve
 activity 19
 stimulation, transcutaneous auricular 137
Valbenazine 173
Valnoctamide 104, 105
Valproate 104, 107, 108, 113
Venlafaxine 106
Ventromedial prefrontal cortex 189
Vesicular monoamine transporter 2 inhibitors 30, 173
Vilazodone 175
Vitamin 196
 B$_6$ (pyridoxine) 64
 D
  acts 198
  low levels of 198
 E 198
 F 95
Voltage-gated potassium channels 14
Vortioxetine 175
Voxel-based measurements 3, 8

W

Wandering lunatic 144, 148
Wnt signal transduction pathway 92, 94

X

Xanthurenic acid 16
X-chromosome 94

Z

Ziprasidone 106, 110, 113
Zuranolone 175

EU GSPR Authorised Reprsentative
Logos Europe, 9 rue Nicolas Poussin
1700, La Rochelle, France
Phone: +33 (0) 6 67 93 73 78
E-mail: contact@logoseurope.eu

www.ingramcontent.com/pod-product-compliance
Ingram Content Group UK Ltd.
Pitfield, Milton Keynes, MK11 3LW, UK
UKHW050455150426
5217IPUK00025B/1695